THE NEUROPSYCHOLOGY OF EVERYDAY LIFE: ISSUES IN DEVELOPMENT AND REHABILITATION

FOUNDATIONS OF NEUROPSYCHOLOGY

Barbara Uzzell, Series Editor

1. Ellis, D.W., Christensen, A.L., eds.: *Neuropsychological Treatment After Brain Injury*, ISBN No. 0-7923-0014-9.

2. Tupper, D.E., Cicerone, K.D., eds.: *The Neuropsychology of Everyday Life: Assessment and Basic Competencies*, ISBN No. 0-7923-0671-6.

3. Tupper, D.E., Cicerone, K.D., eds.: *The Neuropsychology of Everyday Life: Issues in Development and Rehabilitation*, ISBN No. 0-7923-0847-6.

THE NEUROPSYCHOLOGY OF EVERYDAY LIFE:

ISSUES IN DEVELOPMENT AND REHABILITATION

Edited by
DAVID E. TUPPER
Director of Clinical Services
New Medico Rehabilitation and Skilled
Nursing Center of Troy
Troy, New York

Clinical Assistant Professor
Department of Psychiatry
Albany Medical College
Albany, New York

KEITH D. CICERONE
Clinical Director
The Center for Head Injuries
Johnson Rehabilitation Institute
Edison, New Jersey

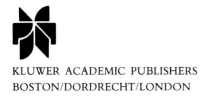

KLUWER ACADEMIC PUBLISHERS
BOSTON/DORDRECHT/LONDON

Distributors

for North America:
Kluwer Academic Publishers
101 Philip Drive
Assinippi Park
Norwell, Massachusetts 02061 USA

for all other countries:
Kluwer Academic Publishers Group
Distribution Centre
Post Office Box 322
3300 AH Dordrecht, THE NETHERLANDS

Library of Congress Cataloging-in-Publication Data
The Neuropsychology of everyday life: issues in development and
   rehabilitation/edited by David E. Tupper and Keith D. Cicerone.
      p.   cm.—(Foundations of neuropsychology; FNPS3)
   Includes index.
   ISBN 0-7923-0847-6
   1. Clinical neuropsychology.   2. Neuropsychology.   3. Brain
damage—Diagnosis.   4. Developmental psychology.   5. Pediatric
neuropsychology.   I. Tupper, David E.   II. Cicerone, Keith D.
III. Series.
   [DNLM: 1. Activities of Daily Living.   2. Neuropsychological
Tests.   3. Neuropsychology   W1 F099K v. 3/WL 103 N49359]
RC386.6.N48N5   1990
616.8—dc20
DNLM/DLC
for Library of Congress

90-4893
CIP

Printed on acid-free paper

Printed in the United States of America

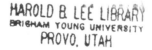

CONTENTS

Contributing Authors   vii

Foreword   ix
JOSEPH D. MATARAZZO

Preface   xiii

1. Introduction: Developmental and Rehabilitative Issues in the Neuropsychology of Everyday Life   1
DAVID E. TUPPER AND KEITH D. CICERONE

I. LIFE SPAN DEVELOPMENTAL NEUROPSYCHOLOGY   15

2. The Neuropsychology of Childhood Learning and School Behavior   17
LOUISE S. KIESSLING

3. The Neuropsychological Determinants of Functional Reading, Writing, and Arithmetic   45
RICHARD GALLAGHER AND URSULA KIRK

4. Cognition and Watching Television   93
JOHN J. BURNS AND DANIEL R. ANDERSON

5. Epilepsy in Children and Adults   109
RICHARD DELANEY AND MARY L. PREVEY

6. Assessment of Everyday Functioning in Normal and Malignant Memory Disordered Elderly   135
HOLLY A. TUOKKO AND DAVID CROCKETT

v

7. Life Span Perspective on Practical Intelligence   183
SHERRY L. WILLIS AND MICHAEL MARSISKE

II. ISSUES IN REHABILITATION   199

8. A Rationale for Family Involvement in Long-Term Traumatic Head Injury Rehabilitation   201
HARVEY E. JACOBS

9. Psychosocial Consequences of Significant Brain Injury   215
MARY PEPPING AND JAMES R. ROUECHE

10. Working: The Key to Normalization After Brain Injury   257
PATRICIA L. PRICE AND WILLIAM L. BAUMANN

11. Neuropsychological Rehabilitation: Treatment of Errors in Everyday Functioning   271
KEITH D. CICERONE AND DAVID E. TUPPER

12. Long-Term Adjustment to Traumatic Brain Injury   293
INGER VIBEKE THOMSEN

Index   311

CONTRIBUTING AUTHORS

Daniel R. Anderson, Ph.D., Dept. of Psychology, University of Massachusetts, Amherst, MA 01003

William L. Baumann, M.S., C.R.C., Program Director, Transitions, Center for Comprehensive Services, 306 West Mill St., P.O. Box 2825, Carbondale, IL 62902

John J. Burns, Ph.D., Dept. of Psychology, University of Massachusetts, Amherst, MA 01003

Keith D. Cicerone, Ph.D., Center for Head Injuries, Johnson Rehabilitation Institute, 2048 Oak Tree Rd., Edison, NJ 08820

David Crockett, Ph.D., Department of Psychiatry, University of British Columbia, Vancouver, B.C., Canada V6T 2B5

Richard Delaney, Ph.D., Psychology Service, V.A. Medical Center, West Haven, CT 06516

Richard Gallagher, Ph.D., Division of Child and Adolescent Psychiatry, Schneider Children's Hospital, Long Island Jewish Medical Center, New Hyde Park, NY 11042

Harvey E. Jacobs, Ph.D., Dept. of Psychiatry and Biobehavioral Sciences, UCLA School of Medicine, Los Angeles, CA 90024

Louise S. Kiessling, M.D., Pediatrics and Family Medicine, Memorial Hospital of Rhode Island, Wood 4, 111 Brewster St., Pawtucket, RI 02860

Ursula Kirk, Ph.D., Teacher's College, Columbia University, 525 West 120th St., Box 142, New York, NY 10027

Michael Marsiske, Department of Human Development and Family Studies, College of Health and Human Development, The Pennsylvania State University, University Park, PA 16802

Joseph D. Matarazzo, Ph.D., Dept. of Medical Psychology, L351, Oregon Health Sciences University, 3181 S.W. Sam Jackson Park Rd., Portland, OR 07201

Mary Pepping, Ph.D., Virginia Mason Clinic, 1100 9th Ave., Seattle, WA 98101

Mary L. Prevey, Ph.D., Psychology Service, V.A. Medical Center, West Spring St., West Haven, CT 06516

Patricia L. Price, M. Ed., C.R.C., Operation Systems Manager, Mentor Head Injury Services, 53 Cummings Park, Woburn, MA 01801

James R. Roueche, M.S., Section of Neuropsychology, Dept. of Neuro-surgery, Presbyterian Hospital, Northeast 13th St. at Lincoln Blvd., Oklahoma City, OK 73104

Inger Vibeke Thomsen, Ph.D., Dept. of Neurology, Rigshospitalet, University Hospital, DK-2100, Copenhagen Ø, Denmark

Holly A. Tuokko, Ph.D., Clinic for Alzheimer's Disease and Related Disorders, U.B.C. Health Sciences Centre Hospital, 2211 Westbrook Mall, Vancouver, B.C., Canada V6T 2B5

David E. Tupper, Ph.D., New Medico Rehabilitation and Skilled Nursing Center of Troy, 100 New Turnpike Rd., Troy, NY 12182

Sherry L. Willis, Ph.D., College of Health and Human Development, The Pennsylvania State University, S-110 Henderson Human Development Bldg., University Park, PA 16802

FOREWORD

For a period of some fifteen years following completion of my internship training in clinical psychology (1950–1951) at the Washington University School of Medicine and my concurrent successful navigation through that school's neuroanatomy course, clinical work in neuropsychology for me and the psychologists of my generation consisted almost exclusively of our trying to help our physician colleagues differentiate patients with neurologic disorders from those with psychiatric disorders. In time, experience led all of us from the several disciplines involved in this enterprise to the conclusion that the crude diagnostic techniques available to us circa 1945–1965 had garnered little valid information on which to base such complex, differential diagnostic decisions.

It now is gratifying to look back and review the remarkable progress that has occurred in the field of clinical neuropsychology in the four decades since I was a graduate student. In the late 1940s such pioneers as Ward Halstead, Alexander Luria, George Yacorzynski, Hans-Lukas Teuber, and Arthur Benton already were involved in clinical studies that, by the late 1960s, would markedly have improved the quality of clinical practice. However, the only psychological tests that the clinical psychologist of my immediate post–Second World War generation had as aids for the diagnosis of neurologically based conditions involving cognitive deficit were such old standbys as the Wechsler-Bellevue, Rorschach, Draw A Person, Bender Gestalt, and Graham Kendall Memory for Designs Test. Given that in those days our hospital colleagues in neurology and psychiatry had little else to help with the difficult diagnostic challenges we and they faced daily, these old standbys, crude and inaccurate as they might have been, were in the minds of all involved better than nothing.

Fortunately, the widespread dissemination circa the middle 1960s by Ralph Reitan of what experience was proving were the more relevant tests developed by his mentor, Ward Halstead, plus the annually increasing numbers of psychologists working full time in medical schools, many of whom were affiliating with the newly being established departments of neurology, helped usher in an era in which by the early 1970s such differential diagnoses by clinical neuropsychologists between neurologic and psychiatric disorders became both more reliable and valid. In fact, during the past two decades in large teaching hospitals throughout the land, there has been almost universal acceptance by neurologists, neurosurgeons, psychiatrists, and that subset of clinical psychologists who are consultants to them that, appropriately supplemented, the Halstead-Reitan or Luria neuropsychological batteries of tests were, and are, infinitely better than any other available psychological test for diagnosing the presence or absence of a brain disease or disorder and, when present for many such cases, even its probable location.

However, for an annually increasing percentage of these cases in which we successfully were called in consultation before the middle 1980s, the improvement in brain imaging techniques (CAT, MRI, PET, etc.) that occurred during the decade of the 1980s shifted clinical practice away from this reliance for *diagnosis* on reasonably good neuropsychological batteries such as the Halstead-Reitan toward these latter, more highly sensitive and accurate imaging techniques. Thus, today the exceptions for which such neuropsychological batteries still remain the diagnostic instrument of choice involve to a great extent individuals who exhibit only the "softer" signs of cognitive deficit—for example, injuries (associated with subjectively defined memory and personality problems) resulting from automobile and other types of head trauma that are not discernible by use of even our best imaging techniques and that increasingly involve litigation.

Such changes in the focus of my own practice are consistent with what my colleagues also report. Early on during the past decade they and I were referred increasing numbers of patients who showed no evidence of brain injury when examined by our best imaging techniques or by standard clinical neurologic examination but who reported an array of *subjective* symptoms of such injury. However, despite the precision of today's imaging techniques, the numbers of such patients with even soft signs are not growing, but, rather, the consultation requests I and others are receiving increasingly involve patients with *unquestionable*, clear-cut laboratory and clinical evidence of brain injury and for whom many of us are asked by attorneys (as frequently for the plaintiff as for the defense) to offer help not in diagnosis but in the assessment of the degree of the *specific functional deficits* associated with everyday living (e.g., driving a car, returning to work) as well as for help in identifying a program geared toward rehabilitating or reinstituting some of that injured individual's cognitive and social adaptive functions that both attorneys agree currently are impaired.

In common with other practitioners I have found that both my education and experience have left me unprepared to make this shift from the responsibilities I feel I relatively comfortably and successfully have been meeting as a specialist in assessment for the past two decades to those associated with a new role, namely, as a consultant to physicians, families, attorneys, workers' compensation personnel, and other constituents who increasingly are asking me to be more precise regarding the functional deficits involved and to help them find rehabilitation programs with the potential to return to a previous level of social-occupational functioning an individual who all agree has become impaired following an injury to the brain.

Thus, when I received the table of contents from the editors of this book with the request that I contribute this foreword, I happily accepted in the hope that I would find in the chapters that were then being commissioned some of that information I so sorely needed, as my practice, in common with that of other neuropsychologists of my generation, had moved from differential diagnosis to the assessment of specific cognitive and functional impairments or referrals for programs and technologies geared toward rehabilitation of patients exhibiting such impairments.

Now that I have read all the contributed chapters I am not disappointed, nor do I feel that other readers will be. The reason is that the editors and authors have brought together in two volumes much of the literature, currently scattered hither and yon, with a good potential to move us from the binary-diagnostic decision of the era of the 1950s and 1960s that involved "Yes there is, no there isn't evidence of a brain injury" to today's more clinically relevant questions such as "Given that there is a brain injury, which specific *functional* competencies related to everyday living are intact and which are impaired?" (*The Neuropsychology of Everyday Life: Assessment and Basic Competencies*) and "Which are the cognitive and social skills training programs currently available in our country with the potential to help in the rehabilitation of individuals with such deficits?" (this volume).

Because of the short history of such ventures into rehabilitation, taken in toto, both the editors and chapter authors appear to me appropriately modest in the claims they are making from their literature reviews (and in their discussions of) the newly emerging rating scales, questionnaires, tests, and other approaches that show promise for the assessment of relevant indices of everyday, real-life functioning, as well as in their descriptions of the intervention and rehabilitation programs that have become available for treatment of the cognitive and social impairments involved. Nevertheless, however modest their current stage of development, having descriptions of these newer assessment and rehabilitation approaches so easily available in two volumes cannot help but increase the quality of the contributions of practitioners of the young, still developing practice of clinical neuropsychology.

Joseph D. Matarazzo, Ph.D.
Oregon Health Sciences University

PREFACE

During the last several years there has been a rapidly evolving emphasis and concern for applied issues in neuropsychology. Much of this emphasis has come from the establishment and acceptance of neuropsychology as a mature discipline, in recognition of its fundamental roles in clinical diagnosis, the study of specific neurobehavioral disorders, and the understanding of basic brain–behavior relationships. Neuropsychology as a discipline is now in a position to examine more complex and professionally related questions and issues. These new issues, also a major focus currently in other areas of professional psychology, include the relationships between neuropsychological test results and complex human performances, the prediction of everyday behaviors and their dysfunctions from neuropsychological instruments, the social-environmental manifestations of specific neurological disabilities, and the relevance of neuropsychological deficits to psychosocial functioning and adaptation in dynamic real-world contexts.

This volume and the previously published volume, *The Neuropsychology of Everyday Life: Assessment and Basic Competencies*, attempt to provide a comprehensive review and synthesis of some of these seminal issues in the continued development of applied neuropsychology. The books survey current knowledge regarding basic theory and methodological concerns and provide reviews of more traditional neuropsychological relationships between test performance and basic competencies. In addition, they develop an appreciation for more functionally related measures and concerns in covering such newly evolving research areas as functional assessment devices, practical cognitive functioning and intelligence, the everyday behavioral competencies of various neurologically disordered clientele, and more psychosocially relevant applications in educational, vocational, and rehabilitative contexts.

Some may call the appearance of this two-volume set premature; some may call its appearance delayed. For us as editors, naturally, we feel that it appears at a particularly fruitful and interesting time for neuropsychology and the study of brain–behavior relations. It appears at a time in which investigators and practitioners alike are struggling with issues deep at the heart of neuropsychology's core—the interrelationship of abilities thought to be related to the function of the brain and aspects of our functioning in the everyday realities of life.

The Neuropsychology of Everyday Life: Assessment and Basic Competencies addresses the relevance of neuropsychological assessment information for predicting everyday behaviors. Chapters in this volume cover methodological considerations about the ecological validity of neuropsychological tests, perspectives on clinical integration and prediction of criterion behaviors, and the development of a variety of new, more "functional" assessment measures. This book also describes underlying cognitive abilities in functional communication, everyday memory, and everyday actions as well as in complex goal-directed behaviors such as activities of daily living and driving. *The Neuropsychology of Everyday Life: Issues in Development and Rehabilitation* then addresses two specific issues related to the neuropsychology of functioning in everyday life. Specifically, one section of this volume covers life span developmental neuropsychology, with chapters directed at major disorders and issues that represent pivotal concerns for real-life outcome and show developmental change. Cognitive disabilities as affecting the rehabilitation of brain injury in everyday task performance are covered in another section, emphasizing everyday living skills and psychosocial functioning during neuropsychological rehabilitation.

Chapter authors are preeminent in their respective topic areas and provide the high level of scholarship and expertise needed to refine further these critical issues in neuropsychology. The books should serve as a landmark reference in the clinical neuropsychological study of more ecologically relevant professional concerns and in the development of more sophisticated practitioners in research and service delivery. Along with both clinical and experimental neuropsychologists, cognitive psychologists, rehabilitation specialists, and others interested in brain–behavior issues as they impact on everyday functioning will find the books of significant interest and use.

We would like to acknowledge our gratitude to all of our contributors who are the "real" people who have produced this two-volume set. We would also like to thank our editors at Kluwer who have assisted us every step of the way. Finally, we would like to thank our families who persevered as much as we have with the completion of these books.

THE NEUROPSYCHOLOGY OF EVERYDAY LIFE: ISSUES IN
DEVELOPMENT AND REHABILITATION

1. INTRODUCTION: DEVELOPMENTAL AND REHABILITATIVE ISSUES IN THE NEUROPSYCHOLOGY OF EVERYDAY LIFE

DAVID E. TUPPER AND KEITH D. CICERONE

INTRODUCTION

In the earlier volume to this set, contributors addressed some of the fundamental concerns and practices currently raised during neuropsychology's maturation into a more ecological science, particularly when neuropsychology is considered an assessment or diagnostic discipline. As neuropsychology moves further into an ecological phase of development, other more specific theoretical and practical issues will be brought to light, and nowhere is this more apparent than in the areas of development and rehabilitation.

Alexander R. Luria, the noted Soviet neuropsychologist, in some of his early writings identified the areas of development and rehabilitation as particularly enlightening for an understanding of neuropsychological processes in daily living (e.g., Luria, 1959), although his was primarily a theoretical interest. In fact, Luria made these two areas—along with the understanding of language-related deficits following brain injury—prominent among his lifelong interests for clinical practice, theory generation, and research in neuropsychology.

In the intervening years since Luria thought about these crucial theoretical aspects of neuropsychology, an increasing number of neuropsychologists have become interested in developmental or pediatric neuropsychology, and more and more neuropsychologists are working in rehabilitative contexts. This book addresses some of the issues relevant to neuropsychology applied in developmental and rehabilitative contexts and outlines how an ecological neuropsychology must especially be concerned with the dynamic interplay inherent in the everyday social reality and functional skills of an individual with a brain injury. This chapter provides a brief overview of the book.

ECOLOGICAL PERSPECTIVES ON NEUROPSYCHOLOGICAL FUNCTIONING

Neuropsychology traditionally uses the *deficit* model of functioning, in that the skill or ability weaknesses demonstrated by an individual following a brain injury are considered of interest in research or clinical assessment and provide a window on the understanding of important elements of the brain–behavior relationship. Rourke (1982) noted that neuropsychology has moved through three separable phases of evolution, from a static enterprise using the brain as the focal point, to a cognitive phase where specific psychological abilities are related to brain function, to a more contemporary phase during which the focus has become the dynamic interplay between the brain and behavioral or psychological processes. The earlier volume in this set introduced the concept of an emerging ecological phase in neuropsychology that emphasizes the dynamic interplay between an individual's brain functioning, psychological capabilities, and environmental resources. Functional assessment devices, practical competencies in daily tasks, and the ecological validity of neuropsychological instruments were all considered. Understanding the brain and behavior in context was emphasized as a key element in an ecological neuropsychology.

One way to view this newer phase of practical applications in neuropsychology is to understand it as a shift to a perspective that emphasizes the *competence*, rather than the deficits, that a brain-injured individual displays. In a competency-based model of functioning, underlying skills and functional changes are understood from the standpoint of their advantage to individuals in the environment in which they must function. Competency is a relative term that relates to one's abilities and not deficits and is variable depending on the environment (Sternberg & Kolligian, 1990); the concept of a deficit implies a fixed, static loss of an ability in all environments. Other psychologists have decried the deficit (or clinical) model (e.g., Albee, 1980), and the development of a competency-based perspective is seen as both more profitable in understanding real-world functioning, as well as more appropriate in understanding the complex relationship between disability and ultimate handicap (Stubbins & Albee, 1984). Use of a competency-based perspective and consideration of the psychosocial impact of deficits are underlying themes in almost all chapters of this volume.

Hence, a competency-based perspective is an additional element of an ecological neuropsychology. Regarding developmental contexts, this book addresses life span developmental neuropsychological issues in a variety of everyday life competencies, and it considers not just the interactions of deficits within various environments during the life span but also the necessary competencies underlying several daily functional tasks. The most apparent application of a competency-based perspective in neuropsychology is in the consideration and application of interventive techniques in the progress of a neurological condition. Ultimately, the goal of neuropsychological intervention is to reduce the experienced level of handicap by individuals with brain injury by fostering increased competence in their ability to carry out daily tasks. A neuropsychology of everyday life thus has to be attuned to developmental and rehabilitative concerns, as well as to issues of ecological validity in the application of research and clinical findings (Acker, 1986; Hart & Hayden, 1986a).

DEVELOPMENT AND CHANGE IN EVERYDAY NEUROPSYCHOLOGICAL COMPETENCIES

As the importance of diagnostic concerns in neuropsychology has diminished (Rourke, 1982), researchers have begun to investigate dynamic aspects of the relationship between the brain and behavior in various environments. Rourke has noted that a dynamic neuropsychology is one that has to be concerned with the development of the brain and its functions, as well as the development of an individual's approach to material to be learned or performed, whether in controlled or more naturalistic settings. In fact, as Vygotsky (1978) earlier proposed, environmental interactions are important in the molding of the brain during development. Simple brain variable-behavioral measurement correlations are no longer viewed as the sole datum of neuropsychology (see also Bakker, 1984). The first section of this book addresses ecological issues during development of various competencies throughout the life span.

The Domains of Neuropsychological Development

Developmental or pediatric neuropsychology has burgeoned in the last decade and is now recognized as a major area of expertise and knowledge within neuropsychology. Many contemporary texts provide a background for the interested reader in clinical and research aspects of pediatric neuropsychology (Hynd & Willis, 1988; Obrzut & Hynd, 1986; Rourke et al., 1983; Spreen et al., 1984). Developmental neuropsychological concerns have also been identified in the adult and older adult populations (Albert & Moss, 1988), and unique issues regarding developmental changes have been raised for individuals throughout the life span. Certainly, differences in focus may exist in studying developmental processes at various points in the life span.

Much of the current focus in developmental neuropsychology has centered on the description of behavioral or cognitive deficit following various types of developmental neurological conditions, and important adult-child and adult–older adult developmental differences have been found. Needless to say, however, the dependent variables used in most of the studies have been changes on neuropsychological tests, and alterations in developmental neuropsychological processes have not been observed frequently or described fully in naturalistic settings or more functional tasks. Examination of neurological influences on emerging developmental competencies or of individual differences on everyday tasks has also not often been performed within neuropsychology.

In the first section of this book, the contributors consider several of these important ecological questions in life span developmental neuropsychology. Not only are pediatric or child developmental issues addressed in the chapters, but because of the importance of understanding everyday functioning in older populations, several chapters also address the impact of changing skills and competencies in the everyday functioning of normal and neurologically impaired adults. Because the important domains of development differ across the life span, some of the ecological issues are applicable throughout the chapters and others are not.

In chapter 2 Louise Kiessling addresses the neurodevelopmental changes that underlie childhood learning and early school performance. For readers not initiated in developmental neuropsychology, this chapter provides an excellent foundation for understanding the complex interactions between neural and behavioral development at young ages. It also points out the importance of the nature of the learning process and neurological foundations for everyday behavioral functioning in one of our frequent daily environments, school. Gallagher and Kirk, in chapter 3, are more specific in describing neuropsychological interactions (both deficits and competencies) in functional academic task performance. They thoroughly analyze neuropsychological underpinnings of reading, writing, and arithmetic performances from a functional perspective.

Next, Burns and Anderson, in chapter 4, discuss the interactions and interplay between neuropsychological skills and a common daily activity for children (and all us adults), watching television. In considering this ecological domain, these authors review the concept that watching television causes brain damage and, fortunately, reach the conclusion that the evidence does not support that concept. Burns and Anderson provide a comprehensive review of the cognitive and neurophysiological activities that we engage in while watching television. The first few chapters of the book, therefore, discuss not only traditional domains in neuropsychological development, such as cognitive developmental processes, but also discuss more ecological competencies in everyday functional tasks.

In a chapter that bridges the life span, Delaney and Prevey describe some of the real-life concerns of individuals with a lifelong neurological disorder. These authors consider the personal and psychosocial impact, as well as the neuropsychological factors, that impinge on the person with chronic epilepsy. Chapter 5 serves as an example of the changing effects of a neurological condition through development.

Of course, as ecological issues continue to be identified throughout development, further research will surface within neuropsychology that has implications for the everyday functioning of normal and disordered individuals (see, for example, Brooks & Baumeister, 1977; DeAngelis, 1989). More complex concerns and processes, such as the role of planning in cognitive development (Friedman, Scholnick, & Cocking, 1987), developmental changes in everyday cognition (Rogoff & Lave, 1984), and individual differences in skills that change during development (Hartlage & Telzrow, 1985), will also be studied within naturalistic contexts in neuropsychology.

Everyday Adult Development

A growing body of recent research in cognitive psychology as well as neuropsychology has pointed out the importance of a life span approach to development, where developing abilities, skills, and cognitive processes are seen as ever-changing and environmentally adaptive during the course of an individual's life, not just during childhood. Thus recent authors have addressed the development of competencies in daily living skills and cognition across the life span into adulthood and late life (Poon, Rubin, & Wilson, 1989; Sternberg & Kolligian, 1990). Indeed, there appears to be a contemporary impetus to study practical living skills and their underlying competencies in an older adult population as the mean age of society increases. Further data on the neuropsychological and psychosocial functioning of various able and disabled geriatric populations will not only provide needed knowledge concerning the developmental processes underlying cognitive competence but should make practical care planning and rehabilitative supports easier to identify. Implementation of appropriate environmental resources would also have a more comprehensive basis.

In chapter 7, Willis and Marsiske review the results of their own work as well as the growing knowledge base on the developmental changes in practical intelligence in older adults. Practical intelligence is generally considered to be a type that reflects our ability to act on our environment with our cognitive skills. Thus it is a very relevant everyday competency (see Sternberg & Wagner, 1986) that needs further investigation from a neuropsychological perspective. Willis and Marsiske emphasize the nature of differences between fluid and crystallized skills in adults and point out, in dynamic fashion, that our abilities may be combined differently across the life span as the nature of our goals and needs change. Thus chapter 7 is a good example of research addressing a foundation of understanding needed for a dynamic neuropsychology.

Everyday development in adulthood from a neuropsychological perspective also needs to be concerned with changes in neurological disorders and neuropsychological processes across the life span. Thus a life span perspective on abnormal processes needs to be part of an ecological neuropsychology (Kerns & Curley, 1985). As already noted, chapter 5 by Delaney and Prevey is concerned with developmental and psychosocial change in epileptic conditions. Tuokko and Crockett, in chapter 6, also address the nature of memory disorder from a psychosocial/adaptive behavior viewpoint in elderly patients.

These authors describe the development of ecologically valid instruments for the assessment and detection of everyday life changes in memory capabilities in elderly patients with malignant memory disorder. These chapters form a representative collection of the type of research that needs to be conducted with normal and disordered adult populations to address everyday life competencies adequately across the life span.

Ecological Settings in Development

The neuropsychological study of practical skills throughout development, as noted in our earlier volume, will necessarily need to be ecobehaviorally oriented and sensitive to the environmental contexts and functional goals of the individual. Barker (1968), in fact, proposed that an ecological approach in psychology needs to address dynamic interactions between the organism, its behavior, and the environmental settings in which the organism participates. Likewise, Bronfenbrenner (1979) argued that an ecology of human development requires a systems approach for analysis, and that a review of the environmental-behavioral context of the individual is a necessary component for study.

Certainly, use of designs that offer much more variability in measuring settings is a recommended tactic in developmental neuropsychological work. Understanding how a given child with a brain injury will respond to school versus home versus play settings, for example, and what environmental stimulus elements or requisite skills affect his or her performance, are important issues to be researched further. Developmental neuropsychology will need to develop methodological techniques for the study of such questions, and a greater concern for psychosocial factors will need to be exploited in a variety of neurological conditions, especially at young ages. In using an ecological approach, a fuller understanding of the impact of such conditions will result.

INTERVENTION AND REHABILITATION NEEDS

A shift in neuropsychology has developed in the last 10 years from a concern with purely diagnostic issues to interventive and rehabilitative issues. Increasing numbers of neuropsychologists are working in rehabilitation settings involved with both psychological and cognitive aspects of the rehabilitation process. The literature on cognitive and neuropsychological treatment interventions has likewise blossomed (Benedict, 1989; Hart & Hayden, 1986b; Horton & Sautter, 1986; Prigatano et al., 1984; Trexler, 1982; Walsh & Greenough, 1976), particularly for individuals with traumatic brain injury. Of course, some controversy remains about the nature of intervention attempts with the brain injured, and well-designed studies with controlled data are only now beginning to emerge.

Many of the issues that confront a neuropsychologist working in a rehabilitative setting are very different from those that operate in other medical settings. In most cases, the important issues raised relate to the prediction or treatment of real-life behavior on the patient's part, a topic for which traditional models of neuropsychology have not provided much assistance. As Heaton and Pendleton (1981) commented, "For many patients who are known to have brain lesions that are not immediately life threatening or grossly incapacitating, the major clinical questions concern living arrangements, employability, prospects for rehabilitation, and the need for specific environmental supports" (p. 807). Thus frequent concerns for the neuropsychologist include assessment of the patient's competencies in everyday life both premorbidly and postmorbidly, assessment of the outcome of cognitive rehabilitative interventions, and measurement of the expected environmental resources of the patient (Chelune, 1985). An ecological neuropsychology related to the rehabilitation process is sorely needed.

The second section of this book addresses some of the practical concerns and needs in neuropsychological intervention. Issues such as the psychosocial and vocational consequences, compensation, and long-term outcome from brain injury are reviewed, and the role of the family as an environmental resource is covered. In addition, although our intent is not to cover the entire area of cognitive rehabilitation, one chapter addresses important elements of an ecological (versus a more traditional componential) perspective in cognitive rehabilitation.

Role of Family Involvement

A major contextual factor that is often overlooked in treatment is the role of the family. Family involvement in the handicap experienced by the person with brain injury is important and may in fact be one of the major determinants of the success or failure of rehabilitative efforts (Gogstad & Kjellman, 1976). Families often alter the level of competency that a person with a brain injury needs to demonstrate at home and in other social situations, and in so doing they affect the outcome of the case from a psychological point of view.

Family members and significant others also act as important factors in the rehabilitation of many types of patients (e.g., Bedrosian, 1981). Along with serving as powerful stimuli for eliciting certain types of behavior from the patient, family members can create an ecological environment conducive to relearning in the rehabilitation process. They can also act to maintain treatment gains by selectively reinforcing adaptive behaviors in the patient (Price, 1979). In chapter 8 Jacobs discusses the role of the family in the long-term rehabilitation of the brain injured, where by necessity family members need to act as important natural ecological forces to effect continued progress in the patient. In the last chapter of the book, Thomsen also touches on the importance of the family in long-term rehabilitation as she addresses the long-term outcome of traumatic brain injury.

Psychosocial Consequences and Outcome

Neuropsychology has yet to benefit from the complete application of an integrated biopsychosocial model in its theorizing (Engel, 1980). Kerns and Curley (1985) noted the beneficial effect of the application of such a model in understanding neurological disorders throughout the life span. As the field of neuropsychological rehabilitation has expanded, greater concern is being focused on the psychosocial outcome of various brain injuries (Lezak, 1987; Oddy et al., 1985), and many ecological and social concerns are being identified. Perhaps in line with the gist of this book, development and application of a *neuropsychosocial* model, in which disorders are considered to be the result of an interaction of neurological, psychological, and social factors, would more convincingly represent the current state of the art in neuropsychology.

Psychosocial outcome following brain injury, especially traumatic brain injury, is reviewed in several chapters. Pepping and Roueche, in chapter 9, discuss some of the results of the Oklahoma Neuropsychological Rehabilitation Program with regard to psychosocial outcome. As noted earlier, Thomsen also reviews the long-term psychosocial outcome of traumatic brain injury, using an interesting methodology stressing naturalistic observation in the home setting. Given the rather significant levels of disability and handicap experienced by the brain injured, even following a comprehensive rehabilitation program, further research is more than justified on a practical and a theoretical level.

It is interesting to note in passing the role of environmental factors in determining psychosocial outcome (see Kettle & Chamberlain, 1989). Much is still to be learned in studying ecological factors that maintain rehabilitative gains. For instance, as Haffey and Johnston (1989) noted, it is often the case that patients perform very differently in the home/discharge environment than they do in the hospital environment, in spite of the plans of well-meaning therapists!

As Luria described in a letter to Oliver Sacks, there may be many other non neuropsychological factors to consider in psychosocial outcome after rehabilitation: "What could we do? What should we do? 'There are no prescriptions,' Luria wrote, 'in a case like this. Do whatever your ingenuity and your heart suggest. There is little or no hope of recovery in his memory. He has feeling, will, sensibilities, moral being—matters of which neuropsychology cannot speak. And it is here, beyond the realm of an impersonal psychology, that you may find ways to touch him, and change him.... Neuropsychologically, there is little or nothing you can do, but in the realm of the Individual, there may be much you can do'" (Sacks, 1985, p. 32).

Practical Treatment of Everyday Task Performance

The new field of cognitive or neuropsychological rehabilitation remains somewhat controversial at present, in spite of the optimism that professionals hold for its benefit for patients. Aside from the difficulties associated with adequate measurement of rehabilitative effectiveness and outcome (see Crovitz, 1989; Diller & Ben-Yishay, 1987; Hart & Hayden, 1986b), a great many ecological concerns can be raised about cognitively based treatment approaches. Issues such as the need for differences in functional treatment techniques in varied patient populations, understanding of the interactions of various cognitive (and emotional) difficulties during dynamic task perform- ance in real-life settings, the role of stimulus and response generalization in rehabilitation, the benefit of process models, and the usefulness of simulation of everyday activities in cognitive rehabilitation, are all fruitful areas for ecological research.

One area addressed in our earlier volume that related to ecologically based rehabilitation endeavors is a need for a better classification and understanding of the psychological and neuropsychological competencies underlying every- day life tasks. Nagele (1985) and Mayer, Keating, and Rapp (1986) have provided models of real-life behaviors that have direct application in the rehabilitation setting. Neuropsychologists may need to cooperate closely with occupational therapists to understand better daily living skills (Morse & Morse, 1988). As noted in our earlier book, these practical models more often revolve around process-based descriptions of competencies and place emphasis on integrated scripts, routines, and goal-motivated activities in everyday behavior. Environmental and task assessment is also part of the expected rehabilitative process (see Fleishman & Quaintance, 1984).

Although some investigators in cognitive rehabilitation still expect to treat components of functioning in isolation, an ecologically valid cognitive reha- bilitation needs to assess the impact of treatment on functional behavior demonstrated by the patient. Therefore, consideration of mechanisms of generalization is a key element in neuropsychological rehabilitation. Hart and Hayden (1986a) have provided a description of some of the important integrated dimensions that should be considered in rehabilitation of informa- tion processing disorders in real life (table 1–1), and these dimensions directly affect the amount of generalization demonstrated by the patient.

Cicerone and Tupper, in chapter 11, describe a rationale for ecologically relevant treatment in neuropsychological rehabilitation. Unlike many models of rehabilitation, the focus in their chapter is on the activities of the therapist during the course of treatment. They make the point that the therapist needs to be concerned explicitly with interventions that provoke generalization of behavior change, and they suggest an outline of the ways in which cognitive rehabilitation can help the patient make connections between activities in the treatment session and better performance in everyday life. Of course, any type of cognitive rehabilitation approach, at this young age in the field's development, still needs to be validated. However, these authors raise im- portant points about the ecological validity of neuropsychological treatment techniques and therapeutic interactions.

Table 1–1. Information-processing dimensions of therapeutic tasks and situations

Dimension	Stimulus characteristics	Response characteristics

Complexity	Density in space
	Rate of presentation
	Amount of sensory integration required
	Familiarity
	Congruence with recently learned
	    information
		Length
		Elaborateness
		Sequential demands
		Automaticity
		Number of responses demanded
		    concurrently (time-sharing)

Autonomy	Activity of search required to obtain
	    necessary information (among
	    competing stimuli)
		Advance planning
		Prioritizing
		Decision making
		Initiative
		Self-evaluation

	Amount of retention required between stimulus and response Amount of manipulation/reorganization of information between stimulus and response	

Stress	Noise
	Distraction
	Interpersonal environment
	Intrapersonal environment
	    (depression, anxiety, fatigue, etc.)
		Performance demands:
		    accuracy, consistency,
		    efficiency, speed
		Demands on endurance

Source: Hart and Hayden, 1986a, p. 40, with permission.

Normalization and Compensation Following Brain Injury

As with all of us, individuals with brain injury strive to lead normal lives in spite of their impairments, and they often are quite adept at developing natural compensations for their areas of deficit, with or without active rehabilitation. In fact, early in the history of neuropsychology it was Kurt Goldstein who remarked about the tendency of brain-injured patients to function as a whole organism and to find ways to adapt and compensate for their deficits (Goldstein, 1939). Such patients attempt to keep their behavior ordered, normalized, and avoid "catastrophic reactions."

To some degree, the amount of normalization that can be experienced by persons with a brain injury depends on their present environment and the stress they are presented with (Hart & Hayden, 1986b). The World Health Organization, in fact, recognized back in 1980 that the experience of handicap for individuals is highly dependent on their social context (World Health Organization, 1980). Measures of long-term outcome following brain injury especially need to assess the social environment to determine the handicap experienced (see Thomsen's chapter).

The concept of the "normalization principle" was developed by Wolfensberger (1972) to encompass culture- and environment-specific adaptation to a deviant condition. Table 1–2 presents the levels on which various systems interact to lead to a normalized experience for the patient. For example, community re-entry is often a socially valued outcome (Condeluci & Gretz-Lasky, 1987). Price and Baumann, in chapter 10, discuss how the vocational rehabilitation process for brain-injured patients affects their redevelopment

Table 1–2. A schema of the expression of the normalization
principle on three levels and two dimensions of action

	Dimensions of action	
Levels of action	INTERACTION	INTERPRETATION
Person	Eliciting, shaping, and maintaining normative skills and habits in persons by means of direct physical and social interaction with them	Presenting, managing, addressing, labeling, and interpreting individual persons in a manner emphasizing their similarities to, rather than differences from, others
Primary and intermediate social systems	Eliciting, shaping, and maintaining normative skills and habits in persons by working indirectly through their primary and intermediate social systems, such as family, classroom, school, work setting, service agency, and neighborhood	Shaping, presenting, and interpretingintermediate social systems surrounding a person or consisting of target persons so that these systems as well as the persons in them are perceived as culturally normative as possible
Societal systems	Eliciting, shaping, and maintaining normative behavior in persons by appropriate shaping of large societal social systems, and structures such as entire school systems, laws, and government	Shaping cultural values, attitudes, and stereotypes so as to clicit maximal feasible cultural acceptance of differences

Source: Wolfensberger, 1972, p. 32, with permission.

of normalized experiences. Return to work is often one of the most visible handicaps for a brain-injured patient, and these authors describe the need for rehabilitation programs to address this real-life handicap.

FURTHER ISSUES IN THE NEUROPSYCHOLOGY OF EVERYDAY LIFE

There remain many further needs to make a neuropsychology of everyday life a reality. Pressures from within and outside of contemporary neuropsychology (e.g., third-party payors, families, and patients) are currently driving a consideration of ecological concerns in neuropsychological assessment and rehabilitation. This volume has discussed developmental and rehabilitative aspects of neuropsychology with an eye toward ecologically valid conceptualizations of processes that would allow us as professionals to make more dynamic predictions and theories about our patients' behavior in varied contexts.

This chapter has reviewed important issues such as the development and change in neuropsychological competencies in everyday life, ecological settings and their effect in development and breakdown, models and factors in an ecologically valid rehabilitation process, and the experience of brain injury. The use of functional assessment devices, the interrelationship of neuropsychological competencies and everyday skills, and the prediction of functional behavior from neuropsychological test instruments, are all major issues that have just begun to be explored in any systematic fashion.

As noted in the earlier volume, the continued development of an ecological neuropsychology will result from a better understanding of the practical needs of individuals functioning in real-world settings. Further investigation is needed to develop and test new methodologies for linking the neurological, the psychological, and the contextual factors into a neuropsychosocial understanding. These books have been presented as a beginning step in that development.

REFERENCES

Acker, M. B. (1986). Relationship between test scores and everyday life functioning. In B. P. Uzzell & Y. Gross (Eds.), *Clinical neuropsychology of intervention* (pp. 85–117). Boston: Martinus Nijhoff.

Albee, G. W. (1980). A competency model must replace the defect model. In L. A. Bond & J. C. Rosen (Eds.), *Competence and coping during adulthood* (pp. 75–104). Hanover, NH: University Press of New England.

Albert, M. S., & Moss, M. B. (Eds.). (1988). *Geriatric neuropsychology*. New York: Guilford Press.

Bakker, D. J. (1984). The brain as a dependent variable. *Journal of Clinical Neuropsychology* 6, 1–16.

Barker, R. G. (1968). *Ecological psychology: Concepts and methods for studying the environment of human behavior*. Stanford, CA: Stanford University Press.

Bedrosian, R. C. (1981). Ecological factors in cognitive therapy: The use of significant others. In G. Emery, S. D. Hollon, & R. C. Bedrosian (Eds.), *New directions in cognitive therapy* (pp. 239–254). New York: Guilford Press.

Benedict, R. H. B. (1989). The effectiveness of cognitive remediation strategies for victims of traumatic head-injury: A review of the literature. *Clinical Psychology Review* 9, 605–626.

Bronfenbrenner, U. (1979). *The ecology of human development: Experiments by nature and design*. Cambridge, MA: Harvard University Press.

Brooks, P. H., & Baumeister, A. A. (1977). A plea for consideration of ecological validity in the experimental psychology of mental retardation. *American Journal of Mental Deficiency* 81, 407–416.

Chelune, G. J. (1985). Toward a neuropsychological model of everyday functioning. *Psychotherapy in Private Practice* 3(3), 39–44.

Condeluci, A., & Gretz-Lasky, S. (1987). Social role valorization: A model for community re-entry. *Journal of Head Trauma Rehabilitation* 2(1), 49–56.

Crovitz, H. F. (1989). Memory retraining: Everyday needs and future prospects. In L. W. Poon, D. C. Rubin, & B. A. Wilson (Eds.), *Everyday cognition in adulthood and late life* (pp. 681–691). Cambridge: Cambridge University Press.

DeAngelis, T. (1989). Controversy marks child witness meeting. *APA Monitor* 20(9), September, 1, 8–9.

Diller, L., & Ben-Yishay, Y. (1987). Analyzing rehabilitation outcomes of persons with head injury. In M. J. Fuhrer (Ed.), *Rehabilitation outcomes: Analysis and measurement* (pp. 209–220). Baltimore: Paul H. Brookes.

Engel, G. E. (1980). The clinical application of the biopsychosocial model. *American Journal of Psychiatry* 137, 535–543.

Fleishman, E. A., & Quaintance, M. K. (1984). *Taxonomies of human performance: The description of human tasks*. Orlando: Academic Press.

Friedman, S. L., Scholnick, E. K., & Cocking, R. R. (Eds.). (1987). *Blueprints for thinking: The role of planning in cognitive development*. Cambridge: Cambridge University Press.

Gogstad, A. C., & Kjellman, A. M. (1976). Rehabilitation prognosis related to clinical and social factors in brain injured of different etiology. *Social Science and Medicine* 10, 283–288.

Goldstein, K. (1939). *The organism: A holistic approach to biology derived from pathological data in man*. New York: American Book Co.

Haffey, W. J., & Johnston, M. V. (1989). An information system to assess the effectiveness of brain injury rehabilitation. In R. L. Wood & P. Eames (Eds.), *Models of brain injury rehabilitation* (pp. 205–233). Baltimore: Johns Hopkins University Press.

Hart, T., & Hayden, M. E. (1986a). The ecological validity of neuropsychological assessment and remediation. In B. P. Uzzell & Y. Gross (Eds.), *Clinical neuropsychology of intervention* (pp. 21–50). Boston: Martinus Nijhoff.

Hart, T., & Hayden, M. E. (1986b). Issues in the evaluation of rehabilitation effects. In M. E. Miner & K. A. Wagner (Eds.), *Neurotrauma: Treatment, rehabilitation, and related issues* (Vol. 1, pp. 197–212). Boston: Butterworths.

Hartlage, L. C., & Telzrow, C. F. (Eds.). (1985). *The neuropsychology of individual differences: A developmental perspective*. New York: Plenum Press.

Heaton, R. K., & Pendleton, M. G. (1981). Use of neuropsychological tests to predict adult patients' everyday functioning. *Journal of Consulting and Clinical Psychology* 49(6), 807–821.

Horton, A. M., Jr., & Sautter, S. W. (1986). Behavioral neuropsychology: Behavioral treatment for the brain-injured. In D. Wedding, A. M. Horton, Jr., & J. Webster (Eds.), *The neuropsychology handbook: Behavioral and clinical perspectives* (pp. 259–277). New York: Springer.

Hynd, G. W., & Willis, W. G. (1988). *Pediatric neuropsychology*. Orlando: Grune & Stratton.

Kerns, R. D., & Curley, A. D. (1985). A biopsychosocial approach to illness and the family: Neurological diseases across the life span. In D. Turk & R. D. Kerns (Eds.), *Health, illness, and families: A life-span perspective* (pp. 146–182). New York: John Wiley.

Kettle, M., & Chamberlain, M. A. (1989). The stroke patient in an urban environment. *Clinical Rehabilitation* 3, 131–138.

Lezak, M. D. (1987). Relationships between personality disorders, social disturbances, and physical disability following traumatic brain injury. *Journal of Head Trauma Rehabilitation* 2(1), 57–69.

Luria, A. R. (1959). The directive function of speech in development and dissolution, parts I and II. *Word* 15, 341–352, 453–464.

Mayer, N. H., Keating, D. J., & Rapp, D. (1986). Skills, routines, and activity patterns of daily living: A functional nested approach. In B. P. Uzzell & Y. Gross (Eds.), *Clinical neuropsychology of intervention* (pp. 205–222). Boston: Martinus Nijhoff.

Morse, P. A., & Morse, A. R. (1988). Functional living skills: Promoting the interaction between neuropsychology and occupational therapy. *Journal of Head Trauma Rehabilitation* 3(1), 33–44.

Nagele, D. A. (1985). Neuropsychological inferences from a tooth brushing task: A model for understanding deficits and making interventions. *Archives of Physical Medicine and Rehabilitation* 66, 558.

Obrzut, J. E., & Hynd, G. W. (Eds.). (1986). *Child neuropsychology* (2 vols.). Orlando: Academic Press.

Oddy, M., Coughlan, T., Tyerman, A., & Jenkins, D. (1985). Social adjustment after closed head injury: A further follow-up seven years after injury. *Journal of Neurology, Neurosurgery, and Psychiatry* 48, 564–568.

Poon, L. W., Rubin, D. C., & Wilson, B. A. (Eds.). (1989). *Everyday cognition in adulthood and late life*. Cambridge: Cambridge University Press.

Price, R. H. (1979). The social ecology of treatment gain. In A. P. Goldstein & F. H. Kanfer (Eds.), *Maximizing treatment gains: Transfer enhancement in psychotherapy* (pp. 383–426). New York: Academic Press.

Prigatano, G. P., Fordyce, D. J., Zeiner, H. K., Roueche, J. R., Pepping, M., & Wood, B. C. (1984). Neuropsychological rehabilitation after closed head injury in young adults. *Journal of Neurology, Neurosurgery, and Psychiatry* 47, 505–513.

Rogoff, B., & Lave, J. (Eds.). (1984). *Everyday cognition: Its development in social context*. Cambridge, MA: Harvard University Press.

Rourke, B. P. (1982). Central processing deficiencies in children: Toward a developmental neuropsychological model. *Journal of Clinical Neuropsychology* 4, 1–18.

Rourke, B. P., Bakker, D. J., Fisk, J. L., & Strang, J. D. (1983). *Child neuropsychology: An introduction to theory, research, and clinical practice*. New York: Guilford.

Sacks, O. (1985). *The man who mistook his wife for a hat*. New York: Summit Books.

Spreen, O., Tupper, D., Risser, A., Tuokko, H., & Edgell, D. (1984). *Human developmental neuropsychology*. New York: Oxford University Press.

Sternberg, R. J., & Kolligian, J., Jr. (Eds.). (1990). *Competence considered*. New Haven, CT: Yale University Press.

Sternberg, R. J., & Wagner, R. K. (Eds.). (1986). *Practical intelligence: Nature and origins of competence in the everyday world*. New York: Cambridge University Press.

Stubbins, J., & Albee, G. W. (1984). Ideologies of clinical and ecological models. *Rehabilitation Literature* 45, 349–352.

Trexler, L. E. (Ed.). (1982). *Cognitive rehabilitation: Conceptualization and intervention*. New York: Plenum.

Vygotsky, L. S. (1978). *Mind in society: The development of higher psychological processes*. Cambridge, MA: Harvard University Press.

Walsh, R. N., & Greenough, W. T. (Eds.). (1976). *Environments as therapy for brain dysfunction*. New York: Plenum.

Wolfensberger, W. (Eds.). (1972). *The principle of normalization in human services*. Toronto: National Institute on Mental Retardation.

World Health Organization. (1980). *International classification of impairments, disabilities, and handicaps*. Geneva: World Health Organization.

I. LIFE SPAN DEVELOPMENTAL NEUROPSYCHOLOGY

2. THE NEUROPSYCHOLOGY OF CHILDHOOD LEARNING AND SCHOOL BEHAVIOR

LOUISE S. KIESSLING

INTRODUCTION

The basis for all childhood learning is the interaction between the environment and the individual, modulated by the developing capacities of the individual. The interaction between capacities—neurological, temperamental, experiential—is expressed over time. Neuropsychology as a discipline endeavors to understand brain–behavior relationships made all the more complex because the underlying neural substrate is continually changing during childhood and adolescence, with hormonal influences greatly adding to the complexity at puberty.

The entire span of growth and development can be divided into periods based on numerous bodies of evidence. One such approach is based on neural growth and myelination as described by Yakovlev & Lecours (1967), another on the description of neuromotor development (Lewis, 1982), a third on Piaget's concepts (Inhelder & Piaget, 1958). They are all equally valid schema, and each describes one facet of normal development. More recently, it has been shown that within each period there are often subtler discontinuities. Progress is not always linear and not always upward.

The purpose of this chapter is to provide information on developmental neuropsychology and what it may tell us about childhood learning and school behavior. Because of space limitations, the chapter will address a selected body of knowledge. Initial discussion will focus on the neural substrate, its development and characteristics, and will include a brief analysis of hormonal interactions with the central nervous system. Next the discussion will focus on what we know about hemispheric specialization in children. This section will be followed by discussion of styles of learning, their neuropsychological basis, and their impact on childhood learning and school behavior.

The competencies necessary for school learning and behavior will be outlined and related to our knowledge of relevant child neuropsychology. Since child neuropsychology is a relatively new field, relevant research will be used to develop the information.

DEVELOPMENTAL PROCESSES OF CHILDHOOD AND NEURAL ORGANIZATION

The process of development implies change over time mediated by changes in the physiology of the individual. Development is episodic with spurts and plateaus. The concept of maturation implies that behavior is a biological function, as Lenneberg (1968) stated in his essay in *The Neuropsychology of Development: A Symposium*: "Throughout childhood, behavioral capacities are constantly changing in accordance with a program that is genetically encoded and that determines the stimuli to which the growing organism shall be susceptible at different times. The notion of the critical period has come of age and may be accepted as a legitimate concept in the study of behavior." Critical to current study of the neuropsychology of children is knowledge of those neural substrates that are responsible for the changes in capacity noted at these times of rapid alterations in specific abilities. What underlies the so-called critical or sensitive periods, the periods when the child is accessible to new learning? Our knowledge is still rudimentary at best 20 years after Lenneberg (1968), but there are indicators of some of the processes that may be occurring.

Neural Development

The most rapid period for brain growth is during the 9 months from conception to birth and for the 2 years following birth. Skull and brain size are at 90% or more of adult levels by age 5 or 6, with very slow further outward growth until full height is achieved in late teens or early 20s (Behrman, Vaughan, & Nelson, 1987; Roche et al., 1987). The central nervous system includes diverse cells of two basic types: neurons, or nerve cells, and glial, or supporting, cells. These arrange themselves into layers such that the cerebral cortex of the adult, the most recently evolved part of the brain, has six layers. Early in development, the nerve cells form in the region around the ventricles, the germinal matrix, and migrate out toward the surface of the cortex. Cell differentiation occurs in the course of migration. Certain glial cells guide the migration of the nerve cells. Other glial cells (oligodendrocytes) form the myelin sheathes around the axons of the nerve cells, giving them a fatty-(lipid-) based insulated covering that greatly enhances neuronal conduction efficiency (Kandel & Schwartz, 1985).

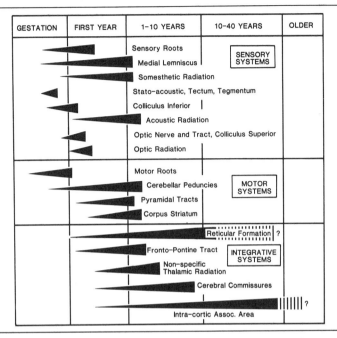

Figure 2–1. Myelogenetic cycles of regional maturation in the brain. (Modified from Spreen et al., 1984, and Yakovlev and Lecours, 1967).

The corpus callosum connects the two hemispheres of the brain. Myelination of the corpus callosum is almost complete by age 10, but myelination of the reticular formation, an area of the brain stem involved in arousal and attention, is not nearly complete until midway through the second decade. Neocortical association areas continue to myelinate in some people at least until the fourth decade and probably beyond, as demonstrated in figure 2–1 (Yakovlev & Lecours, 1967). Neural migration is felt to be complete by about age 5 months, but myelination of the cortex has barely begun at birth (Sarnat, 1987).

It is estimated that the brain has 10^{12} nerve cells, which can be classified into anywhere from 1000 to 10,000 different types with some common elements. In general, the cell body has an axon (with multiple terminals) that is transmitting and dendrite or dendrites that are receptive. Of major importance to the organization of the nervous system is the fact that, because of the multiple ways cells can be connected, a given cell can participate in a variety of different patterns of activity, in both the "on" (activated) and "off" (inhibited) states (Kandel & Schwartz, 1985). The connections between cells are called synapses. According to Sarnat (1987), the initial synaptic connections are always between the axon and dendrite, and synaptogenesis begins in the cortex only when neural migration is complete.

Working with Rhesus monkey brains, Rakic et al. (1986) showed rapidly developing numbers of synapses appearing synchronously in five different areas of the brain up to age 2 to 4 months, succeeded by a rapid falloff in the number of synapses to adult levels by one year. This finding is contrary to their original hypotheses. They had expected to find differing rates of synaptogenesis in different parts of the brain consistent with known patterns of neural migration (Sarnat, 1987) and rates of myelination (Yakovlev & Lecours, 1967). Similar data have been reported in humans (Huttenlocher, 1979; Huttenlocher et al., 1982) with rapid synaptogenesis to ages one to 2½ and then a falloff such that by age 11 onward the number of synapses is consistent with adult levels. However, detailed human studies have shown there is some regional cortical specificity for the timing of maximal synaptic production with maximal synaptogenesis in the visual system early, about one year of age. The overall almost synchronous development of synapses over the entire cortical area may provide the matrix for connections between all parts of the hemispheres (Rakic et al., 1986). It may provide the basis for much of the plasticity seen in the developing brain. These connections are then believed to be modified by learning and other environmental influences (e.g., toxins, emotional deprivation, sensitization, habituation), resulting in selective loss or strengthening of synaptic connections. Finally, throughout the life of the organism the existing synapses are regulated by biochemical and experiential mediation (Kandel & Schwartz, 1985).

Dendrites continue to expand their surface area by growing in stages, called segments, with periodic branching. The process of branching is called arborization. In the human neonate only the lower dendritic segments (orders 1 and 2) are present (Scheibel, 1984), with arborization continuing over time.

An important question of neural organization concerns the processes that subserve discrete capacities. What are the specific processes that underlie a change in capacity? As one approach to this question, Scheibel (1984) has been studying the process of dendritic aborization in adult postmortem brains, showing differences between right and left hemispheres in layer III of the area of neocortex that subserves speech (Broca's is on the left). The left hemisphere shows a greater number of higher-order dendritic segments (4th, 5th, and 6th), but the right hemisphere shows relatively greater length of 2nd- and 3rd-order branches, suggesting differential rates of growth and types of connections, especially in the first few years of life. Scheibel (1984) theorized that these results suggest that the right hemisphere, with its greater length of early developing dendritic segments, is more active during the early postnatal (preverbal) sensory motor stage. He postulated further that the increased late arborization noted for the left hemisphere correlates with the rapidly expanding conceptualization and speech skills from the end of the first year on.

Recently, Goldman-Rakic and her collaborators (Goldman-Rakic et al., 1989) showed, in the Macaque prefrontal cortex, that a dendrite of a pyramidal cell may have closely adjacent synaptic contacts, one symmetrical and dopaminergic and one asymmetrical and, likely of an excitatory nature, possibly responsive to glutamate (or aspartate). They also identified adjacent post-synaptic Tyrosine Hydroxylase immunoreactive boutons. Usually (but not always) symmetrical synaptic contacts are inhibitory; asymmetrical, excitatory (Colonnier, 1981). These researchers suggested that the triadic pattern of a DA-responsive symmetric synapse, Tyrosine Hydroxylase immunoreactive bouton, and a nonstaining asymmetric synapse on dendritic spines of pre-frontal cortex is similar to the pattern found in the caudate nucleus. The finding that two different synaptic contacts converge on the same dendritic spine provides a possible mechanism for modulation of output and will be discussed in the next section. It also suggests a possible unitary basis for the physiological effects of stimulant medication in children with attention deficit hyperactivity disorder and organizational disabilities—a point that will be taken up in the final segment of this chapter.

Neurotransmitters and neuropeptides

Another major component of central nervous function is the group of substances that mediate both slow membrane potential changes in the nerve cell and all-or-none axonal "firing." These are divisible into two main classes, the standard neurotransmitters and the neuropeptides. The former number about eight, including acetylcholine, norepinephrine, epinephrine, dopamine, serotonin (5-HT), glutamate (or aspartate), and GABA (gamma-aminobu-tyric acid). The known neuropeptides, which currently number more than 50 (Krieger, 1985), include the hypothalamic releasing factors, the neurohypo-physeal hormones (vasopressin, oxytocin, the neurophysins), pituitary peptides (such as ACTH and MSH), and centrally acting peptides (such as VIP and cholecystokinin) of which Krieger (1985) lists 14. In the prior section, we mentioned the finding of Goldman-Rakic and her group (1989) that synaptic contacts of two different types (symmetrical and asymmetrical) involving two different transmitters converge on a single dendritic spine. Dopamine is released at the presumed inhibitory (symmetric) terminal, and glutamate (or aspartate) is presumed to be released at the excitatory (asymmetric) terminal. The interplay between these dual contacts implies a mechanism for inhibitory modulation of the output of the unit. Goldman-Rakic and her group (1990) have shown that blocking DA receptors results in a deficit in working or short-term memory.

Whereas standard transmitters are modulators affecting whole projection systems, and accordingly often have large-scale tonic effects, neuropeptides have more discrete distribution in central neuronal populations. And in contrast to standard transmitters whose synthesis, uptake, and recycling occurs in or near axon terminals, synthesis of neuropeptides or their precur-sors occurs in ribosomes of cell bodies. Neurons apparently lack reuptake mechanisms for neuropeptides, and their concentrations are several orders of magnitude lower than those of the neurotransmitters—factors suggesting a more phasic mode of action (Krieger, 1985). Some of the neural transmitters identified in specific areas of fetal brains differ from the transmitters found in those locations in adult brains (Sarnat, 1987). Specifically, parts of the brain stem show evidence of high activity of the enzyme cholinesterase (ChE), which metabolizes acetylcholine during the fetal period but not afterward (Kostovic & Goldman-Rakic, 1983). Substance P, one of the neuropeptides, also shows a pattern of differential activity in brain stem areas, depending on whether newborn or adult brains are studied (Del Fiacco, Dessi, & Levanti, 1984).

Neurophysiological Measures

Studies of glucose metabolism using 2-Deoxy-2 [^{18}F] fluoro-D glucose (^{18}FDG) positron emission tomography performed in nine infants and young children from 5 weeks and younger through 1.5 years have shown developmental progression (Chugani & Phelps, 1986). Although the infants were examined because of questions of neurological disorder (seizures, port wine stains), their studies were analyzed in this report because they were functioning normally at the time of testing and in short-term follow-up (6 to 14 months). Measurement of the rate of glucose metabolism is used to decide which are the more metabolically active parts of the brain. Chugani and Phelps (1986) showed that infants 5 weeks or less in age had the highest rates of glucose metabolism in the sensorimotor cortex, thalamus, midbrain, and vermis of the cerebellum (the phylogenetically oldest part). This finding is consistent with the myelination data presented previously (Yakovlev & Lecours, 1967), as well as with the behavioral data showing the newborn and young infant to be mainly operating at the sensorimotor-subcortical level. By 3 months, there was a general increase in cortical regional glucose metabolism, with more activity also noted in the striatum (basal ganglia) as well. The activity in the cerebellum had increased laterally to the vermis, also consistent with the increasing capacity for the infant to balance, hold its head up, and begin to develop righting reflexes with loss of primitive tonic neck and startle reflexes. The pattern of glucose metabolism more closely resembling that of adults occurred in the children from 7.5 months on (ages 7.5 months, 1 year, and 1.5 years), with high metabolic rates now appearing in the frontal and association cortices. The thalamus shows consistently high glucose utilization at all ages studied, consistent with its role as a switching center.

Thatcher, Walker, and Guidice (1987) showed differential development for the cerebral hemispheres using measures of electroencephalographic coherence and phase. They evaluated 577 children whose ages ranged from 2 months to early adulthood. The cross-sectional study found both continuous growth processes expressed by exponential growth functions and discrete growth spurts coincident with specific anatomical development at specific ages. Right hemisphere development provided a relatively smooth progression from infancy to young adulthood, with the alpha phase reaching 90% of adult values by about 10 years of age. Left hemisphere development was characterized by more episodic development and large changes between age 2 and 4 and 2 and 5 in the mean alpha phase, with the alpha phase reaching 90% of adult values by age 6. The right hemisphere, however, showed a slight growth spurt in EEG alpha phase between 8 and 10 years. The final plateaus appeared during the teen years, coincident with physical maturation. A small, coinciding individual growth spurt in overall head circumference has also been noted at adolescence (Roche et al., 1987).

Thatcher and colleagues (1987) related the timing of these growth spurts, as well as those found earlier by Matousek and Petersen (1973) in their EEG normative studies, to the episodic developmental stages identified by Piaget (Inhelder & Piaget, 1958). These periods of differential growth may actually be related to periods of increased reorganization and integration, mediated by selective loss of some synapses and strengthening of others, regional increases in myelination, maturation of neurotransmitter function, or some combination of these. The periods of reorganization and integration, in turn, are related to some of the inter- and intrahemispheric developmental processes neuropsychology has been identifying; they will be discussed later.

Hormonal Influences

Among the other potent forces at work in the developing organism are the hormonal changes that occur during childhood and adolescence. Hormones have been shown to have roles as organizing factors for the development of sexual dimorphism, but they also act as organizing elements for the CNS and other tissues mediating behavior. From studies of genetic accidents—such as Turner's syndrome (with only one x chromosome, xo as opposed to xx female and xy male) and androgen insensitivity syndromes, in which the receptor for testosterone is missing from the target cells—we have learned that phenotypic female development occurs in the absence of the male hormone. Also from animal studies and studies of diseases caused by human genetic error—such as congenital adrenal hyperplasia, in which an excess of male hormone may occur in female fetuses—we know the fetus will be masculinized by such excess (Kelly, 1985). The hormones act during critical periods or, as Goy and McEwen (1980) prefer to describe it, during "periods of maximal sensitivity." These are periods when the presence of specific hormones results in gender-specific organizational blueprints. Future sensitivity of targeted brain cells to hormones specific to one sex or the other is also determined (Kelly, 1985). During human fetal and neonatal development, between the 12th and 22nd week after conception and again during the first 6 weeks of postnatal life, there are two separate periods when the male testes are more active in androgen secretion. It has been shown that sexual differences originally found in the anatomy of the adult human brain are also present in fetal brains. The corpus callosum is sexually dimorphic in the adult as well as in the fetal brain. Females show larger cross-sectional surface area relative to brain weight of the corpus callosum. This male-female difference develops maximally during weeks 18 to 26 of prenatal life, overlapping the first period of greater androgen production in the male (Kelly, 1985). The effects of hormones on development can occur in three different characteristic patterns. In type I, for the behavioral characteristics to occur, the appropriate hormones must be present during one of the early periods of maximal sensitivity and again at a later stage. In other words, the hormone(s) must be present for organizing the target cells as well as for their later activation. Relative superiority of males on mental rotation and visuospatial tasks that is present early on but enhanced at puberty fits this pattern (Waber, 1977; Witelson, 1976). Type II requires that the specific hormone(s) be present in significant quantities for activation only. The basal amount of hormone(s) available to either sex is enough for organization in the type II situations. An example of a type II case from physiology is that balding can be triggered in females by administration of testosterone. In type III situations the hormone(s) is necessary for organization, as in the differentiation of the human reproductive tract, but is not relevant to activation. An example of a type II situation from neuropsychology is the suggested alterations in female visuospatial processing ability noted in girls who have engaged in intensive exercise in the prepubertal state (Petersen, 1983).

Puberty is the result of interactions between releasing factors produced by neuroendocrine cells of the hypothalamus, pituitary hormones, and the reproductive organs (Kupfermann, 1985). Other studies have shown hormonal effects on axon and dendrite growth and synaptic development, just to list a few (Kelly, 1985). Specific effects for estrogen-progesterone as well as testosterone on nerve cells have also been delineated (Goy & McEwen, 1980). Onset of puberty is generally accepted to be when the child moves from sexual maturation rating 1 (SMR1), or prepuberty, to SMR2, or early puberty (Behrman, Vaughan, & Nelson, 1987). Prior to the onset of puberty, hormonal influences have been changing but overt puberty is believed to be preceded by release of hypothalamic-releasing factors and by secretion of pituitary gonadotropins and growth hormone.

Secretion of these hormones causes an increase in the size of ovaries or testes and triggers the secretory phases of these organs, which begin to produce estrogen and testosterone, respectively. These sex-specific hormones then produce further physical and physiological changes. In addition, the adrenal glands are producing their own androgens that promote added changes, including acne. The ages for SMR2 vary from 10 to 13 in girls and 10.5 to 14.5 in boys. As such, there is considerable overlap at any given age between early and late maturers.

HEMISPHERIC PLASTICITY, DIFFERENTIATION, AND SPECIALIZATION
The cerebral hemispheres in humans have long been known to exert a large amount of control of the motor and sensory functioning of the opposite sides of the body, by way of a system of crossed fiber tracts in addition to the

uncrossed ones. For the last 150 years or so the effects of injury to the left hemisphere have also been known to cause impaired language production in adults, first described by Dax in the early 19th century but more fully studied since Broca in the 1860s (Geschwind, 1984). These two observable facts—as well as much intervening information, one suggesting equality, the other specific laterality to the hemispsheres—raise the issues of plasticity and hemisphere specialization.

A body of data has been gathered from diverse fields showing clear anatomical asymmetries to brain and skull in humans (including fossil and fetal), as well as in other mammals (Galaburda, 1984; LeMay, 1984; LeMay & Culebras, 1972). The asymmetries are developmental (Chi, Dooling, & Gilles, 1977), neurochemical, and architectonic, with the most well documented differences noted in the areas of the sylvian fissure (Galaburda, 1984). The right sylvian fissure is higher and shorter than the left sylvian fissure, and the temporal and parietal areas surrounding it are also larger. One of the most intensely studied areas of the temporal lobes is a flat plate of tissue referred to as planum temporale. Geschwind and Levitsky (1968) found it larger on the left in 65% of autopsied brains. The left planum temporale has also been noted to be larger in 31-week fetuses who also showed a second transverse gyrus on the right (Chi, Dooling, and Gilles, 1977) as is found in adults. This establishes the prenatal anatomical occurrence of hemispheric asymmetry, suggesting early prenatal potential for hemispheric specialization. Lenneberg (1967) theorized that the cerebral hemispheres were functionally equipotential up to at least age 2 to 3, with some plasticity up to puberty. If destruction of tissue occurred before these ages, the innate processes of organization and lateralization would be altered and the brain would reorganize itself. Lenneberg (1967) saw the process of lateralization as a phenomenon of growth and development. Teuber (1967), however, questioned the concept of total plasticity.

Hemispheric Functions

More recent work suggests the hemispheres are probably never equipotential for all cognitive abilities. For example, some subtle language disabilities, particularly with regard to syntactic comprehension and semantic repetition, are noted in right-hemiplegic children who had lesions to the left hemisphere prior to age one, most often before, at, or around birth (Kiessling, Denckla, & Carlton, 1983). The impaired functioning of the right-hemiplegic group, when compared to siblings and left-hemiplegic children with infantile hemiplegia, was noted primarily on tasks of higher-level language functioning—syntactical awareness and the repetition of semantically coherent materials. This finding was consistent with those of Dennis and Kohn (1975) and Rankin, Aram, and Horwitz (1981).

The more basic receptive language capacities as measured by the Peabody Picture Vocabulary Test (Dunn, 1969) were generally intact in the group with left hemisphere lesions. They scored in the average range, although there was a trend toward scores lower than those of siblings or right-brain-damaged children.

In addition to the results regarding receptive vocabulary and complex language functions, a measure of word finding that required recognition of line drawings (Goodglass, Kaplan, & Weintraub, 1976) showed similar but nonsignificant decrements for both hemiplegic groups when compared to controls (Kiessling, Denckla, Carlton, 1983). This task requires perception of the drawing, a right hemisphere function, coupled with semantic output, a left hemispheric function. The data suggested that the Boston Naming Test requires input from both hemispheres.

The Raven's Coloured Progressive Matrices (Raven, 1965) were completed equally well by children with either left or right hemisphere lesions and scoring at average levels using age adjusted norms, suggesting that this test is measuring a reasoning ability that transcends hemispheres because it can be approached by using several strategies. Hecaen and Albert (1978) noted that Raven scores may be affected by injury to either hemisphere. The puzzles appear to require both visuospatial and logical functions. Consequently, a child with impaired visuospatial ability (right-hemisphere-impaired) may solve the problems using a logical strategy (possibly aided by tracing the figures with a finger or using verbal encoding), or one impaired for logical functions (believed to be left hemisphere) may solve the problems by relying entirely on visuospatial congruence relations. If it were necessary to have both hemispheres fully intact for successful completion of these puzzles, one would expect decrements in both left- and right-brain-damaged groups when compared to controls, which was not the case.

Robinson (1981) looked at the issue of early lateralization and summarized data from adult commissurotomy patients and found they were in agreement with the previous results with regard to receptive language. He noted that the right hemisphere can understand short phrases from the vocabulary of the phrase, not from the syntax. Bishop (1981) suggested that the crowding effect may be an important determinant of what functions are preserved after early brain damage. She theorized that some of the lost function after early lesions is a result of competition for synaptic sites, with early-appearing functions such as receptive vocabulary filling the available synaptic sites and "crowding out" late-maturing, more complex functions such as syntactical awareness.

Goldman (1972), working with infant monkeys, described differential recovery of function after trauma to two functionally related parts of the brain. She gave evidence that part of the differential recovery at least depends on whether the *uninjured* area is functionally "committed" or mature at time of injury. If the uninjured area is "committed" or mature, recovery of functions subserved by the injured area will not occur. If the spared area is functionally immature, recovery will occur over time. In the latter case the immature, developing, "uncommitted" neocortex or subcortical structures of the infant would be available to take over functions of the injured area. This recovery would not be possible in an adult animal because most areas would be "mature" or "committed." This may be just one of many mechanisms of reorganization available to mammalian brains after early injury. The possibility of multiple mechanisms is underscored by comparison of these data with the material reported earlier on neural migration, synaptogenesis, and myelination.

The evidence suggests that an element of laterality or specialization exists at birth, at least with regard to language development and physical handedness, most often residing in the left hemisphere. The data suggest preprogramming of potential synaptic connections and potential neurotransmitter specificities according to a sequential program whose timing is individual specific. At the same time, there is a degree of plasticity early in development (Goldman, 1972). There may be a hierarchy such that maximal plasticity is available to regions that mature latest.

The process of maturation from a neurophysiological perspective appears to have differential rates or timetables depending on which part of the central nervous system one is looking at. As discussed before, myelination progresses in different parts of the brain at varying rates. As an example, the auditory-vestibular system myelinates in several phases, first in the brain stem (trapezoid body and superior olive) during intrauterine life from the 5th to the 9th fetal months, then in the inferior colliculi early in the first year, and finally in the acoustic radiations (geniculotemporal projection system) beyond the first postnatal year. This progression contrasts with that of the visual system, in which the colliculi don't begin myelinating until the 9th fetal month, but the entire system is complete by the third postnatal month (Yakovlev & Lecours, 1967). These periods of myelination coincide with the ability to process what sensory data are available to the fetus. Vestibulo-acoustic stimuli are present in utero, while visual stimuli are not available until after birth. Use of the vestibulo-auditory stimuli in an integrated fashion, however, does not appear until well after birth. The hemispheres also show differential changes with regard to the presence of alpha-phase (7–12Hz) waveforms in the EEG (Thatcher, Walker, & Guidice, 1987), with the left maturing in rapid spurts such that 90% of adult levels are present by age 6. The right hemisphere shows steady but slow growth of alpha preponderance, with a small spurt between ages 8 and 10.

The motor and sensory functions have both crossed and ipsilateral representation in each hemisphere. The data support some degree of ipsilateral motor control, which appears to be involved in the better motor skill development seen in childhood hemiplegics as opposed to adult stroke patients. Nass (1985) summarized the material and postulated a role for the corpus callosum, which myelinates about age 10 as previously noted (Yakovlev & Lecours, 1967), in developing inhibition of the mirror movements seen in normal children up to that age.

The developmental pattern of differential hemispheric contribution to somatosensory processing was assessed by Sherman (1985) in her doctoral thesis. These data were presented at the meeting of the International Neuro-psychological Society in 1985. She used a tactuospatial recognition (matching) task of graded complexity with both whole and part-whole matching. Sher-man found across all age levels that whole tactuospatial matching was more accurately performed with the left hand, implying more proficient right hemisphere processing. In contrast, part-whole tasks were performed more efficiently with the right hand, suggesting greater left hemisphere engagement. She used three age-matched groups of normal children—7–8, 10–11, and 13–14—each with 20 boys and 20 girls. The data suggest the degree of laterality for this tactuospatial task is already established by age 7, as no developmental increase in accuracy was noted from ages 7 to 14.

However, there were differences between the groups at different ages. Both 7- to 8 and 13- to 14-year-old groups had significantly greater left hand mean scores for the whole tactuospatial matching task, suggesting greater right hemisphere processing. In contrast, the 10- to 11-year-old group demon-strated a predominant pattern whereby the right hand mean scores were greater, indicating greater left hemisphere engagement for the same task. The data are consistent with some other studies of right hemisphere function that suggest either a plateau or depression at or around 10 to 12 years of age (Carey & Diamond, 1977; Carey & Diamond, 1980; Denckla, Rudel, & Broman, 1980). In this case, use of a left hemisphere strategy occurs preferentially at the 10- to 11-year level with a return to right hemisphere strategy by 13 to 14. Harris (1978) found that boys showed catch-up growth to girls with regard to verbal ability in the 10- to 12-year-old period. This return to right hemisphere strategy then corresponds to the period when boys put their former visuo-spatial skills to more abstract use, suggesting male-female differences as well as maturational ones.

Carey and Diamond (1980) summarized studies of the development of the ability to recognize (encode) unfamiliar faces. Previously, Yin (1970, reported in Carey & Diamond, 1980) had developed evidence from adult lesion studies that right hemisphere specialization for encoding upright faces was a skill distinct from that of the right hemisphere for encoding visual configurations in general. Other researchers had previously shown that image inversion interfered significantly with the subject's ability to encode faces, an effect more pronounced than with any other class of tested visual stimuli (houses, bridges, dog's heads, landscapes, etc.). When compared to normals and patients with other lesions on these tasks, patients with right posterior lesions were significantly impaired only on encoding upright faces. They were no more impared on the encoding of inverted faces or inverted or upright houses than controls, suggesting a very specific deficit and underscoring the usual dichotomy between responses to inverted and upright faces.

These researchers then used the Yin faces and houses tasks to show the de-velopmental progression from 6 years old through adolescence. To summarize, they found that at the younger ages (6 and 8), contrary to adult findings, inversion of faces had no greater effect on accuracy of recognition than inversion of houses did. At the same time, by age 10 there was a rapid improvement in response to orientation of the faces, accounted for by improvement between ages 6 and 10 in encoding upright unfamiliar faces. Thus 9- to 10-year-olds show the adult form of interaction between the materials and their orientation, but younger children do not. There is also a drop in the interactive effect between 12 and 14 because of a decline in performance on upright faces at those ages. By 16 the adult form of performance has returned. Several related studies have shown the dip in performance at age 12 or a plateau from 10 to 13 and true adult performance by age 16.

Carey and Diamond (1977) proposed that these changes are consistent with a developmental hypothesis. They found that children under 10 rely on more superficial, piecemeal cues to encoding unfamiliar faces and take longer to form an adequate representation. This finding suggests that experience with many unfamiliar faces is one aspect of the sharp improvement in the 10-year-old, and supports their contention that it is the relatively invariant relationships of configuration found in all faces that give them their special type of encoding characteristics. Younger children engage the left hemisphere for this task. Further work by Leehey quoted by Carey and Diamond (1980) had shown a right hemisphere advantage for encoding unfamiliar faces that develops around age 9 and again shows a dip in performance between ages 12 and 14, followed by development of an adult form of right hemisphere advantage by 16.

Diamond, Carey, and Back (1983) replicated the relative dip in performance in girls with regard to encoding unfamiliar faces and related it to pubertal status. Generally, girls in the midst of puberty showed a disruption in the ability to encode unfamiliar faces. Comparison with results obtained from prepubescent and postpubescent girls showed that in the disruption of this skill pubertal status, not age specifically, was the critical factor.

Denckla, Rudel, and Broman (1980) found similar developmental curves for normal children carrying out a Map Walking task. Interestingly, dyslexics and other nondyslexic learning disabled children had much poorer performance at younger ages when left hemisphere engagement is felt to be in place for this task. By age 11, the dyslexics showed a more accurate performance than normals, suggesting that as myelination of the callosal system occurs (Yakovlev & Lecours, 1967) a shift from left to right hemisphere processing takes place. A related possibility is that improved right hemisphere integration occurs after the spurt in alpha-phase development noted by Thatcher et al. (1987). Denckla et al. (1980) also postulated that maturation of frontal systems may account for this pattern.

Petersen (1983) took issue with the concept of a decrement or plateau in visuospatial skill development in early adolescence. She postulated that experience may alter hormonal functioning and therefore self-image and timing of maturation. Specifically, early heavy exercise has been noted to alter body habitus and may affect onset of puberty; such girls may also engage in more athletic activities and more visual-spatial activities. Petersen (1983) quoted Newcombe, Bandura, and Taylor as finding the latter in late-maturing girls who were also less feminine and better in math skills.

Petersen (1983) reported a consistent relationship between timing of maturation and spatial performance on the field independence measure. Late-maturing girls showed more field independence (better spatial performance) than early-maturing girls but still less field independence than late-maturing boys, consistent with Waber (1977, 1980). She also reported that in a meta analysis of the literature she found that the sex differences with regard to spatial skills arise prior to early adolescence, as Witelson (1976) and Harris (1978) had reported.

Petersen (1983) used the preceding research to support the theory that pubertal change, in addition to direct hormonal effects on the brain, sets off a series of responses to the change in physical appearance that provide the basis for gender intensification. The period of gender intensification may be upsetting to the child, resulting in alterations of biochemical stability and leading to disruption of normal cognitive growth. It may also promote what is perceived as sex role appropriate feminine behavior such that the girls limit experience with tasks labeled "masculine" (see also Waber, 1980).

Petersen (1983) found no significant effect of pubertal status on any of the cognitive measures but did find a pattern on the field independence task somewhat consistent with the pubertal disruption hypothesis. At each grade (6, 7, and 8) the pubertal group scored lowest when compared with early and late pubertal groups, but the results did not reach significance. Petersen (1983) interpreted their overall findings as inconsistent with a theory of plateau or decline in skills at puberty. The neurophysiological data, however, appear to be consistent with some type of growth spurt followed by a period of neural reorganization, which may be recognized as a plateau of right hemisphere functions. The neurophysiology is noted in the EEG studies of Thatcher et al. (1987).

MATURATIONAL THEORY

Relative to these neurophysiological processess, Waber (1980) summarized many of the earlier arguments in child development that reflect on whether development was biologically or environmentally determined and whether maturation was a proper topic of research. Current thinking in child development has returned to a maturational theory of development but with allowance for modification by environmental factors. For example, in lower mammals, if an eye is stitched shut such that the animal has no visual experience with it, the visual system for that eye will not function when the stitches are removed. If the functioning eye is then removed, however, the previously nonfunctional eye will develop vision (Joseph, 1982). With regard to the development of complex visual processing skills, a series of partially overlapping "critical" or "sensitive" periods was identified in primates (Harwerth et al., 1986). The system appears to be hierarchical, with basic visual functions in the retina (rods and cones) having shorter, earlier sensitive periods, whereas those involving complex central processing have much longer sensitive periods (spatial vision less than 25 months, binocular functions greater than 25 months). These studies were done in Macaque monkeys. A rate of development of the visual system in human infants comparable to that of the Macaque is 4 to 1, suggesting age 8 as the time when spatial vision plasticity ends in humans. This estimate is consistent with the data from children who had prolonged traumatic cataract (Harwerth et al., 1986). Thus experience is necessary for full development of the neural network; and the genetic scheduling of development requires that experience of a given type has to occur in its "expected" epoch if it is to have full effect.

Current child development theory is that cognitive development is the result of environmental factors both positive and negative (parental caring, good nutrition, good instruction, adequate but not excessive exercise, exposure to toxins such as lead, etc.) acting on an intrinsic biological program. The order of development is predetermined, but the rate is individually determined and affected by experience.

Waber (1980) undertook the development of neuropsychological methods to elicit the specific maturational processes at work. The concept of prepared learning is important for developmental research, akin to the idea of the "critical period" referred to by Lenneberg (1968). Prepared learning implies that the learning is tied to the developmental state of the child. Inhelder's conservation training experiments (cited in Waber, 1980) show that the child in the preoperational state of Piaget can be taught certain concrete operational tasks only with great difficulty, whereas a child of the same age who has reached the transitional stage (a state of disequilibrium beyond the pre-operational) will learn the concrete operations readily and will generalize the knowledge to other domains. In this case, the structure needed to assimilate the new learning was available within the transitional but not the preopera-tional child. In the educational setting, the concept of "readiness" would be synonymous with prepared learning. For a skill to be learned easily and effectively, functional organization must be in place. The 4-year-old may want to write his name, but the fine motor coordination must be in place as well as the ability to name the letters of his name, or at least to copy them, before he can easily complete the task. If the neural maturity is not in place, it will take an inordinate amount of training and rehearsal to get the name correct; nor will he, for instance, begin to generalize to learning other letters.

Waber (1980), in searching for methods to quantify the mechanics of matu-ration, correlated advancement in one system with advancement in another and studied the ways in which different patterns of maturation result in different outcomes. Females commonly mature before males. Females have been believed to be more competent verbally, and males show marked superiority as a group on spatial tasks. The question is whether this difference results from biologically determined changes in physiology as a result of puberty or because the pubertal adolescent reacts to the changes of puberty by adhering to specific sex roles (see also Petersen, 1983). Waber questioned whether the differing rates of maturation of males and females were related to the differential abilities apparent after puberty. She studied children at various ages who were in the process of maturing and subdivided the groups by maturation, early or late. (Tanner staging was done by a pediatrician.) She then gave the children a series of tests previously shown to have a sex difference and found that the late maturers scored better than the early maturers on the tests of spatial ability, that is, a male-like pattern. She found no difference in any of the groups for verbal abilities, however. In a second experiment using dichotic listening, she explored the issue of hemispheric lateralization. It was theorized that people in whom language is less well lateralized will have more difficulty with spatial tasks (competition for space, incompatibility of processing style, etc.) than a person with language well lateralized. Waber's (1980) data showed a strong right ear advantage for only the older group of late maturers. The younger groups showed no systematic results. The data are suggestive, not definitive.

Possible mechanisms for the increasing differentiation of the CNS with age include the sex hormones that have receptors on brain cells (Kandel & Schwartz, 1985). High levels of sex steroid hormones in the male fetus at 18 to 22 weeks and in the immediate postnatal period (up to 6 weeks) have an organizing effect on the brain in mammalian species in general, but the effect may be biphasic in some instances, with the new behavior elicited by the second wave of steroid hormone output at puberty. The early pulses are a primer; the last produces an anamnestic response, as it were. As discussed above, this seems to be an example of the type I hormonal pattern where the hormone is first an organizer, later an activator. This may explain the finding that boys show better spatial skills even before puberty (Witelson, 1976; Harris, 1978; Petersen, 1983) but with enhanced skill afterward.

PROCESSING STYLES

Critical to the understanding of childhood learning and school behavior is the interaction of task and its level of difficulty with optimum processing style. Much of our information on right versus left hemisphere task superiority is now felt to reflect intrinsic sensory and associational processing mechanisms within the respective hemispheres and their subcortical projections as opposed to isolated modality-specific sensory processing centers. Nebes (1978) emphasized the need to adequately analyze the components of tasks rather than look for "centers" that encompass specific mental functioning. He pointed out that the type of information processing required to solve the problem may determine which hemisphere is dominant.

Ornstein and co-workers (1980), using an EEG technique paired with the geometrical whole and part–whole matching task employed by Nebes (1978), found part–whole discrimination tasks engaged the left hemisphere, not the right, suggesting the left hemisphere is necessary for analysis and synthesis of these complex geometrical discriminations, despite the fact that this is a visual spatial task (see also Sherman, 1985). They concluded that the more complex the abstraction, the more the left hemisphere is involved. It is not the content of a particular problem but the strategy employed that determines which hemisphere is chiefly involved. The right hemisphere preferentially uses simultaneous, synthetic strategies, the left analytical, sequential and "propositional" (Denny-Brown, 1962).

Rourke (1985) pointed out the need to determine the role in cognition for the subcortical structures and white matter. He postulated that these have significant effects in nonlanguage learning disabilities. Various authors (Goldberg & Costa, 1981; Harris, 1978; Nebes, 1974) summarized the terms ascribed to the processing styles of the major and minor hemispheres: "linguistic/nonlinguistic," "sequential/simultaneous," "symbolic/visual-spatial," "analytic/gestalt," and "propositional/appositional." Ultimately, the major hemisphere, usually the left, best handles sequential analysis of sensory input, and the right, or minor, hemisphere responds more appropriately to stimultaneous, configurational material.

Waber and Holmes (1985, 1986) developed norms for children's performance on the Rey-Osterrieth Complex Figure for both copy and memory state. Their work sheds more light on the developmental progression noted for style of performance, particularly for a difficult visual-spatial task as well as for its memory. They found that the copy form of the Rey is completed in a part-oriented manner until age 10 or so (levels IV and V of their groups, ages 5–14), after which the preponderance of children use a more configurational approach to the copy form, with the whole base rectangle and mid-structure as the salient features. Memory for the design, however, results in more configurational production beginning after age 5. After age 9, almost no one used a part-oriented memory strategy. At age 5 copy and memory forms were equally frequently completed in a part-oriented manner. After age 5 the memory format promoted use of the base rectangle and the midstructure as the salient elements. The developmental progression for organization of the Rey-Osterrieth Complex Figure follows the progression seen for other visual-spatial copy tasks (Beery, 1982). First the base rectangle, then horizontal and vertical crosspieces, and finally diagonals are incorporated into the schema.

The Waber and Holmes (1985, 1986) work shows the importance of task specificity and level of difficulty as determinants of optimal style of processing, based on the developing competency of the child. These results complement those of Carey and Diamond (1980) summarized earlier regarding encoding of unfamiliar faces. There, too, the younger child used a part-oriented strategy, whereas the older child (around age 10) showed a gestalt processing approach suggesting right hemisphere engagement.

Thus processing style is in part determined by task type and difficulty level.

Other factors, such as the ability to use verbal encoding, also affect processing style. This may explain the ability to solve the Raven's Coloured Progressive Matrices at a normal level by children with congenital right hemisphere lesions (Kiessling et al., 1983).

ATTENTION

Selective attention is a necessary component for effective learning and school behavior. The central nervous system mechanisms that mediate attention are complex. In classical neurology, work with Rhesus monkeys implicated frontal systems approximately 100 years ago, but studies in the 1940s focused on the reticular activating system (Mesulam, 1985). More recent work has emphasized the interrelatedness of neocortical, thalamic, and limbic structures as all involved in modulating attention. The reticular formation (RF) was described by Bishop (1958) as a "linked system" running the length of the neuraxis. It includes such major nuclei as nucleus gigantocellularis of the medulla, which figures in pain and escape reactions, or the locus coeruleus of the caudal midbrain, which projects widely to the forebrain and is important in the maintenance of normal waking states. Lesions to this nucleus or its (noradrenergic) projections have been found, for instance, to impair an animal's ability to ignore irrelevant stimuli. The RF receives input from virtually all ascending and descending fiber systems. It appears to have global monitoring functions and to mediate forebrain arousal or "novelty" responses—features necessary but not sufficient for fine modulation of attention.

The thalamus acts as a major relay station between the reticular formation and the cortex. Injury to the intralaminar nuclei and/or the thalamic reticular nucleus can also result in attentional deficits. Finally, limbic structures such as the amygdala (Murray & Mishkin, 1985; Pribram & McGuinness, 1975) and the association areas of the cortex have a role in attention and its fine tuning. Again, specific cortical lesions result in deficits that may be specific. For example, the frontal lobe appears to play an important role in a person's response to complex and novel stimuli. Tests known to be sensitive to attentional disturbances are usually poorly done by people with documented frontal lobe injury, although deficits of directed or focused attention may be more severe in right hemisphere lesions (Mesulam, 1985). Children with attention deficit hyperactivity disorder are also sensitive to at least some of those same tests of frontal lobe function. Chelune and co-workers (1986) standardized the Wisconsin Card Sort Task (a measure of frontal lobe disinhibition) on a normal population of children and also administered the test to a group of attention deficit disordered (ADD) children (DSM III definition). The ADD children had scores consistent with those of normal children at younger ages. That is, 8–9 year-old ADD children score more like normal 6–7-year-olds. This fits some of the maturational deficit theories of ADD. However, improvement in attention brought on by use of dextroamphetamine or methylphenidate in children is felt to be mediated through the catecholamine systems, implicating the thalamus and brain stem reticular activating system (Laufer, Denhoff, & Solomons, 1957).

Clearly, there are multiple locations where the ability to attend can be interfered with. Theoretically, one can postulate multiple mechanisms or sites of action for the stimulant medication as well. The previously cited study (Goldman-Rakic et al., 1989) showing both dopamine (inhibitory) and probable glutamate (or aspartate) terminals (excitatory) closely adjacent on the same dendrite of prefrontal pyramidal cells in monkeys provides an additional site of action for stimulant medications, particularly methylphenidate or pemoline, which act primarily to increase availability of dopamine at synapses. The finding of a similar pattern of synapses in the caudate nucleus suggests these closely related areas may respond similarly. Recent research (Kiessling et al., 1988; Kiessling, 1989) suggested differential effects of dextroamphetamine and methylphenidate in a group of children with attention deficit disorder, with methylphenidate more likely to produce less variability in the computerized EEG of the group as a whole when compared to the effects of placebo or dextroamphetamine.

IMPLICATIONS FOR EDUCATION AND SCHOOL BEHAVIOR

In early childhood learning, "readiness" is an important concept. As described before, "readiness" has a neurophysiological basis, emphasizing the need to assess the child not only intellectually but for maturation. The concept of "readiness" is particularly important to consider before beginning instruction in early academics. The rate of maturation differs from one child to another and can be altered by stress or lack of experience. It is also relatively independent of IQ, so sensitivity to readiness is essential to promote maximal success in early learning. It is important to recognize that physical benchmarks such as loss of first teeth may be related to neuropsychological maturity as they are to physical maturity.

The concept of "readiness" can be extended throughout the school period although it is usually reserved for the preacademic child. In essence, the child progresses through multiple developmental stages that are coupled to underlying neurophysiological and hormonal changes. Optimal performance is more likely to occur if teaching and expectation for learning are geared to the developmental state of the child.

Early cognitive tasks perceived by the child as difficult are best handled by a sequential, analytic style according to the data presented (Carey & Diamond, 1980; Waber & Holmes, 1985, 1986). This applies whether the material is of a linguistic or visual-spatial type. It has implications for the child who has difficulty with sequencing, whose more natural processing style may be configurational. The child with a more gestalt, holistic processing style may have difficulties with deductive reasoning, retaining specific sequential steps to complete a task, and retrieving supportive details to substantiate a conclusion. The result may be the child who fits into subtype 2 of reading disabled groups as described by Rourke and Strang (1983). They postulated that the area compromised is left parieto-occipital in this group. The child with an underlying language deficit, clear left hemisphere impairment, fits into their subtype 1, reading impaired. This group, Rourke and Strang (1983) theorized, may have left temporal lobe impairment. Subtype 3, reading disabled (Rourke & Strang, 1983), describes the child with specific difficulty generating verbal information, word-finding deficits, often associated with impaired short-term memory (in which case the deficit may be more left frontal than temporal). This subtype is similar to a group described by Saffran (1982). Because of contiguity of language output areas to the motor strip, right-sided motor performance of these children is likely to be less efficient than left. Ojemann and Mateer (1979) found areas of syntactical comprehension, naming, and reading between the areas identified for short-term verbal memory and those carrying out phonemic identification. All of these surrounded the final common motor pathway for speech.

The data strongly support a maturational-environmentally interactive view of child development, consistent with a structural theory (Lewis, 1982). They also suggest that a newborn already has genetic preprogramming for differential development of the two homologous hemispheres, as well as for the subcortical structures such as the thalamus, which acts as a relay station. Early childhood learning is of the sensorimotor type with mostly subcortical, reflexive integration for the first month or so. The fetus has already made use of auditory and vestibular stimuli in utero, responding with movement or quieting as the case may be. By 3 months of age, the child has rudimentary associative skills with simple face and voice recognition, ability to make visual and auditory discriminations, and maturing motor skills, changes reflecting the myelination (Yakovlev & Lecours, 1967) and dendritic arborization occuring in the visual, auditory, and motor cortices (Purpura, 1974; Sarnat, 1987). Although the basic processes of learning at the sensorimotor stage are often a result of conditioning, there is the beginning of improved memory ability and a beginning level of logical sequencing by 7 to 9 months when the child acquires object permanence (Lewis, 1982). This timing is consistent with evidence of more active glucose metabolism in the frontal and posterior association areas of the brain (Chugani & Phelps, 1986). This capacity for object permanence and improved memory occurs quite suddenly, implying a discontinuity with immediately preceding capacities.

De Loache (1987) showed evidence for another discontinuity. She reported: "Three year old children who observed an object being hidden in a model knew where to find an analogous object hidden in the corresponding location in a room, but 2.5 year old children did not. The success of the group of older children reveals an advance in their cognitive flexibility: they think of a model in two ways at the same time—both as the thing itself and as a symbol for something else." The data support Kagan (cited in Lewis, 1982), showing multiple periods of discontinuity concomitant with the appearance of many discrete changes, including alterations in processing style (Carey & Diamond, 1980; Waber & Holmes, 1985, 1986) and improved capacity to use verbally mediated logical processing (Thatcher, Walker, & Guidice, 1987). These periods of discontinuity in development seem to be consistent with periods of reorganization and may be preceded by relative plateaus in skill development (Carey & Diamond, 1980; Denckla, Rudel, & Broman, 1980; Waber, 1980.)

Kagan (cited in Lewis, 1982) referred to the switch from a perceptual to a symbolic/linguistic processing mode at about 17 months, which seems consistent with Scheibel's dendritic arborization studies (1984) as well as mye-lination data (Yakovlev & Lecours, 1967) and EEG data (Thatcher, Walker, & Guidice, 1987). We previously presented data on the change from sequential/analytic to a more configurational approach for visual-spatial tasks (Waber & Holmes, 1985, 1986) and face recognition (Carey & Diamond, 1980), which occurs around age 10, consistent with the neurophysiological data. There is a further discontinuity brought out by Diamond, Carey, and Back (1983), Lindgren and Benton (1980), Sherman (1985), and others. The normal child has the haptic ability to make complex perceptual judgments before age 7 but uses differing processing styles that seem age- and complexity-specific depending on the task.

Childhood learning progresses from the sensorimotor to increased use of symbolic and linguistic strategies, coinciding with rapid development of an alpha predominance in the left hemisphere (Thatcher, Walker, & Guidice, 1987). This period of reorganization is coincident with the cutting back and restructuring of synapses (Rakic et al., 1986; Huttenlocher, 1979; Huttenlocher et al., 1982). The child persists in using the piece-by-piece, analytic, sequential style to approach tasks perceived as difficult even when the theoretical optimal style suggested by the material itself is configurational (e.g., unfamiliar face encoding) (Carey & Diamond, 1977, 1980). Experience appears to play a significant role in how the child approaches the task. There is a tendency to process unfamiliar, new information in a more piecemeal fashion, particularly before age 10, but when overlearned the material may become processed in a configurational manner. Memory for visuospatial material becomes con-figurational as early as age 6, certainly by 9 (Waber & Holmes, 1986). With development and maturation, the child shows increasing ability to attend, probably related to continuing myelination of the reticular formation and frontal lobes.

Age 10 or thereabouts has been mentioned several times in this chapter as a transitional or critical age. The reason may be because this is the age when the corpus callosum has usually reached almost full myelination, permitting efficient transfer between the hemispheres. Neuron and synapse loss may also be complete (Huttenlocher, 1979; Rakic & Goldman-Rakic, 1982). Myelina-tion increases the efficiency of neural transmission and thus enhances the capacity for cooperation between hemispheres, permitting the usually better developed part by part strategies (more left hemisphere style) of the 6- to

9-year-old to be improved upon by the configurational strategies of the child 10 and older. It is also the end of the right hemisphere increase in alpha-phase predominance noted by Thatcher et al. (1987). This is also the period when early pubertal changes are appearing.

Where loss and replacement of first teeth is a strong physical maturational marker for readiness for reading (Kiessling, personal observation), there is a close correlation between time of eruption of the second permanent molars and of menarche ($r = 0.62$) (Behrman, Vaughan, & Nelson, 1987). With puberty, the child is neuropsychologically able to use the increasing store of knowledge, apply more complex processing, and make more associations because of the increasing interconnections supplied by continued myelination, maturation of neural transmitter function, and apparent enhancement by hormonal action at receptors in the brain.

Physical maturation has significant neuropsychological effects, as demonstrated by Harris (1978), Petersen (1983), and Waber (1977, 1980). Petersen (1983) and Waber (1977, 1980) both found evidence that late maturers performed better on a field independence task than early maturers, and Waber (1980) found late-maturing boys performed better than late-maturing girls. Harris (1978) presented extensive data describing sex-specific differences in learning. The exact role of societal and peer pressure in forming these sex differences is hard to quantify (Petersen, 1983), but evidence that the sex steroids have receptors on brain cells suggests a significant role for them in brain maturation and activity (Kandel & Schwartz, 1985).

The learning and reasoning capacities for a 12-year-old will be related both to cognitive capacity as measured by IQ and to pubertal state. Since a 12-year-old can be anywhere from prepubertal to postpubertal, a group of them may include children still working at the concrete operational stage of Piaget as well as others capable of formal operations—the contrast between a child at an "empirico-deductive" stage and one at the "hypothetical-deductive" stage.

With regard to academic skill development, the early school-aged child should have adequate left hemisphere linguistic skills to ensure success with early reading, spelling, and arithmetic. The ability to rapidly name the alphabet by age 6 (Jansky & De Hirsch, 1973) is a good prognostic indicator for early reading. Word finding or naming is a left hemisphere skill strongly related to reading success (Wolfe, 1979). Syntactic competence is another left hemisphere skill related to reading success (Kiessling, Denckla, & Carlton, 1983). The above skills are deficient in the subtype 1, reading-impaired children described by Rourke and Strang (1983). Spelling is highly dependent on sequencing (subtype 2, Rourke & Strang, 1983), also a left hemisphere strategy, and spelling deficits have been related to early left hemisphere injury (Wood & Carey, 1979).

Early on, arithmetic skill is related to number naming, a left hemisphere skill, but overall mathematical ability has strong right hemisphere, stimultaneous configurational components, particularly geometry, and measures of field independence and spatial rotation (Waber, 1977, 1980). Kiessling et al. (1983) found a strong relationship between left hand (right brain) function measured by the Annett Pegboard (Annett, 1970) and scores on the arithmetic section of the Wide Range Achievement Test in a mixed normal and hemiplegic population.

The organization of written material is particularly sensitive to problems with attention and impulsivity. This suggests frontal lobe/reticular activating system involvement because marked improvement in written work is noted in stimulant-treated children with attention deficit hyperactivity disorder (Kiessling, unpublished data). The data of Goldman-Rakic et al. (1989) previously mentioned, indicating the presence of (symmetrical) dopamine- and (unsymmetrical) probably glutamate-containing terminals on the same dendritic spine on a prefrontal pyramidal cell, suggest a general mechanism whereby catecholaminergic inhibitory control could be exerted directly on units involved in the scheduling of motor output. The Wisconsin Card Sort Test (Chelune et al., 1986) is sensitive to ADD as is the Trail Making Test (Lezak, 1983).

Superimposed on the natural developmental readiness for learning are the specific strengths and weaknesses of the individual child. The vast majority of individuals have relative strengths and weaknesses, whether because of subtle genetic preprogramming differences, minor insults to the brain early on, lack of appropriate experience at the sensitive times, or conversely, especially rich experience at sensitive times. The range of individual differences is wide. Through use of developmental neuropsychological assessment, it is possible to elucidate learning strengths and weaknesses as well as learning style. These can then be related to the task at hand as well as to the developmental state of the individual and the individual's processing style. Programs of education and remediation appropriate to the individual may be suggested by the test results. Multiple theories and approaches were discussed in four recent volumes (Obruzt & Hynd, 1986; Rourke, 1985; Spreen et al., 1984).

Combination of the methods of brain imaging—MRI, PET scanning (Chugani & Phelps, 1986), biochemical studies and selective EEG studies (Duffy et al., 1980 a, b; John, 1977; Thatcher, Walker, & Guidice, 1987)—coupled with neuropsychological assessment have the potential to further enhance our knowledge of both normal and pathological child development.

REFERENCES

Annett, M. (1970). The growth of manual preference and speed. *British Journal of Psychology* 61, 545–558.

Beery, K. E. (1982). *Revised administration, scoring and teaching manual for the developmental test of visual-motor integration.* Cleveland: Modern Curriculum Press.

Behrman, R. E., Vaughan, V. C., & Nelson, W. E. (1987). *Textbook of pediatrics* (13 ed.). Philadelphia: WB Saunders.

Bishop, D. V. M. (1981). Plasticity and specificity of language localization in the developing brain. *Developmental Medicine & Child Neurology* 23, 251–255.

Bishop, G. H. (1958). The place of the cortex in a reticular system. In H. H. Jasper, L. D. Proctor,

R. S. Knighton, W. C. Noshay, & R. T. Costello (Eds.), *Reticular formation of the brain* (pp. 413–421). Boston: Little, Brown.

Carey, S., & Diamond, R. (1977). From piecemeal to configurational representation of faces. *Science* 195, 312–314.

Carey, S., & Diamond, R. (1980). Face encoding. In D. Caplan (Ed.), *Biological studies of mental processes* (pp. 60–93). Cambridge, MA: MIT Press.

Chi, J. G., Dooling, E. C., & Gilles, F. H. (1977). Gyral development of the human brain. *Annals of Neurology* 1, 86–93.

Chelune, G. J., Ferguson, W., Koon, R., & Dickey, T. O. (1986). Frontal lobe disinhibition in attention deficit disorder. *Child Psychiatry and Human Development* 16 (4), 221–234.

Chugani, H. T., & Phelps, M. E. (1986). Maturational changes in cerebral function in infants determined by FDG positron emission tomography. *Science* 231, 840–843.

Colonnier, M. (1981). The electron-microscopic analysis of the neuronal organization of the cerebral cortex. In F. O. Schmitt, F. G. Worden, G. Adelman, & S. G. Dennis (Eds.), *The organization of the cerebral cortex* (pp. 125–152). Cambridge, MA: MIT Press.

Del Fiacco, M., Dessi, M. L., & Levanti, M. C. (1984). Topographical localization of substance P in the human post-mortem brainstem. An immunohistochemical study in the newborn and adult tissue. *Neuroscience* 12, 591–611.

De Loache, J. S. (1987). Rapid change in the symbolic functioning of very young children. *Science* 238, 1556–1557.

Denckla, M. B., Rudel, R., & Broman, M. (1980). The development of a spatial orientation skill in normal, learning disabled and neurologically impaired children. In D. Caplan (Ed.), *Biological studies of mental processes* (pp. 44–59). Cambridge, MA: MIT Press.

Dennis, M., & Kohn, B. (1975). Comprehension of syntax in infantile hemiplegia after cerebral hemidecortication: Left hemisphere superiority. *Brain and Language* 2, 472–482.

Denny-Brown, D. (1962). Discussion, fourth session, A. In V. B. Mountcastle (Ed.), *Interhemispheric relations and cerebral dominance* (pp. 224–252). Baltimore: Johns Hopkins Press.

Diamond, R., Carey, S., & Back, K. J. (1983). Genetic influence on the development of spatial skills during early adolescence. *Cognition* 13, 167–185.

Duffy, F. H., Denckla, M. B., Bartels, P. H., & Sandini, G. (1980). Dyslexia: Regional differences in brain electrical activity mapping. *Annals of Neurology* 7, 412–420.

Duffy, F. H., Denckla, M. B., Bartels, P. H., Sandini, G., & Kiessling, L. S. (1980). Dyslexia: Automated diagnosis by computerized classifications of brain electrical activity. *Annals of Neurology* 7, 421–428.

Dunn, L. M. (1969). *Expanded manual for the Peabody Picture Vocabulary Test*. Circle Pines, MN: American Guidance Service.

Galaburda, A. M. (1984). Anatomical asymmetries. In N. Geschwind & A. M. Galaburda (Eds.), *Cerebral dominance: The biological foundations* (pp. 11–25). Cambridge, MA: Harvard University Press.

Galaburda, A. M., LeMay, M., Kemper, T. L., & Geschwind, N. (1978). Right-left asymmetries in the brain. *Science* 199, 852–856.

Geschwind, N. (1984). Historical introduction. In N. Geschwind & A. M. Galaburda (Eds.), *Cerebral dominance: The biological foundations* (pp. 1–8). Cambridge, MA: Harvard University Press.

Geschwind, N., & Levitsky, W. (1968). Left-right asymmetry in temporal speech region. *Science* 161, 186–187.

Goldberg, E., & Costa, L. D. (1981). Hemisphere differences in the acquisition and use of descriptive systems. *Brain and Language* 14, 144–173.

Goldman, P. S. (1972). Developmental determinants of cortical plasticity. *Acta Neurobiologica. Exp.* 32, 495–511.

Goldman-Rakic, P. S., Leranth, C., Williams, S. M., Mons, N., & Geffard, M. (1989). Dopamine synaptic complex with pyramidal neurons in primate cerebral cortex. *Proceedings National Academy of Science* 86, 9015–9019.

Goldman-Rakic, P. S., & Sarvoguchi, T. (1990). The workings of working memory. *The Journal of NIH Research* 2, 42–43.

Goodglass, H., Kaplan, E., & Weintraub, D. (1976). *The Boston Naming Test, experimental edition*. Boston, MA: Aphasia Unit, VA Hospital, Huntington Avenue.

Goy, R. W., & McEwen, B. S. (1980). *Sexual differentiation of the brain*. (Based on a Work Session of the Neurosciences Research Program). Cambridge, MA: MIT Press.

Harris, L. J. (1978). Sex differences in spatial ability: Possible environmental, genetic, and neurological factors. In M. Kinsbourne (Ed.), *Asymmetrical function of the brain*. Cambridge: Cambridge University Press.

Harwerth, R. S., Smith, E. L., III, Duncan, G. S., Crawford, M. L. J., & von Norden, G. K. (1986). Multiple sensitive periods in the development of the primate visual system. *Science* 232, 235–238.

Hecaen, H., & Albert, M. L. (1978). *Human neuropsychology*. New York: Wiley.

Huttenlocher, P. R. (1979). Synaptic density in human frontal cortex: Developmental changes and effects of aging. *Brain Research* 163, 195–205.

Huttenlocher, P. R., deCourten, C., Garey, L. J., & Van Der Loos, H. (1982). Synaptogenesis in human visual cortex—Evidence for synapse elimination during normal development. *Neuroscience Letters* 33, 247–252.

Inhelder, B., & Piaget, J. (1958). *The growth of logical thinking: From childhood to adolescence* (A. Parsons & S. Milgram, Trans.). New York: Basic Books.

Jansky, J., & De Hirsch, K. (1973). *Preventing reading failure*. New York: Harper & Row.

John, E. R. (1977). *Neurometrics: Clinical applications of quantitative electrophysiology*. Hillsdale, NJ: Lawrence Erlbaum.

Joseph, R. (1982). The neuropsychology of development: Hemisphere laterality, limbic language, and the origin of thought. *Journal of Clinical Psychology* 38 (1), 4–33.

Kandel, E. R., & Schwartz, J. H. (1985). *Principles of neural science*. New York: Elsevier.

Kelly, D. D. (1985). Sexual differentiation of the nervous system. In E. R. Kandel and J. H. Schwartz (Eds.), *Principles of neural science*. New York: Elsevier.

Kiessling, L. S. (1989). Attention deficit hyperactivity disorder. In G. Adelman (Ed.), *Neuroscience year* (Supplement 1 to the *Encyclopedia of neuroscience*). Boston: Birkhauser.

Kiessling, L. S., Denckla, M. B., & Carlton, M. (1983). Evidence for differential hemispheric function in children with hemiplegic cerebral palsy. *Developmental Medicine and Child Neurology* 25, 727–734.

Kiessling, L., Wagner, R., Thompson, L., Riccitelli, A., & Davies, R. (1988). Differential effects of methylphenidate and dextroamphetamine on a group of attention deficit disordered children. *Developmental Medicine and Child Neurology Supplement No. 57*, 30, (5), p. 23.

Kostovic, I., & Goldman-Rakic, P. S. (1983). Transient cholinesterase staining in the mediodorsal nucleus of the thalamus and its connections in the developing human and monkey brain. *The Journal of Comparative Neurology* 219, 431–447.

Krieger, D. T. (1985). Brain peptides: What, where and why? In P. H. Ableson, E. Butz, & S. H. Snyder (Eds.), *Neuroscience* (pp. 309–331). Washington, D.C.: American Association for the Advancement of Science.

Kupfermann, I. (1985). Hypothalamus and limbic system I: Peptidergic neurons, homeostasis and emotional behavior. In E. R. Kandel & J. H. Schwartz (Eds.), *Principles of neural science* (pp. 612–625). New York: Elsevier.

Laufer, M. W., Denhoff, E., & Solomons, G. (1957). Hyperkinetic impulse disorder in children's behavior problems. *Psychosomatic Medicine* 19 (1), 38–49.

LeMay, M. (1977). Asymmetries of the skull and handedness. *Journal of the Neurological Sciences* 32, 243–253.

LeMay, M. (1984). Radiological, developmental, and fossil asymmetries. In N. Geschwind & A. M. Galaburda (Eds.), *Cerebral dominance: Biological foundations* (pp. 26–42). Cambridge, MA: Harvard University Press.

LeMay, M., & Culebras, A. (1972). Human brain: Morphological differences in the hemispheres demonstrable by carotoid arteriography. *New England Journal of Medicine* 287, 168–170.

Lenneberg, E. H. (1967). *Biological foundations of language*. New York: Wiley.

Lenneberg, E. H. (1968). The effect of age on the outcome of central nervous system disease in children. In R. L. Isaacson (Ed.), *The neuropsychology of development: A symposium* (pp. 147–170). New York: Wiley.

Lewis, M. (1982). *Clinical aspects of child development* (2nd ed.). Philadelphia: Lea & Febiger.

Lezak, M. (1983). *Neuropsychological assessment* (2nd ed.). New York: Oxford University Press.

Lindgren, S., & Benton, A. (1980). Developmental patterns of visuospatial judgments. *Journal of Pediatric Psychology* 5 (2), 217–225.

Matousek, M., & Petersen, I. (1973). Frequency analysis of the EEG in normal children and adolescents. In P. Kellaway & I. Petersen (Eds.), *Automation of clinical electroencephalography* (pp. 75–102). New York: Raven Press.

Mesulam, M.-M., (1985). *Principles of behavioral neurology*. Philadelphia: Davis.

Murray, E. A., & Mishkin, M.(1985). Amygdalectomy impairs crossmodal association in monkeys. *Science* 228, 604–606.

Nass, R. (1985). Mirror movement asymmetries in congenital hemiparesis: The inhibition hypothesis revisited. *Neurology* 35 (7), 1059–1062.

Nebes, R. D. (1974). Dominance of the minor hemisphere in commissurotomized man for the perception of part-whole relationships. In M. Kinsbourne & W. L. Smith (Eds.), *Hemispheric disconnection and cerebral function* (pp. 155–164). Springfield, IL: Charles C Thomas.

Nebes, R. D. (1978). Direct examination of cognitive function in the right and left hemispheres. In M. Kinsbourne (Ed.), *Asymmetrical function of the brain* (pp. 99–137). Cambridge, MA: Cambridge University Press.

Obrzut, J. E., & Hynd, G. W. (Eds.). (1986). *Child neuropsychology: Volumes I and II*. Orlando, FL: Academic Press.

Ojemann, G. A., & Mateer, C. (1979). Human language cortex: Localization of memory, syntax and sequential motor-phonemic identification systems. *Science* 205: 1401–1403.

Ornstein, R., Johnstone, J., Herron, J., & Swencionis, C. (1980). Differential right hemisphere engagement in visuospatial tasks. *Neuropsychologia* 18, 49–64.

Petersen, A. C. (1983). Pubertal change and cognition. In J. Brooks-Gunn and A. C. Petersen (Eds.), *Girls at puberty* (pp. 179–198). New York: Plenum Press.

Pribram, K. H., & McGuinness, D. (1975). Arousal, activation, and effort in the control of attention. *Psychological Review* 82 (2), 221–234.

Purpura, D. P. (1974). Dendritic spine "dysgenesis" and mental retardation. *Science* 186, 1126–1128.

Rakic, P., Bourgeois, J.-P., Eckenhoff, M. F., Zecevic, N., & Goldman-Rakic, P. S. (1986). Concurrent overproduction of synapses in diverse regions of the primate cerebral cortex. *Science* 232, 232–235.

Rakic, P., & Goldman-Rakic, P. S. (1982). *Development and modifiability of the cerebral cortex*. *Neurosciences Research Program Bulletin* (Cambridge, MA: MIT Press) 20 (4), 429–611.

Rankin, J. M., Aram, D. M., & Horwitz, S. J. (1981). Language ability in right and left hemiplegic children. *Brain and Language* 14, 292–306.

Raven, J. C. (1965). *The coloured progressive matrices*. New York: Psychological Corporation.

Robinson, R. O. (1981). Equal recovery in child and adult brain? *Developmental Medicine and Child Neurology* 23, 379–383.

Roche, A. F., Mukherjee, D., Guo, S., & Moore, W. M. (1987). Head circumference reference data: Birth to 18 years. *Pediatrics* 79 (5), 706–712.

Rourke, B. P. (Ed.). (1985). *Neuropsychology of learning disabilities: Essentials of subtype analysis*. New York: Guilford.

Rourke, B. P., & Strang, D. (1983). Subtypes of reading and arithmetical disabilities: A neuropsychological analysis. In M. Rutter (Ed.), *Developmental neuropsychiatry* (pp. 473–488). New York: Guilford.

Saffran, E. M. (1982). Neuropsychological approaches to the study of language. *British Journal of Psychology* 73, 317–337.

Sarnat, H. B. (1987). Disturbances of late neuronal migrations in the perinatal period. *American Journal of Diseases of Children* 141 (9), 969–980.

Scheibel, A. B. (1984). Dendritic correlates of human speech. In N. Geschwind & A. M. Galaburda (Eds.), *Cerebral dominance: The biological foundations* (pp. 43–52). Cambridge, MA: Harvard University Press.

Sherman, B. R. (1985). Lateralized tactuospatial recognition patterns in children and young adolescents. (Doctoral dissertation, Boston College, October 1984.) *Dissertation Abstracts International*, Pub # 85–10691, 46 (3) Book B.

Spreen, O., Tupper, D., Risser, A., Tuokko, H., & Edgell, D. (1984). *Human developmental neuropsychology*. New York: Oxford.

Teuber, H.-L. (1967). Lacunae and research approaches to them. In F. L. Darley & C. H. Millikan (Eds.), *Brain mechanisms underlying speech and language*. New York: Grune & Stratton.

Thatcher, R. W., Walker, R. A., & Guidice, S. (1987). Human cerebral hemispheres develop at different rates and ages. *Science* 236, 1110–1113.

Waber, D. (1977). Sex differences in mental abilities, hemispheric lateralization and rate of physical growth at adolescence. *Developmental Psychology* 13 (1), 29–38.

Waber, D. P. (1980). Maturation: Thoughts on renewing an old acquaintanceship. In D. Caplan (Ed.), *Biological studies of mental processes* (pp. 8–26). Cambridge, MA: MIT Press.

Waber, D. P., & Holmes, J. M. (1985). Assessing children's copy productions of the Rey-Osterrieth complex figure. *Journal of Clinical and Experimental Neuropsychology* 7, 264–280.

Waber, D. P., & Holmes, J. M. (1986). Assessing children's memory productions of the Rey-Osterrieth complex figure. *Journal of Clinical and Experimental Neuropsychology* 8, 563–580.

Witelson, S. F. (1976). Sex and the single hemisphere for spatial processing. *Science* 193, 425–427.

Wolfe, M. (1979). The relationship of disorders of word-finding and reading in children and aphasics. Unpublished doctoral dissertation, Graduate School of Education of Harvard University.

Wood, B. T., & Carey, S. (1979). Language deficits after apparent clinical recovery from childhood aphasia. *Annals of Neurology* 6, 405–409.

Yakovlev, P. I., & Lecours, A. R. (1967). The myelogenetic cycles of regional maturation of the brain. In A. Minkowski (Ed.), *Regional development of the brain in early life* (pp. 3–70). Oxford: Blackwell.

3. THE NEUROPSYCHOLOGICAL DETERMINANTS OF FUNCTIONAL READING, WRITING, AND ARITHMETIC

RICHARD GALLAGHER AND URSULA KIRK

INTRODUCTION

The neuropsychological aspects of reading, writing, and mathematical disorders have received considerable attention from the beginning of the modern study of brain–behavior relationships. Both Broca's and Wernicke's first papers discussed aspects of at least one of these disorders when they analyzed their aphasic patients. With subsequent study, the broad outlines of the neuroanatomical basis of disorders in these skills have become well understood. More recently, unusual cases have been thoroughly assessed and critical substrates for specific components of reading, writing, and arithmetic are being identified. This information has fleshed out the skeletal understanding of the association between brain damage and disruption of these important skills. Additionally, advances in the neuropsychological study of children have provided insight into the impact of early brain dysfunction on limited acquisition of reading, writing, and mathematical skills. From the combined advances in the study of acquired deficiencies and developmental dysfunctions, a new awareness of how the brain supports the functional activities of these important skills has begun to emerge.

This chapter reviews recent literature on acquired and developmental disorders to provide a foundation for understanding the neuropsychological determinants of functional reading, writing, and mathematics. The chapter also reviews the epidemiology of acquired reading, writing, and mathematical disorders to indicate the likelihood of encountering such deficits. It is hoped that this review will afford the neuropsychological professional with an understanding of how day-to-day reading, writing, and mathematical functioning can become disrupted, how likely it is that the capabilities will become disrupted given particular forms of brain dysfunction, and how likely it is that these functions will recover over the course of time.

READING DISORDERS: ALEXIA

The term used for a reading disorder that develops as the result of acquired brain damage is alexia. This condition refers to the situation in which people show deficits in comprehension of written material. The term refers primarily to deficits in the capacity to comprehend letters, words, and sentences, although other written symbols such as numbers may also be incomprehensible.

Within the last 10 years, two classification systems for the alexias have been applied in case studies. The first classification system is the traditional system adopted as early as 1891 by Dejerine to distinguish between those conditions in which reading deficits exist by themselves: alexia with agraphia and alexia without agraphia, respectively. The second, more recent system discriminates among forms of alexia on the basis of reading errors. This latter approach has developed out of the field of psycholinguistics and relies on analysis of the cognitive components of reading.

The Traditional System

Alexia without agraphia

This condition exists when a person's comprehension of written material is severely disrupted but the capacity to write is nearly normal. Spelling and written communication is adequate, but the person is unable to read what has just been written. Because of the nature of the lesions observed in such cases, other deficits are usually found with this syndrome. Specifically, the person almost always has visual field cuts of the right hemifield of each eye. This condition contributes to problems in design copying, naming of objects seen, and color naming. Oral language is usually intact, although mild anomia may be present.

Anatomically, the condition occurs when the angular gyrus of the left parietotemporal region is disconnected from visual input from both the right and left eyes. The angular gyrus seems essential for reading, as it mediates the association of verbal labels with written words and letters. Severing this region from visual input prevents the recognition of the names of the symbols perceived. Symbols can be matched on visual characteristics, but their meaning is not understood. Written spelling and writing are possible because the lexicon is available to the hands through indirect connections between the angular gyrus and the frontal, motor regions.

Lesions that cause this disorder are localized to the left hemisphere in path-

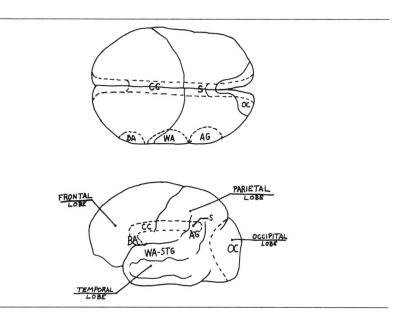

Figure 3–1. Side and horizontal views of the left cerebral hemisphere with major areas of concern highlighted and labeled. Legend: BA, Broca's areas; CC corpus callosum; WA-STG, Wernicke's area/superior temporal gyrus; AG, angular gyrus; S, splenium of the corpus callosum; OC, occipital cortex.

ways between the angular gyrus and the left visual cortex of the occipital lobe (see figure 3–1). They are most often accompanied by lesions of the posterior third of the corpus callosum (Ajax, 1968; Greenblatt, 1973, 1976; Momose et al., 1986; Nicole, Nardi, & Fortuna, 1982) that disrupt visual input from the intact right hemisphere to the angular gyrus in the left hemisphere.

Alexia with agraphia

When writing disorders accompany reading deficiencies, the lesions as well as the functional disturbances are greater than when reading disturbances occur alone. Two forms of the disorder are present: (1) that occurring with only mild general language disturbances and (2) that associated with aphasic disorders.

Parietal alexia describes the narrower condition in which only mild language disturbances are present. In this condition, letters and words cannot be read, and spontaneous writing, writing to dictation, and copying letters are severely disordered. This condition is associated with lesions of the left angular gyrus. In this condition, the source of dysfunction is not poor access to an intact lexicon, as it is in alexia without agraphia, but an area of storage for the lexicon (i.e., the angular gyrus) that is disrupted through damage. Associated problems include acalculia, right-left disorientation, impaired finger recognition, hemianopsia, and apraxia; consequences of general parietal lobe damage. However, oral language is generally intact.

Alexia associated with aphasia

Reading disorders that accompany broader language disorders are typically found with receptive or Wernicke's aphasia. Prior to the most recent studies, these reading disorders were thought to parallel the nature of the receptive language disorders: word substitutions in reading (paralexias) and paraphasias or word substitutions in speech were both present and of equivalent frequency. The level of reading comprehension deficits matched the level of deficits in receptive language comprehension. These deficits were attributed to a disconnection between the lexicon (stored in the angular gyrus) and the auditory association areas in the temporal lobes. The model was based on the assumption that accurate reading required subtle auditorization of the words. However, recent case studies implied that levels of language comprehension disorder and reading comprehension disorder may be different (Heilman et al., 1979; Kirschner & Webb, 1982).

Heilman and colleagues (1979) reported on three cases in which receptive or global aphasia was present without alexia. One patient had a lesion limited to the temporal lobe; the other two had lesions that appeared to include the angular gyrus. In one of these latter cases, right hemisphere mechanisms may have facilitated reading, as the patient lost the skill to read when a second stroke occurred in the right hemisphere. These cases imply that lesions in Wernicke's area alone may not disrupt reading. Kirschner and Webb (1982) drew the conclusion from their case studies that there is partial independence of brain mechanisms for auditory and visual language comprehension. In their three cases, they observed greater impairment of reading comprehension than auditory comprehension with lesions in the posterior portion of the superior temporal lobe and adjacent sections of the angular gyrus in the inferior parietal lobe. Thus the reading disabilities found in Wernicke's aphasics do not appear to be the consequences of lesions to auditory cortex alone, but they may result from damage that extends to posterior regions of the temporal lobe and closely adjacent regions of the parietal lobe including the angular gyrus.

Although reading disorders are associated with Broca's aphasia, patients can often read many words, especially those that elicit visual images (e.g., concrete nouns). However, reading errors occur because the person is unable to read single letters. Words seem to be recognized as wholes and cannot be decoded. As with the speech disorder in Broca's aphasia, word category influences reading comprehension. The person is able to read nouns better than function words and adjectives. The reason why specific words go uncomprehended is uncertain, although studies imply that subvocalization which activates motor speech areas (Broca's area) may be important in reading infrequent words (Duffy et al., 1980a). Therefore, reading may be disrupted by lesions that limit access to words through motor mediators.

The Psycholinguistic System

A psycholinguistic taxonomy has developed based on the forms of reading errors made by the patients studied. This effort has helped delineate more specifically the brain–behavior relationships in alexia. Four forms have been described: (1) phonological alexia, (2) surface dyslexia, (3) deep dyslexia, and (4) letter-by-letter reading (cf. Friedman & Albert, 1985).

Phonological alexia

A person with phonological alexia is capable of reading many words and may actually appear competent in reading when evaluated using only single words that are frequently encountered. However, reading of text becomes difficult because words of low frequency cannot be decoded. Specific problems occur with words that follow rules of phonemic decoding so that low frequency words or pseudo-words that follow phonemic rules cannot be read. For example, the phonological alexic is unable to read pseudo-words like *bace* or infrequent words like *pact*. Mistakes made are often real words that grossly match the correct word in visual characteristics of length and shape.

It has been proposed that the remnants of normal reading are present because the person still has one reading system available that allows direct access to the lexicon through visual association. Coslett, Gonzalez-Rothi, and Heilman

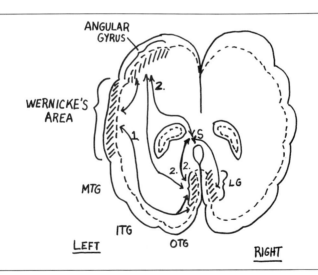

Figure 3–2. Coronal section of the brain at the level of Wernicke's area to show connections and lesion sites thought responsible for phonological and surface alexia. The dotted lines indicate that the angular gyrus, splenium, fusiform gyrus, and lingual gyrus are posterior to Wernicke's area (see figure 3–1 for relative position). Legend: MTG, middle temporal gyrus; ITG, inferior temporal gyrus; OTG, fusiform gyrus; LG, lingual gyrus; S, Splenium. #1. Lesions to this pathway are responsible for phonological alexia. #2. Lesions in these dorsal and medial pathways are responsible for surface alexia.

(1985) found evidence that such a dissociation between the phonological reading system and a visual, whole-word or lexical reading system can occur. Lesions that account for disturbance of the phonological system alone affect ventral pathways from the inferior association areas of the left hemisphere to Wernicke's area and disconnect these two cortical areas (see figure 3–2). Rapscak, Rothi, and Heilman (1987) described a patient with lesions in the posterior inferior left temporal lobe and underlying white matter. This condition disconnected Wernicke's area from the association fibers of the longitudinal fasciculus of the visual cortex and seemed responsible for phonological alexia. In this case, dorsal connections from the visual cortex to the angular gyrus remained intact, possibly accounting for the reading of familiar words based on visual matching. Thus the possibility exists that the phonological system of reading is mediated by connections between visual cortex and Wernicke's area. Auditory decoding may require visual perception, auditorization of the phonemes, and, through connections between Wernicke's area and the angular gyrus, comparison of the decoded words with the stored lexicon to determine if the word is known, and if so, what it means.

Significantly, phonological alexia may be accompanied by writing disturbances and aphasia or it may occur without agraphia or aphasia (Friedman & Albert, 1985).

Surface dyslexia

Surface dyslexia describes the deficiency encountered when the direct reading system is impaired, but the phonetic reading system remains intact. In this condition, familiar and unfamiliar words are decoded according to grapheme-to-phoneme-conversion rules. As long as words follow the expected pattern, the patient can read and understand them. Reading impairment emerges when words do not follow such conversion rules. Reported paralexias consist of phonetic transcriptions of words without any correction based on the lexical store. For example, words such as *laugh, peace,* or *gnat* are neither pronounced correctly nor interpreted meaningfully (Coltheart, 1980; Coltheart et al., 1983; Marshall & Newcombe, 1973; Prior & McCorriston, 1985; Coslett, Gonzalez-Rothi, & Heilman, 1985). Additionally, some authors have noted that the labored decoding of words that is required leads to errors in word meaning. Homophones (words that sound the same but have different meaning) are frequently misinterpreted. Thus the person may confuse *soul* for *sole* (Coslett, Gonzalez-Rothi, & Heilman, 1985) or *beggin* for *begin* (Marshall & Newcombe, 1973). As a result, semantic aspects of comprehension are disturbed.

This form of acquired disturbance may be due to lesions that are medial and dorsal to the lesions that disrupt the phonological reading system. In many case studies some form of visual field defect is reported because the left visual radiations are disrupted as are dorsal connections between the visual cortex and angular gyrus (Deloche, Andrewsky, & Desi, 1982; Marshall & Newcombe, 1973; Prior & McCorriston, 1985; Rapscak, Gonzalez-Rothi, & Heilman,

1987) (see figure 3–2). However, there is no consensus on the neuroanatomy of the condition. Recently, Prior and McCorriston (1985) suggested that the characteristics of surface dyslexia simply reflect a regression to a more immature form of reading. Their study of immature normal readers revealed that during normal reading development these forms of errors occur at a high frequency in young children but decrease as reading proficiency increases. Prior and McCorriston raise the possibility that surface dyslexia may simply be a deterioration to a less adept form of reading rather than a true neuropsychological condition with a specific cortical basis.

Deep dyslexia

Deep dyslexia is distinguished by the occurrence of semantic paralexias in which words from the same semantic category are substituted for the target word (e.g., *child* is read as *boy*, Roeltgen, 1987). Other forms of reading errors have been associated with this cardinal feature, including visual paralexias (e.g., word substitutions based on the appearance of the words), an inability to decode written words phonetically, and derivational errors in which the error shares the same base morpheme as the target word—e.g., *confident* for *confidence* (Roeltgen, 1987). Additionally, the persons share similar characteristics of residual reading abilities. High-imagery words can often be read and are more easily read than low-imagery words. Other words that can be read depend on word class. Nouns can be read more easily than adjectives, adjectives more easily than verbs, and content words more easily than function words. It appears that as words become abstract, they become more difficult to read. Comprehension is often good for passages, because the person gains meaning and guesses at the few words that cannot be read.

The lesions associated with deep dyslexia have not been specified adequately although the characteristic difficulties are similar to those observed in Broca's aphasia. However, the sites of lesions are not always located in the traditional area associated with that form of aphasia. Roeltgen (1987) described a patient who was evaluated on the Western Aphasia Battery. Along with the aphasic symptoms, the patient demonstrated reading deficits associated with deep dyslexia. When the site of the lesion was investigated, using CAT scan analysis three years postcerebral infarct, damage was evident in the posterior portion of the left temporal sulcus, the angular gyrus, and portions medial to these structures towards the lateral ventricle. Broca's area was spared. Thus precise localization of the symptoms of deep dyslexia remains unclear. Coslett, Gonzalez-Rothi, and Heilman (1985) also described a deep dyslexic who had mixed transcortical aphasia due to a "watershed infarct" in the areas surrounding the lateral ventricle. These findings suggest that the lesions associated with deep dyslexia may be subcortical in nature.

Significantly, the remnants of reading reported in deep dyslexia may result from spared left hemisphere structures or right hemisphere mediation of reading. The person described by Roeltgen (1987) lost the capacity to read any words following a second left hemisphere infarct that incorporated sections of the left frontal temporal juncture. In contrast, Heilman and co-workers (1979) found a patient with effective reading comprehension following a left hemisphere stroke who lost his reading skills following a second stroke in the right hemisphere.

Letter-by-letter reading

Descriptions of this disorder indicate that the person reads by identifying individual letters, stating them aloud, and then forming the word based on the recognition of the letters and their meaningful sequence. Many terms have been used to label this pattern of reading style, including spelling dyslexia (Kinsbourne & Warrington, 1962; Prior & McCorriston, 1985) and dynamic spelling dyslexia (Horner & Massey, 1986) despite the fact that spelling is not disrupted. For practical purposes, the person reads in a slow, labored fashion, and, although able to comprehend, finds reading a chore that becomes harder as word length increases.

The neuroanatomy of this disorder is unclear, but most research indicates that these symptoms are consistent with alexia without agraphia or pure alexia. It is likely, therefore, that the lesions involve the left occipital region and the splenium of the corpus callosum, which disconnects the visual association cortex and the angular gyrus.

Correspondence Between Classical and Psycholinguistic Systems

In their review of alexia, Friedman and Albert (1985) raised tentative ideas about the interrelationships between syndromes defined in the classical taxonomy and the psycholinguistic taxonomy. Their views have been supported by subsequent studies that suggest that the types defined by the newer framework can be subsumed within the classical system.

Friedman and Albert (1985) indicated that in all cases studied, letter-by-letter reading was similar to alexia without agraphia. Studies previous to and subsequent to their review (Horner & Massey, 1986; Nicole, Nardi, & Fortuna, 1982; Prior & McCorriston, 1985) reported similar shared characteristics, skill profiles, and lesion sites: intact writing and spoken language, with lesions involving a disconnection between angular gyrus and visual input.

Phonological alexia seems to form a subset of alexia with agraphia (Sartori, Barry, & Job, 1984) in which visual input is disconnected from the phonological decoding system in the temporoparietal junction. The patient described by Rapscak, Gonzalez-Rothi, and Heilman (1987) replicated this pattern.

However, phonological alexia can also form a subset of aphasic alexia. This occurs when lesions extend beyond regions that mediate lexical knowledge, causing aphasia, but leave the dorsal and medial connections between the visual cortex and the angular gyrus, the direct reading route (Coslett, Gonzalez-Rothi, & Heilman, 1985), intact, allowing for reading based on visual characteristics (Rapscak, Gonzalez-Rothi, & Heilman, 1987).

Surface alexia forms a subset of alexia with agraphia. Lesions involve at least the dorsal and medial radiations of the visual cortex of the left hemisphere. Reading remains possible through two mechanisms: (1) some sparing of the angular gyrus and intact connections between the phonological system in the temporal lobe and the visual cortex through ventral pathways (Rapcsak, Gonzalaz-Rothi, & Heilman, 1987; Prior & McCorriston, 1983) or (2) through right hemisphere reading mechanisms (Coslett, Gonzalez-Rothi, & Heilman, 1985).

Finally, deep dyslexia is highly correlated with the alexia associated with Broca's aphasia. The words that can be read depend on word class as indicated in the reading disturbances reported in Broca's aphasia. However, reading difficulties are not always present in Broca's aphasia. It may require more extensive lesions than those that produce Broca's aphasia for this disorder to occur. The condition is rare, so case reports are few. However, as previously noted from studies by Roeltgen (1987) of Broca's aphasia and Coslett and collaborators (1985) of transcortical aphasia, subcortical factors appear to be responsible for the reading disturbance. Whatever resolution emerges from future research, it would appear that deep dyslexia is associated with some form of aphasic alexia.

Developmental dyslexia

Reviews of alexia highlight the neuropsychological aspects of reading dysfunction once the ability to read has been acquired. However, the neuropsychological study of reading acquisition is important for a full understanding of functional reading. A discussion is in order of dyslexia in children who exhibit delays in reading achievement or in adults who have a documented history of failure to acquire normal reading. As in alexia, the review highlights the importance of the left hemisphere but also provides insight into the role that right hemisphere mediation may play in reading acquisition.

Within the last 20 years, both the study of dyslexia and models of dyslexia have changed dramatically. Initially, research designs compared groups of reading-disabled children with matched children of equal intellectual ability who had acquired reading skills at an average pace. The groups of children were compared on a single variable believed to be important in reading acquisition. This research revealed that dyslexic children were deficient in a number of specific skills, including auditory discrimination, visual perception, visual motor coordination, and the integration of auditory perception and visual perception (cf. Hynd & Cohen, 1983). With each new discovery, authors claimed the key to dyslexia had been found. Despite much discourse and model building, the field was disorganized because theoreticians were in conflict about the single most important factor that hindered reading acquisition.

Two trends emerged that advanced the field beyond this state of disarray. The first took the lead from research on alexia and studied the linguistic characteristics of disabled readers. The second analyzed groups of dyslexic children on a broad array of skills to determine if consistent clusters of neuropsychological deficits existed within the population.

Studies linking acquired adult disorders with developmental dyslexia have analyzed the component skills found deficient in damaged adults within populations of dyslexic readers and children of average reading skill. The research has emphasized four major areas of concern: expressive aspects of language, general auditory processing, phonological processing, and the capacity to process information in sequences.

Denckla (1972a, b), working to determine if developmental dyslexia shared characteristics of adult aphasia and alexia as suggested by Critchley (1970), analyzed the color-naming skills of disabled readers relative to average readers. She found that disabled readers were less capable than average readers in naming colors under time pressure. This suggested that developmentally dyslexic children share a form of dysnomia with alexic adults. Further studies revealed that dyslexic children throughout the age range showed slowed access to names relative to their intellectually matched peers (Denckla & Rudel, 1974, 1976a, b), suggesting that reading disabilities were correlated with a deficiency in the rapid attachment of labels to sensory stimuli. This pattern is similar to that found for alexia without agraphia, suggesting that left hemisphere mechanisms are highly significant in reading acquisition. Recent research suggests this naming weakness in dyslexics may not be limited to visual stimuli. Hutchinson (1983), among others, reported that finger localization, which requires labeling of tactile sensation, was less accurate in reading-disabled children than in normal and language-disordered children who are not dyslexic. Wolf and Goodglass (1986) highlighted the importance of naming in their longitudinal study of three groups of children from kindergarten to the end of second grade (average readers, severely impaired readers, and bilingual readers). Confrontation naming scores in kindergarten predicted grade 2 reading comprehension scores and discriminated between severely impaired readers and those who had achieved a functional capacity to gain meaning from written material. Thus severely impaired readers have confrontational naming deficits, another pattern found in aphasic and alexic adults.

Tallal conducted a series of studies on the auditory processing of language-disabled children, all of whom had reading disabilities. The language-disordered children not only demonstrated deficits in receptive and expressive language skills but also showed generalized differences in auditory processing. Specifically, they demonstrated a slowed brain stem response to auditory input that seemed to contribute to difficulty processing brief auditory clues that are followed in rapid succession by other equally brief auditory cues (Tallal & Stark, 1983). This pattern occurred in the reading-disabled children who had severe receptive and expressive disorders but not in the reading-disabled children without other language impairments (Tallal & Stark, 1981; Stark & Tallal, 1981), suggesting that at least some forms of reading disabilities are associated with severe language impairments and auditory processing weaknesses (Doehring et al., 1981).

In another series of studies, children with reading disabilities who did not have weaknesses in basic auditory discrimination demonstrated difficulties in their ability to identify and abstract phonemes from the stream of speech (cf. Mann, 1986; Wagner, 1986). Groups of reading-disabled children have problems identifying words when the speech perception system is stressed under conditions of high background noise (Bradley, Schankeweiler, & Mann, 1983) and also have difficulty on tasks that stress awareness of phonemes (Bradley & Bryant, 1978). They appear less adept than good readers at analyzing spoken words for their phonetic segments. In longitudinal studies across the years, a deficit in phonemic awareness when reading is beginning to be acquired has been found to be highly correlated with later reading achievement. Two other aspects of phonological processing have also proven to be highly correlated with reading achievement in longitudinal studies and in comparisons of reading-disabled students with average achievers. The children with poor reading skills had problems with decoding of written words phonologically and with retaining phonetic components in working memory. Good readers were more adept at rapidly accessing phonetic rules for word analysis and at retaining phonetic segments in short-term memory (Mann, 1986; Wagner, 1986). The neuropsychological aspects of phonological processing have not been well delineated, but they have traditionally been considered quintessential functions of the left hemisphere (Rudel, 1985).

Another function important for language comprehension that is disrupted in acquired alexia is memory for sequences and analysis of sequences, especially language sequences. Meaning varies at the letter and word level when order of stimuli changes, so that sequential processing is essential for decoding written language (e.g., *net* has a different meaning than *ten*) and reading comprehension (e.g., "the boy hit the ball" is different from "the ball hit the boy") (Rudel, 1985). That this language-related skill is deficient in reading-disabled children has been demonstrated in numerous studies with a variety of stimuli. Reading-disabled children have shorter memory spans for sequential material, including digits, words in sentences, unrelated words, and block tapping sequences (Bakker, 1973; Stark & Tallal, 1979; Stark & Tallal, 1981). Matching sequences of light flashes or replicating them are difficult tasks for reading-disabled children relative to normals and even for learning-disabled children without reading disability (Denckla, Rudel, & Broman, 1981; Gordon, 1980; Rudel, 1985).

Thus reading-disabled children have been found to be deficient in a series of language-related tasks on which alexic and aphasic adults are also deficient. This research has provided support for models of dyslexia based on language impairments (cf. Vellutino, 1979) and has focused neuropsychological investigation on the importance of left hemisphere activity.

Despite the advances this research has provided, it is not comprehensive enough to account for all forms of dyslexia and all the component skills essential for reading acquisition (Rudel, 1985). Other research studies were designed to develop a taxonomy of reading disabilities by assessing a wide variety of skills. The results of these studies showed that, although language-based dysfunctions dominated the skill profiles of the majority of children, a significant group had problems with visual-spatial processing in the presence of adequate language skills. This pattern was especially evident in the young reading-disabled population. As a result of this research, it became clear that components mediated by the right hemisphere must be considered in order to understand functional reading.

Reading Disability Subtypes

The basis for the current understanding of dyslexia subtypes is Boder's (1971, 1973) classification research and the results of studies from four other neuropsychology laboratories. The evidence converges on a set of factors that contribute to developmental reading disorders.

Boder (1971, 1973) evaluated reading-disabled children on the basis of reading and spelling errors. One group of children was observed to make reading and spelling errors that broke the rules for converting sounds to letters and letter combinations. These children were categorized as dysphonetic readers, readers who showed poor awareness of phonetic rules. They composed the vast majority (67%) of the population of disabled readers studied. Reading errors were primarily semantic paralexias; reading style seemed to follow a whole word as opposed to a decoding approach. In contrast, a smaller group of children (10%) made reading and spelling errors that showed good knowledge of phoneme-to-grapheme conversion rules, but they had difficulty with words that were irregular in their spelling. These children did not effectively retain visual images of words nor read irregular words as wholes. Because they showed impairments in the visual imagery of words, they were called dysidetic readers. Finally, the remainder of the group, who formed a larger proportion of the population (23%), made a mixture of errors, so they were called dysphonetic-dysidetic readers. These children had severe reading disabilities, for neither a competent auditory linguistic reading system nor a competent visual reading system was available to them.

Mattis, French, and Rapin (1975) examined the skills of 82 dyslexic children to challenge the prevailing assumption that reading disabilities were the result of a homogeneous disorder. They defined dyslexia operationally as characterized by a reading recognition score two or more years below the age-appropriate level, average IQ, and no history of psychosis or school truancy. Because the subjects were older (10–12 years) than many children who face reading difficulties (the definition required at least a two-year lag in skills), the subtypes that emerged may not apply to younger children with early reading acquisition difficulties. The analysis proved useful because it supported the hypothesis that dyslexia cannot be attributed to a single neuropsychological source. Specifically, three major subtypes were revealed: (1) a language disorder, (2) an articulatory graphomotor dyscoordination disorder, and (3) a visual-spatial perceptual disorder. The language disorder, demonstrated by 39% of the sample, was characterized by expressive deficits, including anomia and poor imitative speech, and receptive problems in comprehension and speech-sound discrimination accompanied by normal functioning in motor performance, verbal intelligence, and nonverbal problem solving. Thirty-seven percent of the sample had an articulatory-graphomotor dyscoordination manifested by poor sound blending and weak graphomotor skills, but good receptive language skills. Finally, a visual-spatial perceptual disorder was apparent in 16% of the children who performed poorly on tests of visual retention, visual-spatial conceptualization, and visual-spatial problem solving. Of a subset of children who showed no evidence of brain damage (i.e., developmental dyslexics), 28% were language disordered, 48% had articulatory graphomotor dyscoordination, and 14% had visual-spatial perceptual deficiencies.

In a cross-validation study of 163 dyslexic children (Mattis, 1978), the same three subtypes emerged but at different rates, possibly because of the younger age of the sample (modal age of 8 to 10). The majority of children demonstrated the language disorder (63%), only 10% showed articulatory graphomotor dyscoordination, and 5% showed a visual-spatial perceptual disorder. In addition, 9% had mixed deficits, and 16% seemed to have a sequencing disorder manifested by inaccurate sequential memory for digits and sentences.

Denckla (1979) concluded from her research and clinical experience with dyslexia that there are six subtypes present in school-aged children. Because the majority of children showed some form of language disorder, Denckla pointed to an underlying deficiency in "left hemisphere mediated skills" (Denckla, 1979) as the most frequent determinant of pure dyslexia. Similar to Mattis and colleagues (1975 and 1978), Denckla reported a global mixed language disorder in which comprehension and expression were poor (6%), an articulatory graphomotor dyscoordination syndrome (12%), an anomic repetition disorder (54%), a dysphonemic-sequencing disorder (13%) in which errors of sequence in naming and memory were present, and a verbal learning disorder characterized by inadequate memory for sequences and paired associates. She reported that 5% showed deficits that may have been due to poor skills on tasks mediated by the right hemisphere. These children performed spatial tasks with analytic strategies that hindered their performance on Block Design and the Rey-Osterreith complex figure. This group also had deficits in left-handed, but not right-handed, motor tasks, implicating problems in the right hemisphere.

Both research groups noted the similarities in their classification systems and suggested that the independent corroboration of the series of language disorder syndromes (e.g., global mixed, articulatory graphomotor, anomia, repetition) provided evidence that left hemisphere mediated functions play a critical role in the acquisition of reading and are often implicated in reading dysfunction. Despite the differences in the percentage of children with visual-spatial deficits, the results of both research efforts indicated that both left and right hemisphere dysfunctions can contribute to dyslexia.

Studies by Rourke summarized in two reports (1981, 1983) led to similar conclusions regarding the heterogeneity of dyslexia. Relying on sophisticated statistical analysis of a comprehensive battery of tests (i.e., the Halstead Reitan Series or Reitan-Indiana series in conjunction with the WISC-R, language-related tasks, and reading tasks), Rourke and his colleagues found three sub-types of retarded readers that were very similar to those just described. Three distinct ability/disability clusters were especially evident in a young group of dyslexics (7 to 9 years of age) and similar patterns were indicated in 9- to 14-year-olds. Significantly, upon the completion of longitudinal studies of retarded readers, the investigators found that those who advanced or caught up in reading skills were those with right hemisphere deficiencies. These were children with visual-spatial problems as well as left-handed sensory and motor performance deficiencies. This pattern suggested to Rourke that reading disabilities change as development progresses. He concluded that right hemisphere deficiencies, related to visual-spatial perceptual disorders, are particularly important in the early stages of reading when the child must learn to recognize the configuration of letters and words. As in the other studies, those with language-based deficiencies form the majority of the population, but a significant minority demonstrated problems in skills mediated by the right hemisphere.

Doehring and co-workers (1981) undertook a comprehensive neuropsycho-logical assessment of 72 dyslexic children (the Halstead-Reitan Battery, WISC-R, reading tests, and neurolinguistic evaluations) to investigate subtypes. Factor analysis classified the majority of subjects into three clusters: (1) type 0, wherein deficient oral reading was present, but silent reading was intact and associated language disorders of articulation errors, dysnomia, and weak verbal memory were present; (2) type A, characterized by difficulties in asso-ciating auditory and visual information as indicated by poor sound-letter association in reading, and (3) type S, where spatial disabilities were present and reading was hindered by slow recognition of letter sequences as pro-nounceable units.

Doehring et al. concluded that although their results did not correspond directly with previous typologies, there were similarities between the type 0 and type S groups and previously identified subgroups (Mattis et al., 1975; Denckla, 1979). Language disorders were evident in the type 0 group—anomia, verbal learning problems, and articulatory graphomotor dyscoordination— and characteristics of the visual-spatial perceptual disorders were found in the type S subjects. The auditory-visual integration problems noted in the per-formance of the type A group represented a hitherto unsuspected basis for reading disabilities.

Taken together, the results of the studies provide convergent evidence that identifiable and distinct patterns of neuropsychological deficits contribute to reading retardation and that further study of left and right hemisphere mechanisms, as well as integrative mechanisms (Rudel, 1985), is warranted.

Another series of studies (Lyon & Watson, 1981; Lyon et al., 1981; Lyon, Stewart, & Friedman, 1982; Lyon, 1985) focused on integrating neuropsychological profiles with types of reading deficits. This research also provided preliminary indications about how to develop prescriptive educational programs for students with different profile types.

The first set of studies explored the neuropsychological and reading profiles of 11- and 12-year-old students (Lyon, 1985). The performance of a sample of reading-disabled students on a series of auditory receptive, auditory expressive, visual-spatial, visual-motor integration, and visual memory measures was compared to that of normal readers. Differences from normal scores were established for each measure. When these differences were subjected to cluster analysis, six distinct subtypes emerged and were later replicated in a second sample of reading-disabled students (Lyon & Watson, 1981). As in the previous studies, some of the groups showed auditory-linguistic deficits, some showed general language deficits, some showed visual-spatial deficits, and one showed a mixture of auditory and visual perceptual problems. Each subtype made characteristic reading and spelling errors. Subtypes 1 and 2, comprising 22% of the sample, showed deficits in both linguistic and visual-spatial tasks, but the children who composed subtype 1 were more deficient in these skills than were the children in subtype 2. Although most of the reading and spelling errors made by the children in subtype 1 were primarily visual in nature, phonetic errors were also observed. As would be expected, the children in subtype 1 who displayed combined skill deficits had the lowest reading, spelling, and reading comprehension skills. Thirty-two percent of the sample showed only visual-spatial deficits (subtype 4); the reading errors of this group occurred primarily on phonetically irregular words. This group's spelling errors usually followed phonetic rules. The reading comprehension of this group was fairly stong, as most words could be read and the group had good language comprehension skills. Two other subtypes (24%) demonstrated effective skills on visual tasks but had some form of auditory-linguistic deficits relative to the performance of good readers. Consistent with the earlier research, a global language disorder was observed in students (subtype 5) who made dysphonetic errors in reading and spelling and had very poor reading comprehension. Another group showed poor auditory comprehension and sound blending skills but had effective expressive linguistic abilities. This group also made dysphonetic reading and spelling errors and had poor reading comprehension. Finally, a sixth subtype was comprised of students with low reading skills who showed no neuropsychological dysfunctions in the auditory-linguistic or visual-perceptual realms. The reading problems of this group were attributed either to lack of motivation or to inefficient teaching.

These studies contributed to the understanding of reading disabilities by making specific associations between reading and spelling problems and neuropsychological deficits. That students with auditory-linguistic weaknesses showed problems with phonetic aspects of reading and spelling emphasizes the connection between word attack skills and auditory processing; that students with visual-perceptual inefficiencies demonstrated errors on the visual aspects of words affirms the relationship between effective reading of phonetically irregular words and visual perception; that students with a combination of auditory-linguistic and visual-perceptual difficulties had both phonetic decoding inefficiencies and visual analysis errors attests to the essential but differential contributions made by both systems to reading acquisition. Additionally, the research highlights the importance of linguistic proficiency for reading comprehension; all subtypes with low auditory-linguistic skills showed major problems with comprehension, whereas the subtype characterized by visual-perceptual disorders exhibited effective comprehension.

Subsequent studies of younger (7 to 9-year-old) reading-disabled students compared to normal readers found similar clusterings, with the exception of subtype 2—relatively mild combined auditory and visual deficits. One subtype (18%) was composed of children with visual-spatial and visual-motor integration problems in the presence of effective auditory and linguistic skills. As expected, those students were poor in reading and spelling on phonetically irregular words but had relatively good reading comprehension. Another subtype (10%) had mixed auditory-linguistic and visual problems with correlated problems in phonetic word attack, reading phonetically irregular words, and comprehension. A global language disorder in the presence of effective visual-spatial skills was found in 10%. This group had poor comprehension and dramatically poor word attack accuracy. Another group had severe auditory-linguistic skills in the presence of slight visual-perceptual weaknesses. These children used letter-by-letter decoding and had the greatest difficulty in comprehension because words were read as minute pieces and reading was laboriously slow. Finally, 12% showed reading weaknesses but no neuropsychological deficits relative to normals.

Thus the research by Lyon and colleagues indicates that a pattern of skills profiles and associated reading and spelling behaviors exists and is stable across reading development.

The studies do not result in consistent subtypes, but, despite variations, several conclusions are warranted. First, reading and spelling disabilities cannot be explained by deficits in a single neuropsychological function. When a broad spectrum of skills are reviewed, several distinct types of deficits are found. Second, all studies report a high frequency of language skill deficits in the population of retarded readers. This implies that left hemisphere mediation of a number of capacities is critical for efficient reading. Third, despite the importance of language skills in learning to read, the research reveals that nonverbal deficits are present in a small proportion of reading-disabled children. These findings implicate posterior right hemisphere mechanisms in reading acquisition. Finally, when developmental trends are investigated, the pattern of disabilities changes. More nonverbal dysfunctions are found in younger than in older disabled readers, suggesting that neuropsychological skills required for learning to read differ from those that contribute to reading to learn.

Neuroanatomy and Brain Activity in Dyslexia

The direct study of brain mechanisms in developmental reading disability has relied heavily on correlational analysis and inferences drawn from those analyses rather than on hard neurological evidence. Therefore, the knowledge is highly speculative. Most of the research has relied on indirect measures of brain activity as monitored by the electroencephalogram, enhanced electro-encephalograms, or, in a few cases, observation of regional cerebral blood flow. This research has shown unusual left hemisphere activity in the majority of subjects studied. Right hemisphere variations were observed in subjects who showed a visual-perceptual basis for reading disability. The research supports the view that the activity of the left hemisphere is important for reading. It also provides evidence that differential patterns of reading disturbances as noted in subtype taxonomies have a basis in cortical functioning.

Studies of the electrical activity of the brain have shown that dyslexic children do not have expected patterns of activation. At rest, there is an excess of slow theta waves over the left hemisphere, specifically noted over the angular gyrus (Rebert, Wexler, & Sproul, 1978). In another study (Duffy, Burechfeld, & Lombroso, 1979), dyslexic children demonstrated slow wave activity over the left hemisphere during a language processing task, whereas average readers showed heightened fast wave activity in the same regions.

Advanced computer analysis of electroencephalogram data, brain electrical activity mapping (BEAM), has stressed the differences in activation patterns (Duffy et al., 1980a, b). The first study compared eight dyslexic boys to ten normal readers who were matched for IQ and socioeconomic status on their performance in a variety of tasks, which were expected to activate the left hemisphere alone (linguistic tasks), the right hemisphere alone (spatial or musical tasks), or both hemispheres simultaneously (visual-verbal associational learning). The groups showed different activation patterns on all tasks. The greatest activation differences were noted in four areas, three which fell in the major language areas of the left hemisphere. Average readers reacted to the tasks with suppression of resting alpha-wave activity, whereas dyslexics showed no change in this resting activity in the supplementary motor areas of both hemispheres, Broca's area, the left temporal lobe, and the left temporal-parietal-occipital junction that incorporates Wernicke's area and portions of the angular gyrus. Thus three areas associated with language and reading were not activated appropriately during cognitive tasks in the dyslexic population. The patterns seem stable in the dyslexic population, for they were replicated in a subsequent study with 24 other subjects (Duffy et al., 1980b).

After categorizing groups of readers according to Boder's taxonomy, Fried and colleagues (1981) found electrophysiological differences between normal readers and dyslexics and among groups of dyslexics. Specifically, those children who demonstrated the dysphonetic form of reading disability showed different activation patterns over the left hemisphere when compared to normal readers, dysidetic dyslexics, and dyslexics with combined dysphonetic and dysidetic errors. The results suggest that the left hemisphere may be significant in the linguistic form of dyslexia.

A single study examined regional cerebral blood flow analysis while developmentally dyslexic adults were reading. The results of the study documented the connection between reading disability subtype and neurophysiological activity. Hynd and colleagues (1987) studied a surface dyslexic who made errors on irregular words that did not follow phonetic rules and a deep dyslexic who made semantic paralexias and could not decode words by applying phonetic rules.

While reading an unfamiliar passage, the surface dyslexic showed appropriate activation of the left hemisphere (most often associated with phonetic processing) but low activation of the right hemisphere (most often associated with visual-spatial analysis). The underactivation of the right hemisphere was consistent with the type of reading errors observed that resulted from inappropriate use of the direct, visual reading route used for decoding irregular words. In contrast, the deep dyslexic showed low activation levels of both hemispheres relative to controls during reading. The study highlights the bilateral aspects of brain activity in normal readers as indicated by increased blood flow in both hemispheres during reading. However, it also stressed the specific nature of neurophysiological deficits and types of reading disability. Right hemisphere mediation must be considered in models of reading and reading disability, especially when errors are based on the visual aspects of words.

Structural correlations that connect brain differences to differential reading acquisition have also been documented (Galaburda et al. 1985). In most right-handed people, the medial surface of the left temporal lobe (planum temporale) is wider and the posterior portion of the left hemisphere longer than corresponding regions of the right hemisphere. However, in several studies of reading-disabled children the normal pattern has not been observed. As a group, dyslexics showed the reverse pattern, a wider and longer posterior right hemisphere than left hemisphere (Galaburda & Kemper, 1979). Even more significant information has been obtained when the brains of dyslexics have been investigated on a cellular level. Although the research is not definitive because the number of subjects is low and appropriate controls have not been analyzed, the data provide strong indications of the importance of structural integrity of the posterior left hemisphere to reading acquisition. Galaburda and colleagues (Galaburda & Eidelberg, 1982; Galaburda & Kemper, 1979; Galaburda et al., 1985) performed brain autopsies on six developmentally dyslexic adults who had died from causes other than brain trauma. For the most part, gross structural variations from the norm were not noted, but the cellular organization and composition of the brains were different, especially in the left temporal regions and thalamic regions medial to the left temporoparietal junction. The cortical layers expected to be achieved through normal development were often disrupted, and neural cells were found to be misplaced, poorly developed in size, and low in number (Galaburda & Eidelberg, 1982; Galaburda & Kemper, 1979; Galaburda et al., 1985). As a result, the expected connections among nerve cells within this region of the brain and between this region of the brain and other regions were not present and nonneural glial cells were prevalent. It could be suspected, then, that the persons studied could not read effectively because the appropriate cortical structure and connections were not present to support reading at least as mediated by the linguistic system of the left hemisphere.

These studies suggest that variations in the physical activity and structure of the brain are highly related to variations in reading skill. That the observed variations in structure and activity occur in areas suspected of mediating skills supports the view that specific reading disturbances are linked to specific brain dysfunctions. This premise enhances our models of neuropsychology and focuses future research study.

Implications of Research for Day-to-Day Reading

The information reviewed on acquired and developmental reading disorders suggests that reading has many neuropsychological components. Reading is influenced by the location of brain damage or dysfunction, the extent of damage or dysfunction, and the age at which the damage or dysfunction is encountered. However, the information only implies a broad impact on reading. It does not clearly indicate how disabled a person will be in day-to-day functioning given a particular location and form of damage or dysfunction. Very little exploration of this issue has been conducted, especially with acquired lesions, for several reasons. First, in the area of acquired damage, much more concern has focused on other essential skills, including language use and comprehension, locomotion, praxis, and problem solving. In this context, reading has been considered to be an unessential skill for maintaining activities of daily living. Second, studies of reading disorders among brain-damaged adults have focused on broad measures of reading skills in order to delineate the brain mechanisms behind specific reading components. The field of study has simply not been active long enough for evidence to be compiled on how disruption of each component influences daily reading. Thus, for example, it is not known how frequently phonological paralexias must occur before a person is unable to read a newspaper or read directions for cooking or rely on road signs. Third, developmental literature, as well as literature on acquired disorders, has contained only a few longitudinal studies. As a result, it is not known what level of reading proficiency will be reached in adulthood by children who demonstrate a particular type of reading error at age 11. Nor is it clear if developmentally dyslexic children continue to improve, stagnate, or deteriorate once formal instruction is complete. Longitudinal recovery studies on acquired alexias are even more rare. Therefore, because of limitations, it is only possible to provide speculation about the connection between specific neuropsychological dysfunctions and functional reading. Two sources of information do provide hints about the impact of specific disorders. However, before these sources of information are reviewed, it is important to define functional reading.

Reading can be defined as the capacity to gain meaning from written language. As already noted, reading is composed of several components in two systems for attaining meaning. A direct, or lexical, reading route requires visual analysis of the word, abstract letter identification, recognition of the cluster as a word, semantic analysis, and retention in memory to be integrated with the stream of words read (Coltheart, 1984; Rapscak et al., 1987). The indirect route, or phonological reading, requires visual feature analysis of the word and abstract letter identification followed by grapheme parcing (a process in which the word is segmented into units that receive phonemic assignments) and blending of graphemes, which is then followed by a process in which the decoded word is matched to the lexicon for semantic analysis (cf. Patterson, Marshall, & Coltheart, 1985). Disruption of any of the steps in either system can disrupt the entire reading process.

For the purposes of functional reading, the main concern is comprehension and how different disorders influence comprehension. Comprehension varies from one reading task to another. For example, comprehending a single-word traffic sign or reading a menu necessitates less skill than comprehension of a newspaper, which in turn is different from a technical manual or novel. It is uncertain what reading levels are required for day-to-day living, but Chall (1979) and others (cf. Johnson, 1987) agree that an eighth grade reading level is barely sufficient in modern Western societies. Based on this level of skill, few persons reported on in the literature are functional readers, but some patients show the capacity to read signs, brief passages, and brief texts. How functional reading is achieved depends on the components of reading that are disturbed by the neuropsychological dysfunction and how extensively other language processes are involved.

The sources of data providing clues on functional reading and neuropsychology come from close study of case studies on acquired alexia and Lyons' study of the educational validation of dyslexic subtypes. Both sources supply indications of how different forms of dysfunction have a differential impact on reading achievement and, in the case of acquired alexia, how different disorders recover over time.

In alexia without agraphia, studies that report minimal data on comprehension suggest that patients are able to comprehend single words or brief passages but that reading of sentences or paragraphs becomes nearly impossible because of their reading capacity. Specifically, patients read in a letter-by-letter fashion, spelling words out loud one letter at a time. This is a tedious process that stresses the damaged person's energy, patience, and memory. At times, letter-by-letter decoding can take several minutes for a single word (Coltheart, 1984). Prior and McCorriston (1983) reported on one patient who achieved a relatively high score of 12 years on a single-word reading test (Schonell Test) but complained of being unable to read because of tedium. When tested on text, he could only grasp a vague idea of the meaning because he recognized only a few key words. This man's level of comprehension is significantly different from his premorbid functioning. A second person with a lower single-word reading score (8 years old) and lower premorbid reading achievement could not even grasp a vague idea from text.

Horner and Massey (1986) report on a person who is capable of reading letter-by-letter with good comprehension for the deciphered words. However, this man found comprehension of text impossible because of memory weaknesses. Other researchers report similar problems for this form of alexia (Henderson et al., 1985; Nicole, Nardi, & Fortuna, 1982; Rosati et al., 1984), suggesting that functional reading is nearly impossible with the exception of brief messages or signs. The functional reading deficits in letter-by-letter reading remain present as long as the condition exists.

The question for understanding long-term consequences then becomes focused on how quickly alexia without agraphia recovers. The answer seems to depend on the source of the lesion. In a review of studies, Greenblatt (1983) indicated that most cases of alexia without agraphia resulted from infarcts of the posterior cerebral artery that supplies the left occipital cortex and the splenium of the corpus collosum. For these cases, recovery seems limited. For example, Horner and Massey (1986) reported no change in their patient nine months after the patient's stroke occurred. Further, many of the original studies that have documented alexia without agraphia have evaluated patients and found it to be present years after the stroke (cf. Friedman & Albert, 1985). Ruptures of arterial venous malformations in the same region result in disturbances noticed years after the study (Rosati et al., 1984). Other less frequent sources of lesion that have lasting effects include closed head injury, abcesses, and excision of tumors that intrude upon the cortical regions of concern (Greenblatt, 1983; Newcombe et al., 1974). When hematomas have been found to be the source of the reading disorder, their removal has often resulted in rapid improvement (Henderson et al., 1985) once pressure effects were removed. Recovery over a 6-month period has been found for an excised tumor that did not occupy the cortical region (Newcombe et al., 1974), but this recovery was only documented for single-word reading. Thus, although there is recovery documented, the cause of the majority of cases in the literature, stroke, is one that creates long-term disruption of functional reading.

The alexias that include agraphia vary in the comprehension deficits noted depending on the reading system that is disturbed. Although not conclusive, studies suggest that comprehension is poor when the direct, lexical reading route is disturbed as in surface dyslexia. That persons with this disorder can read regular words through phonetic decoding leaves them with no capacity to read numerous irregular words. Therefore, their comprehension is determined by the number of irregular words encountered, a frequent event in English. Thus the majority of cases reported indicate poor single-word comprehension and nearly absent passage comprehension (Bub, Cancelliere, & Kertesz, 1985; Newcombe & Marshall, 1985; Prior & McCorriston, 1981; Saffran, 1985). Even in cases in which "good" comprehension is reported, persons are only able to determine the meaning of single words and reach only 47% accuracy at the highest level while showing little passage comprehension (Kay & Patterson, 1985). Only one case study reported excellent reading comprehension (96% accuracy in word meaning; Goldblum, 1985). Thus surface dyslexia is characterized by severely limited functional reading.

In contrast, comprehension in phonological alexia in which the direct reading route works well and the phonetic reading route is impaired is generally good for words and passages. Persons with this disorder can read regular and irregular words as long as they are familiar, and they demonstrate problems only when required to phonetically decode unfamiliar words. Comprehension of passages can be good because the person is able to use the surrounding context in which an unfamilar word is embedded to guess at the meaning of the word. Thus infrequent gaps are present as the person reads, but a grasp of meaning can be achieved. Sartori, Barry, and Job (1984) reviewed 16 cases of phonological dyslexia and found that 11 could read at least 80% of the words contained in the list. Rapscak et al. (1987) reported a case in which there were no complaints about reading and the person was able to complete the reading sections of the Western Aphasia Battery without error.

Recovery of lost skills in surface and in phonological alexias is sparsely documented. What is indicated in surface dyslexia suggests that closed head injuries and surgical excision have lasting effects (cf. Patterson et al., 1985). With the exception of one case (Rapscak et al., 1987), no indication is provided on recovery in phonological dyslexia. However, it can be suspected that strokes, closed head injury, and other lesions that damage tissue in the cerebral region of concern will have consistent effects.

Comprehension in alexias associated with aphasia is correlated with the language comprehension skills of the person. In Broca's aphasia, paralexias are found but comprehension is often intact, especially for text. However, the paralexias may determine the meaning that the person derives. In deep dyslexia, a possible associate of Broca's aphasia, patients can judge meaning based on their paralexia, which can hinder comprehension of a sentence. Additionally, inability to read function words can handicap text comprehension. However, despite these problems comprehension can be functional as the person grasps nouns, verbs, and, frequently, modifiers, so that the basic idea is understood (Coslett et al., 1985; Roeltgen, 1987). With Wernicke's aphasia, when reading is disturbed comprehension is generally not functional (Benson, 1979), although reading can be functional when the angular gyrus is relatively spared (Benson, 1985; Heilman et al., 1979; Kirschner & Webb, 1982). Recovery of skills that are usually lost through cerebral vascular accident is usually slow or nonexistent in alexia associated with Wernicke's aphasia and global aphasias, but can recover relatively quickly (over one year's time) in Broca's aphasia (Benson, 1985). However, one of the few longitudinal studies of recovery reported that over half the sample of aphasics had persistent reading problems evaluated an average 6 years after their stroke (Siirtola, Narva, & Siirtola, 1977).

Functional Reading and Developmental Dyslexia

As stated earlier, longitudinal studies of children with developmental dyslexia have not been conducted. As a result, it is not known how severe disorders must be before functional literacy is hindered. However, studies of adults with reading disabilities suggest that functional reading is hard to attain if any of the component skills are deficient. Johnson (1987) studied a sample of 62 reading-disabled adults who attended remediation programs at Northwestern University. The people had attained some level of reading competence but were generally slow and often made errors, which made reading comprehension for passages and text an exhausting process. Those who used reading in their daily lives did so with great expense to their energy levels and time, thus hindering job performance and emotional ease. These people found functional reading for job performance a chore if any component of reading was inefficient, even though they often had high intelligence.

Research by Lyon and his colleagues highlights the neuropsychological components that influence text comprehension. Those children who had purely visual reading errors and disorders suggestive of right hemisphere dysfunction had fairly strong reading comprehension. They had the best reading comprehension among the disabled subtypes at both age levels studied. When the phonetic system was disturbed alone or in combination with other language disorders or neuropsychological skills assumed to be mediated by the left hemisphere, reading comprehension was poor. Finally, when both visual and linguistic-phonetic weaknesses were observed, reading comprehension was extremely poor.

Johnson's (1987) anecdotal reports suggest that the pattern holds throughout adulthood. Those with generalized language disorders and combined language and visual problems reported the most severe frustration in reading and writing. Despite high intelligence in many cases, these people could not hold jobs that required reading or written communication. In contrast, visual problems were found in the minority, and persons with these problems reported that their reading was much less disrupted. They were frustrated because they complained of reversing words and letters, but they often stated that they were reading slowly and with repetition to check their responses.

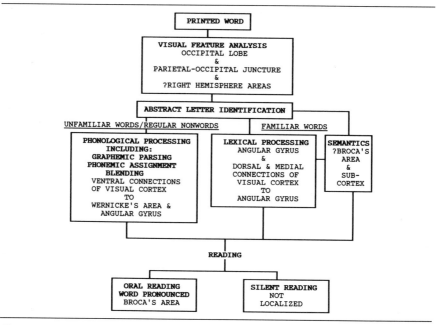

Figure 3–3. Schematic representation of components of reading and their possible anatomic substrates. Based on papers by Coltheart (1984), Coslett et al. (1985), Rapscak et al. (1987), and Roeltgen (1987).

Summary of Implications

Overall, the information to date suggests that functional reading has variable neuropsychological determinants, depending upon the time of its evaluation. A model of functional reading and the suspected anatomic location of the components is presented in figure 3–3. To attain functional reading skills through the education process, it seems best to have an intact capacity to remember and discriminate among visual symbols in the early stages of learning. This process seems best facilitated by the activity of the right hemisphere. To continue beyond this early phase, the visual perceptual and visual memory skills must be supplemented by language-related skills mediated by the left hemisphere. These skills include word fluency, access to names, auditory processing, phonological processing, sequential processing, and semantic processing. The best understanding is that this process involves at least the temporal and parietal regions of the left hemisphere (Duffy et al., 1979). To maintain functional reading, clinical studies suggest that both frontal and parietotemporal regions of the left hemisphere should remain intact. The angular gyrus of the parietotemporal region is essential. If this is damaged, reading becomes nearly impossible for all practical purposes and people are able to read letter by letter in a slow, labored process that allows effective reading of only the briefest messages. When disruptions occur surrounding this region, reading deficits become less extensive, but skills do not match demands of a literate life. If there is loss of access to the direct reading route, as in surface dyslexia, practical comprehension is nearly lost. In contrast, comprehension can be effective if the direct reading route is spared in phonological alexia. When disorders spread to language comprehension regions as in Wernicke's aphasia, reading comprehension is also nearly lost. Thus functional reading appears to be a fragile skill that, once acquired, becomes easily disrupted by many neurological disorders of the left hemisphere.

WRITING DISORDERS

Just as neuropsychological perspectives on reading have changed, discussions of adult writing disorders contain two classification systems, a traditional version and a recent version based on analysis of cognitive components (Roeltgen, 1985). The recently developed system is less well established than the modern version of reading disorders, but it is just as valuable, for it has highlighted the component skills and component structures necessary for functional writing. Our discussion now turns to a description of disorders found, their anatomical substrate, and their impact on day-to-day functioning. The discussion is briefer because less attention has focused on writing disorders (Margolin, 1984) and because reading and spelling disorders in children have, for all practical purposes, been clustered together. Thus since neuropsychological aspects of developmental spelling disorders have been covered in the previous section, this section primarily focuses on disorders subsequent to their acquisition.

Writing is a complex activity that requires the cognitive formulation of words to be produced, the execution of motor movements to produce the letters on the page in the appropriate order, and spatial orientation. It can be disrupted in many ways because of its complexity, and disorders are broadly categorized as affecting the linguistic, motor, or spatial elements.

Traditional Nosology

The traditional classification system describes five disorders differentiated on the basis of the associated neuropsychological deficits present: (1) pure agraphia, (2) aphasic agraphias, (3) agraphia with alexia, (4) apraxic agraphia, and (5) spatial agraphia. Pure agraphia, aphasic agraphia, and agraphia with alexia include conditions in which the linguistic components of writing are disrupted. They share the characteristic that spelling and word selection are in error but formation of letters and their spacing is accurate. They are different because associated disorders are different.

Pure agraphia, as the name implies, describes the condition in which spelling and writing errors abound, but other linguistic processes, including speaking, comprehension, repetition, and reading, remain intact. The condition is rarely encountered, in less than 2% of the cases in a recent survey of 90 aphasic patients (Mazzochi & Vignolo, 1979). Lesion location for most reported cases is in the region of the left superior parietal lobule (Vignolo, 1983). However, the condition has also been reported with lesions in the posterior perisylvian region (Rosati & DeBastiani, 1979), Exner's area in the second frontal convolution (cf. Roeltgen, 1985), subcortical regions of the caudate and adjacent external capsule (Laine & Marttila, 1981), all in the left hemisphere, with one documented case resulting from a right hemisphere lesion in the superior-posterior parietal-occipital lobule (Gonzalez–Rothi, Roeltgen, & Kovistra, 1987).

Aphasic agraphia consists of writing disturbances in the presence of aphasia. It has been documented in all forms of aphasia (cf. Benson, 1979; Clark & Grossfield, 1983; Kaplan & Goodglass, 1981; Kirschner & Webb, 1982; Leishner, 1983; Roeltgen, 1985; Roeltgen, Gonzalez-Rothi, & Heilman, 1986), although its form varies with the nature of the aphasic disorder. In most cases, the nature of spelling and writing disturbances follows the characteristics of that person's aphasic disorder. Thus, in those with Broca's aphasia, some persons are deficient in selection of letters utilized in a word if they exhibit speaking difficulties with single-word pronunciation and selection, whereas others write agrammatic sentences containing correctly spelled words if their aphasia is characterized by accurate word production but telegraphic statements (Kaplan & Goodglass, 1981). Persons with Wernicke's aphasia present written statements that appear to be grammatically correct, but their word selection of correctly spelled words is often incomprehensible. Additionally, when asked to spell words to dictation, many "words" written are either phonemic or semantic substitutions for the desired word (Kaplan & Goodglass, 1981; Kirschner & Webb, 1982). Transcortical aphasias—motor, sensory, and mixed—are associated with written communication that is generally correct but sometimes includes semantic substitutions for the desired word (Clark & Grossfield, 1983; Roeltgen et al., 1986).

Agraphia with alexia has been reviewed earlier. As noted, it is a common feature acompanying left parietal lobe lesions that include the angular gyrus. Affected individuals read with great difficulty and spell many words incorrectly in spontaneous writing and writing to dictation.

A person is described as having apraxic agraphia when the motor aspects of writing are disturbed but spelling remains intact when motor movements are simple. As a result, persons with the disturbance write words incorrectly, but they spell words correctly if given the opportunity to use anagram letters, such as plastic letters or letter-blocks, or, at times, orally spell. To exist in its pure form, the disturbance of function would have to be limited to motor movements for letter formation but exclude the language problems and other motor deficiencies. It is assumed that a very discrete lesion would be required (Margolin, 1984) but how discrete and in what location cannot be determined, for only two specific cases have been reported. Coslett et al. (1986) reported on a patient who could perform movements to commands with the right hand, and could copy designs, but could not write words spontaneously or to dictation. This subject had multiple small lesions that were localized to the left hemisphere superior posterior internal capsule and superior parietal lobule and the right hemisphere posterior corona radiata. Another patient reported by Baxter and Warrington (1986) had a similar pattern of skills, no difficulties copying figures or letter, and no deficiencies in oral spelling (not evaluated in Coslett et al.'s subject, although type-written spelling was intact), but had severe impairments in writing letters or words spontaneously or to dictation. The presumed cause was a large mass originating in the medial left parietal-occipital region and extending through the corpus callosum to the right hemisphere.

When apraxic agraphia exists with other disturbances, individual case reports indicate discrete regional lesions, but the lesions show no consistent pattern from case to case. They include left and right hemisphere lesions of frontal and posterior regions (cf. Margolin, 1984; Margolin & Wing, 1983). However, when apraxic agraphia without general apraxia has been documented, lesions in the parietal lobe of either the right or left hemisphere seem to be responsible (Margolin & Binder, 1984; Roeltgen & Heilman, 1983).

Micrographia is one of many forms of writing disturbances that are manifestations of generalized motor disorders. In this condition, spelling is accurate, but handwriting is small and becomes progressively smaller as the person continues to write. As a result, written statements include words that may be of an appropriate size at the beginning of a line but quickly decrease to minute approximations of words. Speed of handwriting is also low. Micrographia is found in persons with Parkinsonism and is often the first sign of that disease. Analysis of micrographic writing indicates that it is the result of gradual decreases in the force applied to the writing instrument (Margolin & Wing, 1983) that make it hard for the person to maintain letters of an appropriate height. Margolin and Wing (1983) suggest that micrographia is a written reflection of the generalized deficiency that Parkinsonian patients have in maintaining enough force to execute motor movements. Thus effective motor execution for handwriting requires intact extrapyramidal tracts through the basal ganglia. Of course, other motor disorders will affect handwriting, but they are not selective and are beyond the scope of this chapter. A recent review of apraxia by Heilman and Gonzalez-Rothi (1985) discussed these disorders and their influence on writing.

Spatial agraphia is found when perceptual skills are disrupted. Writing is characterized by inappropriate spacing between individual letters, inappropriate formation of letters (including too few or too many elements or strokes), and writing that deviates from the horizontal and is often restricted to the right side of the page (Margolin, 1984; Roeltgen, 1985). Spelling is usually accurate when written words can be deciphered, but it is clearly intact when reviewed using oral responses. This disorder is found with parietal or parietal-occipital lesions of the right hemisphere. Significantly, the disruption in writing seems the result of inaccuracies in interpreting visual feedback, for normal subjects will create similar mistakes when visual review of their handwriting is blocked (Margolin, 1984).

The Cognitive Neuropsychology or Psycholinguistic System

A modern system has developed to determine what component skills are necessary for spelling and to account for noted variations in types of errors produced by agraphic patients. Cognitive science has contributed the idea that written and oral spelling are complex processes that are best understood when the component skills utilized in their completion are elaborated. Cognitive neuroscience has sought to link ideas about component skills with anatomical investigations to delineate the neurological substrate for component skills.

In the cognitive models of spelling, each of which contains several components, two major stages are proposed (Villa & Romani, 1987; Margolin, 1984; Roeltgen, 1985). First, the generation of a graphemic representation for a word occurs. This is the process of determining what letters should be utilized. In the second stage, the processes of planning a motor program to create the grapheme through the selected output mode (e.g., writing, oral spelling, typewriting) and executing the necessary motor movements are activated. Between the stages, a memory component has been proposed to act as a temporary store of the graphemic representation whereas motor programs for creating it are determined. This component has been called the orthographic buffer (Margolin, 1984) or the graphemic buffer (Caramazza et al., 1987). During the first stage, composed primarily of linguistic components, disruption to those components results in different forms of linguistic agraphia. The second stage requires motor and spatial components, and lesions to structures that mediate these processes result in apraxic agraphias and spatial agraphias. Delineation of the linguistic components has been the main focus of recent research, so our discussion will highlight those. The understanding of motor and spatial components is consistent with information already discussed, so no further elaboration is necessary. Clear selective disruption of the graphemic buffer has been documented in one case (Caramazza et al., 1987), so mneumonic aspects of agraphia are also presented.

Linguistic agraphias

Analyses of the spelling errors made by agraphic patients indicate that the misspelled productions of target words often resemble the desired words in one of three ways: visual appearance, phonology, or semantics. The analyses also indicate that a particular person is prone to make the same kinds of errors for all misspelled words (Beauvois & Derouesne, 1981; Shallice, 1981). These observations have been utilized to categorize patients into clusters that are similar to the clusters described in the psycholinguistic model of the alexias. Four types have been proposed: (1) phonological agraphia, (2) deep agraphia, (3) lexical agraphia, and (4) semantic agraphia.

PHONOLOGICAL AGRAPHIA. When a word is to be spelled, it is assumed that the auditory input activates either a visual association or a phonemic association that is then decoded and converted into letter choices. Models of spelling suggest that accomplished spellers primarily rely on the visual or lexical association to guide letter choices (Ellis, 1982; Margolin, 1984; Roeltgen, 1985). However, when a word is unfamiliar and follows the rules for phoneme-to-grapheme conversion, the phonological system utilizes the rules to segment the word and select graphemes to represent the discrete segments.

Breakdown in this system results in phonological agraphia manifested by spelling errors on words that are unfamiliar but phonologically regular and an inability to spell pronouncible nonsense words (e.g., *tup, kip*). The errors that persons with this disorder produce for real words often share the visual appearance of the real word but differ in their pronunciation (e.g., *coay* for *coat, foos* for *food* [from Clark & Grossfeld, 1983], and *wadder* for *wallet* [from Roeltgen, 1985]. Spelling is preserved for familiar words that are regular (e.g., *dog*) and irregular (e.g., *laugh*) because it is assumed that a visual, lexical association is used to facilitate spelling. For familiar words that are regular the visual image is remembered because that is the preferred system for associations and it is easily accessed because of repetitive use. Irregular familiar words are correctly spelled because the only means to remember their spelling is through storage of their appearance.

The lesions responsible for phonological agraphia have been widespread throughout the left hemisphere (Bob & Kertesz, 1982; Nolan & Caramazza, 1982; Roeltgen et al., 1983; Roeltgen & Heilman, 1984; Shallice, 1981), but Roeltgen (1985) reported that they all share at least one aspect in common: The supramarginal gyrus or the insula medial to it is incorporated in the lesions. One patient who had no other language impairments had a small lesion confined to the insula and possibly the supramarginal gyrus lateral to it. Lesions are usually due to cerebral vascular accidents that affect posterior branches of the middle cerebral artery that supplies the insula and the supramarginal gyrus.

Associated neuropsychological disorders include aphasia, alexia, acalculia, and apraxia. Of the patients studied carefully, the majority had phonological alexia, but this is not necessary as at least one demonstrated lexical alexia and another had no alexia. It is assumed from these patients that phonological reading centers are adjacent to the phonological spelling center, but they can be differentially organized (Roeltgen, 1985).

DEEP AGRAPHIA. A special subset of patients with phonological agraphia have been reported as having deep agraphia. Similar to lesions with deep dyslexia, word class and imageability of words affect proficiency of spelling using the lexical spelling route (Bob & Kertesz, 1982; Nolan & Caramazza, 1983; Roeltgen, 1985). This pattern of performance indicates that nouns are spelled better than adjectives and verbs, which are all spelled better than function words. Additionally, nouns of high imageability, such as *dog*, are spelled better than abstract nouns such as *law* (Roeltgen, 1985). It is possible that the strong visual association of concrete nouns facilitates access to the visual appearance of their labels. Errors made are often semantic paragraphias of the target word (e.g., *funny* for *happy* [from Bub & Kertesz, 1982]. Nonsense words cannot be spelled at all.

The characteristics of deep agraphia indicate that it is a form of phonological agraphia with more extensive impairments to include misspelling of more words based on their imageability and class. Lesions responsible for deep agraphia are more extensive than lesions for phonological agraphia but also incorporate the supramarginal gyrus or insula medial to it (Roeltgen, 1985). Stroke has been the cause for the lesions found. Accompanying deficits include Broca's aphasia and alexia, usually of the deep dyslexic type.

LEXICAL AGRAPHIA. Preserved spelling of regular words and pronounceable nonsense words in the presence of acquired spelling disturbances of irregular words is present in cases of lexical agraphia. In such disorders, the visual word image or lexical store is disrupted and the person becomes a phonetic speller. Thus *laugh* may be spelled as *laff.* The condition is much less frequent than phonological agraphia, estimated to be one-third as common by Roeltgen (1985). This fact is probably the result of the location of the lesion that seems responsible and the ways in which such lesions are sustained. Specifically, the cases analyzed showed commonalities in that the angular gyrus and the parietal-occipital lobule adjacent to it contained lesions (Roeltgen & Heilman, 1984, Roeltgen, 1985). Because the angular gyrus and adjacent regions do not receive their blood supply from one specific artery, they will not be damaged by a single occlusion. Responsible lesions have included occlusion of vessels between the internal carotid and the posterior cerebral artery, hemorrhages, tumors, and degenerative diseases. Such sources of disorder are encountered less frequently than are the primary sources of lesions in phonological agraphia. Additionally, lexical agraphia may be a more acute phenomenon that changes rapidly, in that the majority of cases reported have been acute and the majority of cases of phonological agraphia are reported in chronic cases. This fact may decrease detection of lexical agraphia, for its presence may be more transient than phonological agraphia.

The disorders that accompany lexical agraphia have included aphasia, all fluent forms (anomia, Wernicke's, and transcortical sensory), alexia, both phonological and lexical, acalculia with right-left disorientation, and ideo-motor apraxia (Roeltgen, 1985).

SEMANTIC AGRAPHIA. Five patients have been described who were capable of spelling words, relying on the lexical writing route, but could not incorporate meaning into their word selection. They had misspellings of many words that looked like the correctly spelled word, such as *now* for *knows* and *scen* for *seen,* thus showing signs of phonological agraphia. In addition, however, they showed a separation of semantic processes from lexical systems. This was demonstrated in their frequent inability to select the correct word when asked to spell homophones, words that have the same sound but different meanings (Roeltgen, Gonzalez-Rothi, & Heilman, 1986). For example, when asked to spell the word *not* and read the sentence "He is not here," to clarify its meaning, patients often wrote *knot*. Similar problems were found for other word pairs such as *dough/doe*, *bowled/bold*, and *where/wear*. The persons often spelled the words correctly even if they were irregular, but they selected the word with the wrong meaning. Thus the lexical system was intact as demonstrated by the accuracy of spelling for irregular words, but selection of the word to be spelled was disrupted.

The patients showed other linguistic characteristics. They all demonstrated forms of transcortical aphasia with intact repetition but impaired comprehension. Although their lesions did not overlap or share a specific location, they all fell in left hemisphere areas previously documented as hindering comprehension, including the watershed distribution, the internal capsule and caudate nucleus, and the thalamus. Roeltgen et al. (1986) suggested that the persons shared a functional similarity rather than a specific anatomic locus, suggesting that comprehension and semantics, as opposed to visual appearance and phonological characteristics, are broadly represented in the cortex and subcortex.

Associated features of semantic agraphia other than impaired comprehension also include alexia with poor comprehension, acalculia, finger agnosia, apraxia, and nonfluent speech.

Mneumonic agraphia

For spelling to occur, the chosen word must be briefly stored in memory and, once its representation is chosen, that representation must be stored while motoric planning is conducted for oro-motor musculature (for oral spelling), for pen or pencil movement (for written spelling), or for finger movements (for typing or anagram spelling). The working memory that stores the representation while motor planning occurs has been called the graphemic buffer (Caramazza et al., 1987) or the orthographic buffer (Margolin, 1984).

One case was reported that provides evidence that this component can be selectively impaired (Caramazza et al., 1987). The patient had suffered a cerebral vascular accident of the left hemisphere in the surface and deep structures of the pre- and postrolandic regions. He was normally functioning in all language tasks that did not require reading or writing, including repetition tasks and complex comprehension tasks. He showed no generalized memory disturbance, so the memory problems noted were limited to the spelling task. With reading, he could not read nonsense words. For spelling, he made many mistakes on both familiar words and nonsense words that were pronounceable. These errors were noted for oral and written spelling, in response to dictation and delayed copy, and also for writing names of common objects shown in line drawings. In other words, whenever a memory for the word to be presented was required, he showed spelling errors. In addition, as the length of the test words increased, his spelling difficulties increased. This suggested deterioration of a visual memory image that was degraded by the time he had completed the execution of initial and medial graphemes. That he could spell familiar words and nonsense words indicated that neither the lexical system nor the phonological system was a source of agraphia.

Models of Functional Spelling

The case study data presented provide indications that many components are present within a functional spelling system. Within the first stage, the generation of a graphic representation occurs. As indicated by the three forms of linguistic agraphia—phonetic, lexical, and semantic—parallel sources of information are available to generate words in spelled form. It appears that the lexical system is preferred, but if it is impaired, the phonological system can be engaged to generate models of words; and if both of those systems are defective, semantic information can influence spelling. Once the spelled form

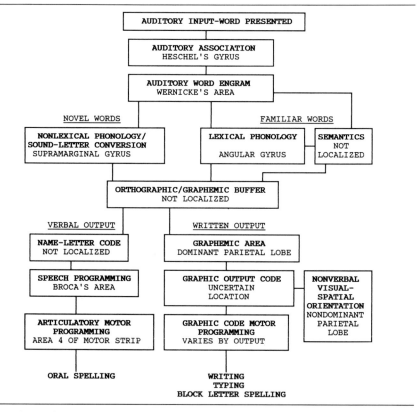

Figure 3–4. Schematic representation of components of spelling and their possible anatomic substrates. Based on similar models from Caramazza et al. (1987), Margolin (1984), and Roeltgen (1985).

is generated, the image is stored in the orthographic buffer while motor programs are developed to guide the movements necessary for execution. These movements are influenced by information systems that determine location of letters and guide motor execution for letter formation.

Three schematic models of the spelling system have been proposed by Caramazza et al. (1987), Margolin (1984), and Roeltgen (1985). Aspects of each of these models have been incorporated in the diagram in figure 3–4. The model highlights the previous discussion and indicates the likely anatomic substrate for each component, if known.

Determinants of functional writing

Written expression for day-to-day activity varies with the task to be completed. A shopping list requires less proficiency than completing an essay or writing a poem. Whether a person is capable depends on the error standards set for word selection and spelling accuracy. Many of the cases of linguistic agraphia studied had high levels of accuracy in spelling but made selective errors. Whether these persons could be described as achieving functional levels depends on the reader's tolerance for mistakes. Clearly, for formal communication, the persons should be considered ineffective, but for the completion of notes to friends or relatives, notes to themselves, and shopping lists, for example, these patients may be effective. For example, in Roeltgen and Heilman's study (1984), three of four persons with phonological agraphia spelled the majority of nouns correctly (95% or more) although they had many errors on other words, for an average rate of accuracy of 56% for regular words and 59% for irregular words. The fourth patient spelled fewer than half the words presented to him correctly. Despite relatively good accuracy on nouns, however, it may be hard to decipher what these patients write, for their mistakes are not phonetically accurate and often do not approach resemblance to the target word (e.g., *gom* for *limb*, p. 815). Those patients with lexical agraphia were significantly lower in accuracy for spelling irregular words (four patients averaged 42% correct) but much better on regularly spelled words (72% of regular words). These patients may be more communicative, however, for their errors usually sound like the target word. Patients with deep agraphia present confusing errors, as misspellings are often semantic substitutions for the target word. Thus, although spelled correctly, their errors may not communicate accurately (e.g., *child* for *boy*).

The effectiveness of writing in sentences and paragraphs for patients with agraphia depends upon the level of generalized language disturbance present. Most of the patients reported have been aphasic. Their written communication has generally reflected their verbal expression (Benson, 1979). Nearly all cases are reported to be mildly anomic, so that word selection during writing can be arduous (cf. Roeltgen & Heilman, 1984). When Broca's aphasia is present, written communication is generally telegraphic but understandable as long as the misspelled words are decipherable. Patients with Wernicke's aphasia write with less effectiveness, as their word selection is often incomprehensible. Spelling errors only add to the confusion for the reader (Benson, 1979).

The persistence of agraphia seems to depend on the nature of the causal lesion. For those cases resulting from ischemic cerebral vascular accidents, agraphia was discovered up to several years after the initial injury (cf. Roeltgen & Heilman, 1984). Because cases studied at different time periods have not been reported, however, it is not known if the number of agraphic errors changes after injury. Patients that experience agraphia due to tumor and hemorrhage usually had some recovery of skills if damaged tissue was removed. This latter situation has been reported most often in lexical agraphia, so it is found to be one of the least persistent forms. Studies designed with a longitudinal analysis need to be performed to attain a better understanding of the lasting impact of agraphia.

Developmental determinants

Developmental studies have not selectively focused on spelling, because children who spell poorly are usually poor readers. However, several studies provide indications that two major systems are present for spelling accuracy: a phonological system and a lexical system that relies upon visual memory. Semantics may play an independent role as children can tell the meaning of a word presented to them even when they cannot read it aloud (noted by Bradley, 1983). A series of studies by Bradley and colleagues indicate that children initially rely on a phonetic approach to spell words and shift to the use of visual cues to spell irregular words at ages above 7. This shift may require effective visual memory skills, since those that spelled irregular words incorrectly also did poorly on tasks of visual memory (Bradley, 1983). However, Rourke and colleagues (Rourke, 1983) found different correlates of phonetically accurate spelling in the studies of children with poor spelling scores. Children whose errors in spelling resulted in words that reflected the words' sounds but not their appearance were not found different on visual memory tasks. Instead, they were found to be different from normal spellers in their knowledge of information. This finding suggested that they may have a limit in their capacity to learn new information, including information related to variations from the phoneme-to-grapheme conversion rules. Children who spell words in a phonetically inaccurate way are similar to phonetically inaccurate readers. They have less well developed language and auditory processing skills than normals and poor spellers who make phonetically accurate misspellings (Rourke, 1983).

How noted variations in spelling proficiency during development are linked to local brain activity has not been determined because selectively poor spellers have not been as thoroughly studied as poor readers. Thus the neuropsychological components of developmental dysgraphia need further study. Written expression in sentences and paragraphs is assumed to be correlated with general language skills, but the neuropsychological aspects of its development remain unclear.

MATHEMATICS

Mathematical thinking is the most complex of the skills considered in this chapter. It necessitates the capacity to read and write numbers as meaningful symbols, the knowledge of operational signs, access and memory for the facts required to correctly perform an operation on numbers, logical processing of rules remembered, application of rules in the appropriate sequence, and concentration to complete all these steps in a timely fashion. The accurate application of mathematical thought thus requires many cognitive skills and is therefore one of the most easily disrupted functions when any form of brain damage is present (Grafman et al., 1982). This sensitivity is documented by the observation that the arithmetic subtest of the Wechsler Adult Intelligence Scale is one of the subtests most likely to be suppressed in the presence of any form of damage (Lezak, 1983).

Despite its sensitivity to the effects of damage, mathematical reasoning and its disruption has received the smallest amount of attention of the functions reviewed here. No comprehensive model of its component skills has been widely discussed, although one has been proposed by McCloskey, Caramazza, and Basili (1985). Thus classification of disorders relies on a broad distinction among disruption of the linguistic components of calculation (in other words, alexia and agraphia for numbers), disturbance of the spatial organization of written calculation, and disorders in the logical application of facts and rules, referred to as anarithmia. Developmental calculation disorders have received only recent investigation, so their neuropsychological understanding is limited.

Acquired Disorders

The classification of acquired arithmetic disorders is based on the distinction among the linguistic elements, spatial elements, and calculation elements. Patients have been encountered who demonstrate alexia and/or agraphia for numbers selectively (Deloche & Seron, 1984), disturbances of placement of numbers in space, and problems applying numerical operations or remembering facts (Grafman et al., 1982; McCloskey, Caramazza, & Basili, 1985). McCloskey et al. (1985) presented a model incorporating cognitive skills that are essential for effective calculation and received partial confirmation through case study. Levin and Spiers (1985) recently reviewed the literature on acalculia that remains current as recent studies do not alter their conclusions. These papers form the basis of the model of functional mathematics.

Linguistic Elements

McCloskey et al. (1985) proposed that there are two cognitive systems in mathematical processing: the number processing system and the calculation system. Both systems contain steps that require reading and writing. In the number processing system a number comprehension system and number production system exist. These systems have separate procedures for processing verbal numbers (e.g., *eighty-two*) and Arabic numbers (e.g., *82*). The comprehension of verbal numbers incorporates syntactical processing to facilitate reading and understanding of value based on word order, phonological processing for the understanding of spoken numbers, and graphemic processing for comprehension of written number words. Arabic number comprehension requires syntactical mechanisms applied after lexical processing mechanisms allow for the reading of numerals. Production of numbers that are verbal requires mechanisms for syntactical processing and separate phonological and graphemic mechanisms to produce spoken number words or written number words. Syntactical mechanisms and lexical production mechanisms are present to produce Arabic numbers. Finally, linguistic ele-

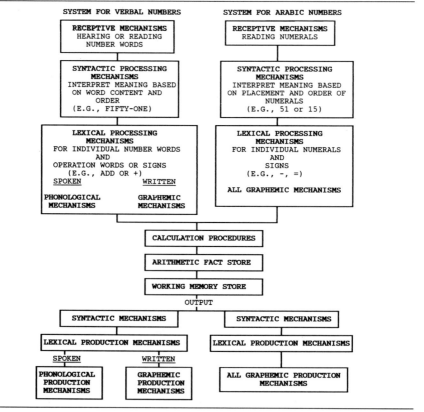

Figure 3–5. Schematic representation of components of calculation. Anatomic localization cannot be stated with clarity for any component. A working memory is proposed for storage of intermediate results in multistep problems (e.g., 140 × 2 = ?) and storage of results before output mechanisms are activated. Based on McCloskey et al. (1985).

ments are present in the calculation system for the comprehension of operational words, such as *add* and operational signs and the production of such words and signs. A schematic representation of the component steps is presented in figure 3–5.

A review of cases documents that distinctions can be made among the components proposed. Comprehension of numbers and their production can be dissociated. McCloskey et al. (1985) reported on cases documented by Benson and Denckla in 1969 and Singer and Low in 1933 in which number alexia was absent but forms of number agraphia and number anomia were present. With one patient, that of Benson and Denckla, verbal and Arabic numbers were inaccurately produced in response to questions, but multiple choice problems could be completed when the numbers were written or spoken by the examiner. The other patient presented paragraphias for Arabic numbers. This patient wrote "20042" when asked to write "two hundred forty-two" (McCloskey et al., 1985). More specific dissociations between processing for Arabic and verbal numbers were also reported by McCloskey et al. (1985) in their own patient population and historical patients. One patient could comprehend Arabic numbers but not verbal numbers in written form, and another patient could comprehend written number-words but not numerals. So alexia for numbers can be selective for the form of presentation. Other patients produced the correct answer to problems in one form but were incorrect for another form of output. One historical patient of Berger in 1926 correctly wrote the Arabic numerals but said the wrong word, and another said the correct word but wrote the wrong numerals (e.g., said "fifty" correctly while writing "32"; McCloskey et al., 1985, p. 177). Thus agraphia or anomia for numbers can be selectively present conditions.

Number comprehension disorders may also depend on the system required for processing. McCloskey et al. (1985) reported on a patient who could comprehend written number-words (e.g., *six*) but not spoken number-words. Thus comprehension was intact for processing graphemes but not phonemes. For number-words, the person was alexic but not receptively aphasic.

In the production of numbers, McCloskey et al. (1985) also indicated that number graphemes and number syntax may be dissociated. They provided examples of patients who wrote the correct digits when writing to dictation but had the wrong meaning. For example, as noted previously, a patient wrote "20042" when aurally presented with the request to write "two hundred forty-two." Another patient showed an opposite problem, producing numbers of the correct magnitude but the wrong digits. When asked to write "two hundred twenty-one" the person wrote "215." These cases highlight that agraphic errors encountered may be present for selective aspects of numbers. Alexic errors that are similar can also be found. A patient reported in this study read individual digits incorrectly, but his answers were the correct magnitude. For example, he said "fifty-five thousand" when presented with "37,000" and said "fifty" when the stimulus was "40" (McCloskey et al., 1985, p. 187).

Two patients reported by Ferro and Bothelho (1980) had agraphia and alexia for operational signs but could read and write numerals and number-words. Thus they showed selective linguistic defects for operational signs. These patients could copy the signs, so visual perception and motor movements did not account for their selective mathematical alexia and agraphia. They could also perform calculations presented orally and respond with correct answers, indicating that they were not aphasic for operational words. These patients provide evidence confirming the presence of operational sign comprehension and production components for the lexical mode of presentation.

That these linguistic components have been found to be selectively disrupted provides confirmation that the general model proposed by McCloskey and colleagues has heuristic value. However, localization of lesions responsible for the separate components has yet to be determined. The review by Levin and Spiers (1985) indicates that linguistic aspects of calculation are most often disrupted by left hemispheric lesions. Slightly over one-third of unselected samples of patients with left hemispheric damage have alexia or agraphia for numbers. Posterior left hemispheric lesions seem most responsible, for over 80% of patients evaluated by Hecaen and Angelergues in 1962 (quoted in Boller & Grafman, 1983) with left temporo-occipital lesions were alexic for numbers. Selective right hemisphere damage has been found to be accompanied by alexia or agraphia for numbers in only 2 to 8% of cases studied (Boller & Grafman, 1983; Levin & Spiers, 1985). Review also indicated that alexia for numbers and agraphia for numbers in numeral form can be present in the absence of word alexia or agraphia. As many as 20% of patients studied in historical reviews by Henschen and Hecaen, Angelergues, and Houllier had alexia for numbers in the absence of word alexia or agraphia for words (Levin & Spiers, 1985). Although most alexic or agraphic patients studied had alexia or agraphia for both words and numbers, many (between 22 and 53%) who could not read or produce written words could read and write numbers. These findings suggest that the locations of lesions responsible for number alexia and number agraphia are in different places from those responsible for word alexia and agraphia. The left parietal lobe had been strongly implicated in selective disruption of numbers, and the parietal and temporo-occipital locations have been suggested for alexia of numerical signs (Levin & Spiers, 1985).

Research by Deloche and Seron (1984) provides some indications how components may be selectively disrupted and what variable locations may be responsible. These authors studied the process of transcoding words into numerals and numerals into words in samples of aphasic patients. Their research suggests that lesions responsible for syntactical disruptions of number reading and writing may correspond to locations responsible for Broca's aphasia, while lexical disruptions may occur with location of lesions in areas that cause Wernicke's aphasia. Deloche and Seron have differentiated between stack errors and stack position errors. *Stack* refers to the column of numerals representing the digits ranked from 0 to 9. *Position* refers to the place from right to left in which a digit is located to indicate ones, tens, hundreds, and so on. A *stack error* refers to a replacement of one numeral in the same position for another; e.g., "7" is read or written when "8" is meant. A *stack position* error occurs when the correct numeral is read but its locations is wrong; e.g., "5" is said or written when the target number is "50" or "500."

Several error patterns were noted by Deloche and Seron. First, errors made by aphasics usually fell into one of the two groups described. Second, a particular patient usually made the same type of error. Finally, the error type encountered correlated with the type of aphasia reported. Those with Broca's aphasia usually made stack position errors and often left out function words. For example, they might read "6" as "60" and say "eight fifty-seven" for "857", leaving out the "hundred." Thus Broca's aphasics were agrammatic and made what could be considered to be syntactic errors. Wernicke's aphasics made stack errors (e.g., "5" for "7") but stated the stack correctly; thus they maintained the syntax but not lexical elements. This research suggests that the distinction between lexical and syntactic processes proposed by McCloskey and associates may correspond to an anterior-posterior distinction in neuroanatomy. Further study like this research may help elaborate the location of lesions for selective disruption of components, as has been done in the dissociation of phonological and surface alexia, for example.

Spatial Elements

Accurate mathematical calculation requires that the numerals to be manipulated are aligned correctly or placed in the correct location from right to left. To produce a correct response, a person must keep all "ones" to the right, and all "tens" one column over, and so on. In other words, spatial elements are required in the calculation system. For example, to add, a person must carry value from one column of figures to the next, and in multiplication the second row of a product in the intermediate steps for multiplying by a two–digit number must be moved over one place from the first row. Selective disruption of spatial elements causing calculation errors has been documented. For example, McCloskey et al. (1985) reported that patients who failed to carry consistently (e.g., $607 + 495 = 1002$) did not carry at all (e.g., $607 + 495 = 10912$) and did not move intermediate products (e.g., $37 \times 24 = 148 + 74 = 222$, instead of $37 \times 24 = 148 + 740 = 888$). Although these and other patients performed oral calculations successfully and obtained the correct sums for the digits used, problems with alignment disrupted their final answers. At times, spatial transposition of numbers occurs that results in errors, though the person retains the ability to complete the operations. As a result, "24" may be read as "42" and the sum of "24 + 3" may be written as "45."

Lesions that have been associated with this form of acalculia have included both right and left hemisphere centers, although the majority of patients with

right parieto-occipital damage have this disorder, but less than 5% of patients
with left hemisphere damage show such a problem (Boller & Grafman, 1983).

Disruption of operational elements

The model proposed by McCloskey and colleagues indicates that the calculation system incorporates comprehension and production of operational signs
along with two other components: calculation procedures and an arithmetic
fact store. They indicate that the calculation procedures involve the logical
manipulation of steps that follow learned rules. Arithmetic facts include mem-
orized results of numbers combined through an operation. Carrying value is
an example of a calculation procedure, and "2 + 2 = 4" is an arithmetic fact.

The review of patients by McCloskey and colleagues found that arithmetic
facts and calculations can be separately disrupted. One patient made errors
in retrieving facts for addition and other operations while providing clear
description of the four basic operations. Other patients performed calculation procedures without error but frequently made errors on the facts, especially for multiplication. Often, their errors were either adjacent to the correct
response (e.g., "49" for "48") or the wrong multiple of a particular number
(e.g., "8 × 6 = 56"). This finding suggested that the selection of numbers was
jumbled. Other patients showed good knowledge of facts but made errors in
the procedures. For example, one patient made errors in carrying value, while
others mixed elements of addition procedures with multiplication procedures.

The types of disorders included in the calculation system that exclude alexia
and agraphia for operational signs have historically been called anarithmia.
Persons with such disorders have been found to have lesions bilaterally represented in posterior and anterior regions of the brain (Grafman et al., 1982;
Levin & Spiers, 1985). Grafman and co-workers (1982) have studied the frequency with which calculation disturbances occur in the absence of alexia or
agraphia in persons with lesions limited to either the left anterior, left posterior, right anterior, or right posterior regions of the brain. Their results
indicate that all brain-damaged groups performed worse than controls when
confronted by problems involving all four operations. Pairwise comparisons
of the brain-damaged groups found that those with left hemisphere damage
were more impaired than those with right hemisphere lesions and that left
posterior lesions resulted in significantly more errors than any other form of
lesion. The persons with left posterior damage continued to show more errors
even when factors of decreased intelligence and aphasic disturbance were
controlled statistically. Thus, although calculation disturbances are found
with lesions throughout the brain, they are more likely and of greater severity
with left posterior damage. Grafman et al. (1982) highlight the correspond-
ence of their findings with other data that indicate greater EEG alteration of
the left hemisphere when arithmetic is performed and that the calculation
skills of the right hemisphere have been found to be negligible in comis-
surotomy patients.

Gerstmann's Syndrome

A collection of neuropsychological deficits, beginning with reports by Gerstmann summarized in 1940 (Gerstmann, 1940), have been proposed to compose a syndrome. The disorder includes acalculia (which type has not been determined), finger agnosia, left–right disorientation, and agraphia. It has been proposed to result from lesions of the left angular gyrus. Despite its prevalence in the literature, however, it is not certain that the syndrome is selective or simply the effect of general aphasia. It has not been reported in patients with focal lesions (Roeltgen, Sevush, & Heilman, 1983). Thus the disorder is controversial.

Recently, however, a strictly defined case was presented with a focal lesion. Roeltgen and associates (1983) reported on a patient who was not aphasic on extensive exam and did not have constructional apraxia. This patient showed all the signs of Gerstmann's syndrome with a lesion of the angular gyrus extending into the edge of the supramarginal gyrus and the superior parietal lobule. The results seemed to support the idea of a selective syndrome with selective lesions. The errors noted in mathematics were of calculation procedures. Thus this study suggested that disruption of the calculation system may be localized to the posterior left hemisphere.

Recovery and Functional Performance

Information on recovery of skills when mathematical thinking is disrupted is scanty. Many patients have been studied years after their initial lesion, suggesting that problems can be persistent, but longitudinal data must be gathered to answer the question of recovery of function. Additionally, cases must be studied on the basis of type of lesion, as the data from alexia and agraphia indicate that lesion type influences recovery. To date, patients with many forms of lesions have been clustered together to form study groups.

Case review suggests that functional performance of mathematics depends on the breadth of the disturbance. Disruption of spatial elements may be overcome if the person alters the orientation of the numerals written (Levin & Spiers, 1985). Linguistic elements may be totally disrupted, or the person may be able to perform calculations because only selective disturbances are present and the person is able to work with Arabic numbers or number-words in written or spoken form (McCloskey et al., 1985). Mathematics may be functional through the use of supplements such as calculators. If disruption in spatial elements and linguistic elements is limited, persons with these disorders could probably function using calculators if they read numerals, but this hypothesis needs to be evaluated through research. When nonlinguistic elements of the calculation system are disturbed, functional performance may be achieved through the use of calculators or tables of values. Certainly, problems with arithmetic facts could be overcome this way. Whether disturbed operations could be altered through supplemental help probably depends on the capacity of the person to follow procedures in a step-by-step fashion. If the person can learn to enter information into the calculator and complete all steps in the right order, calculation may be possible. Because of these possibilities, acquired disorders in arithmetic may be the most easily overcome of the functions discussed.

Developmental Disorders

The disruption of learning in mathematics probably depends on many skills, for arithmetic is a complex process that requires many steps. The research by Rourke and colleagues on the neuropsychological correlates of selective mathematical disturbance in children without known brain lesions provides the best hypothesis for understanding brain–behavior relationships in learning mathematics. Their studies indicate that many children with reading and spelling difficulties also have arithmetic disabilities, indicating that the skills required for acquisition overlap greatly (Strang & Rourke, 1985). However, mathematical learning may require selective skills independent of the linguistic facility necessary for reading and writing.

The research focused on three groups of children: (1) a group that was 2 years below grade level in reading, spelling, and mathematics; (2) a group that was significantly more deficient in spelling and reading than in mathematics; and (3) a group that had mathematics scores significantly below their reading and spelling performance. The results indicated that the groups varied greatly in associated neuropsychological profiles. Children who exhibited relatively good mathematical performance in relation to reading and spelling were found to be less effective on measures of verbal and auditory perceptual skills. They also exhibited a pattern of relative inefficiency in completing psychomotor tasks using the right hand when compared to the left hand. In contrast, the children with poor mathematical skills in relation to reading and spelling had somewhat low visual-perceptual skills, poor performance when using their left hand for complex psychomotor tasks, and marked impairment on left-sided tactile perception of stimuli. Thus, the groups showed very different ability/disability patterns.

The data suggest that those children with deficiencies in all three subjects measured, who are more deficient in reading and spelling than mathematics, do not perform functions mediated by the left hemisphere well. In contrast, those with selective calculation disturbances seem to have problems completing tasks mediated by the right hemisphere (Strang & Rourke, 1983). Error analysis supports this possibility, in that the children with selective mathematical deficiencies made errors related to spatial organization and visual detail and also errors described as related to impaired reasoning. The neuropsychological profile suggested that the children may have problems in learning because of two processes that may be related to right hemisphere functioning. These children were low in nonverbal sensory-motor skills that may facilitate learning about concrete properties such as number, proportional size, and relative value. They also showed problems in judgment and concept formation considered by some researchers to require an intact right hemisphere for their appropriate development (Strang & Rourke, 1983). Thus, for acquisition of effective mathematical skills, children seem to require intact linguistic systems and also intact nonverbal systems to facilitate calculation and comprehension of number concepts. Of course, much more study is required to evaluate these very preliminary hypotheses, as they are based on a relative paucity of data.

CONCLUSIONS

It is clear from this discussion that reading, writing, and mathematical calculation are highly complex tasks that require the integration of numerous component skills for effective performance. The neuropsychological study of their disruption has advanced from the level of descriptions of broad variations in skill performance to the point of localizing lesions responsible for mediating specific component skills. This advancement has occurred through the integration of cognitive psychology and the neurosciences. The discussion of reading highlights how fruitful this integration has been. The efforts utilized in dissecting the reading process have helped in developing models for research in writing and arithmetic that are now being pursued. It is believed that these models will provide the framework for groundbreaking research in writing and arithmetic. Although the data to date highlight the importance of the skills mediated by the left hemisphere in each of the functions reviewed, it seems certain that future research will only expand our awareness that functional skills are not easily localized and are complexly represented in the brain. Holding such recognition in conjunction with knowledge of the necessary component skills for competence can only enhance our capacity to facilitate the daily performance of these skills for the able and disabled. Thus detailed analysis is a worthy goal that can provide scientific as well as practical benefits.

REFERENCES

Ajax, E. T. (1976). Dyslexia without agraphia. *Archives of Neurology* 17, 645–652.
Bakker, D. J. (1973). Hemispheric specialization and stages in the learning to read process. *Bulletin of the Orton Society* 23, 15–27.
Basso, A., Taborelli, A., & Vignolo, L. A. (1978). Dissociated disorders of speaking and writing in aphasia. *Journal of Neurology, Neurosurgery, and Psychiatry* 41, 556–563.
Baxter, D. M., & Warrington, E. K. (1986). Ideational agraphia: A single case study. *Journal of Neurology, Neurosurgery, and Psychiatry* 49, 369–374.
Beauvois, M. F., & Derouesne, J. (1981). Lexical or orthographic agraphia. *Brain* 104, 2–49.
Benson, D. F. (1979). *Aphasia, alexia, and agraphia.* New York: Churchill Livingstone.
Benson, F. (1985). Aphasia. In K. M. Heilman & E. Valenstein (Eds.), *Clinical neuropsychology: 2nd edition.* New York: Oxford University Press.
Boder, E. (1971). Developmental dyslexia: Prevailing diagnostic concepts and a new diagnostic approach. In H. Myklebust (Ed.), *Progress in learning disabilities.* New York: Grune & Stratton.
Boder, E. (1973). Developmental dyslexia: A diagnostic approach based on three atypical reading patterns. *Developmental Medicine and Child Neurology* 15, 663–687.
Boller, F., & Grafman, J. (1983). Acalculia: Historical development and current significance. *Brain and Cognition* 2, 205–223.
Bradley, L. (1983). The organization of visual, phonological, and motor strategies in learning to read and to spell. In U. Kirk (Ed.), *Neuropsychology of language, reading, and spelling.* New York: Academic Press.

Bradley, P. & Bryant, P. (1978). Difficulties in auditory organization as a possible cause of reading backwardness. *Nature* 271, 746–747.

Bradley, S., Schankeweiler, D., & Mann V. (1983). Speech perception and memory coding in relation to reading ability. *Journal of Experimental Child Psychology* 35, 345–367.

Bub, D., Cancelliere, A., & Kertesz, A. (1985). Whole-word and analytic translation of spelling to sound in a non-semantic reader. In K. E. Patterson, J. C. Marshall, & M. Coltheart (Eds.), *Surface dyslexia: Neuropsychological and cognitive studies of phonological reading.* Hillsdale, NJ: Lawrence Erlbaum.

Bub, D., & Kertesz, A. (1982). Deep agraphia. *Brain and Language* 17, 146–165.

Caramazza, A., Miceli, G., Villa, G., & Romani, C. (1987). The role of the graphemic buffer in spelling: Evidence from a case of acquired dysgraphia. *Cognition* 26, 59–85.

Chall, J. S. (1979). The great debate: Ten years later, with a modest proposal for reading stages. In L. B. Resnick & P. A. Weaver (Eds.), *Theory and practice of early reading.* Hillsdale, NJ: Lawrence Erlbaum.

Clark, L. W., & Grossfeld, M. L. (1983). Nature of spelling errors in transcortical sensory aphasia: A case study. *Brain and Language* 18, 47–56.

Coltheart, M. (1980). Deep dyslexia: A review of the syndrome. In M. Coltheart, K. Patterson, & J. C. Marshall (Eds.), *Deep dyslexia.* London: Routledge & Kegan Paul.

Coltheart, M. (1984). Acquired dyslexias and normal reading. In R. N. Malatesha & H. A. Whitaker (Eds.), *Dyslexia: A global issue.* The Hague: Martinus Nijhoff.

Coltheart, M., Masterson, S., Byng, S., Prior, M., & Riddoch, J. (1983). Surface dyslexia. *Quarterly Journal of Experimental Psychology* 35A, 469–495.

Coslett, H. B., Gonzalez-Rothi, L., & Heilman, K. M. (1985). Reading: dissociation of the lexical and phonologic mechanisms. *Brain and Language* 24, 20–35.

Coslett, H. B., Gonzalez-Rothi, L. J., Valenstein, E., & Heilman, K. M. (1986). Dissociations of writing and praxis: Two cases in point. *Brain and Language* 28, 357–368.

Critchley, M. (1970). *The dyslexic child.* Springfield, IL: Charles C Thomas.

Deloche, G., Andrewsky, E., & Desi, M. (1982) Surface dysgraphia: A case report and some theoretical implications to reading models. *Brain and Language* 15, 12–31.

Deloche, G., & Seron, X. (1984). Some linguistic components of acalculia. In F. C. Rose (Ed.), *Advances in neurology: Progress in aphasiology.* New York: Raven Press.

Denckla, M. B. (1972). Color-naming defects in dyslexic boys. *Cortex* 8(2), 164–176.

Denckla, M. B. (1972). Performance on color tasks in kindergarten children. *Cortex* 8(2), 177–190.

Denckla, M. (1979). Childhood learning disabilities. In K. M. Heilman & E. Valenstein, *Clinical neuropsychology: 1st edition.* New York: Oxford University Press.

Denckla, M. B., & Rudel, R. (1974). Rapid "automatized" naming of pictured objects, colors, letters and numbers by normal children. *Cortex* 10, 186–202.

Denckla, M. B., & Rudel, R. G. (1976a). Naming of object-drawings by dyslexic and other learning disabled children. *Brain and Language* 3, 1–15.

Denckla, M. B., & Rudel, R. G. (1976b). Rapid "automatized" naming (R.A.N.): Dyslexia differentiated from other learning disabilities. *Neuropsychologia* 16, 471–479.

Denckla, M. B., Rudel, R. G., & Broman, M. (1981). Tests that discriminate between dyslexia and other learning disabled boys. *Brain and Language* 13, 118–129.

Doehring, D. G., Trites, R. L., Patel, P. G., & Fiedorowicz, C. A. M. (1981). *Reading disabilities: The interaction of reading, language, and neuropsychological deficits.* New York: Academic Press.

Duffy, F. H., Burchfield, J. L., & Lombroso, C. T. (1979). Brain electrical activity mapping (BEAM): A method for extending the clinical utility of EEG and evoked potential data. *Annals of Neurology* 5, 309–321.

Duffy, F. H., Denckla, M. B., Bartels, P. H., & Sandini, G. (1980a). Dyslexia: Regional differences in brain electrical activity by topographic mapping. *Annals of Neurology* 7, 412–420.

Duffy, F. H., Denckla, M. D., Bartels, P. H., Sandini, G., & Kiessling, L. S. (1980b). Dyslexia: Automated diagnosis by computerized classification of brain electrical activity. *Annals of Neurology* 7, 421–428.

Eidelberg, D., & Galaburda, A. M. (1982). Symmetry and asymmetry in the human posterior thalamus—I: Cytoarchitectonic analysis in normal persons. *Archives of Neurology* 39, 325–332.

Ellis, A. W. (1982). Spelling and writing (and reading and speaking). In A. W. Ellis (Ed.), *Normality and pathology in cognitive functions*. London: Academic Press.

Ferro, J. M., & Bothelho, M. A. S. (1980). Alexia for arithmetical signs: A cause of disrupted calculation. *Cortex* 16, 175–180.

Fried, I., Tanguay, P. E., Boder, E., Doubleday, C., & Greensite, M. (1981). Developmental dyslexia: Electrophysiological evidence of clinical subgroups. *Brain and Language* 12, 14–22.

Friedman, R. B., & Albert, M. L. (1985). Alexia. In K. M. Heilman & E. Valenstein (Eds.), *Clinical neuropsychology: 2nd Edition*. New York: Oxford University Press.

Galaburda, A. M., & Eidelberg, D. (1982). Symmetry and asymmetry in the human posterior thalamus—II: Thalamic lesions in a case of developmental dyslexia. *Archives of Neurology* 39, 333–336.

Galaburda, A. M., & Kemper, T.L. (1979). Cytoarchitectonic abnormalities in developmental dyslexia: A case study. *Annals of Neurology* 6, 94–100.

Galaburda, A. M., LeMay, M., Kemper, T. L., & Geschwind, N. (1978). Right-left asymmetries in the brain: Structural differences between the hemispheres may underlie cerebral dominance. *Science* 199, 852–856.

Galaburda, A. M., Sanides, R., & Geschwind, N. (1978). Human brain: Cytoarchitectonic left-right asymmetries in the temporal speech region. *Archives of Neurology* 35, 812–817.

Galaburda, A. M., Sherman, G. F., Rosen, G. D., Aboitiz, F., & Geschwind, N. (1985). Developmental dyslexia: Four consecutive patients with cerebral anomalies. *Annals of Neurology* 18, 222–233.

Gerstmann, J. (1940). Syndrome of finger agnosia, disorientation for right and left, agraphia, and acalculia. *Archives of Neurology and Psychiatry* 44, 398–408.

Goldblum, M. C. (1985). Word comprehension in surface dyslexia. In K. E. Patterson, J. C. Marshall, & Coltheart M. (Eds.), *Surface dyslexia: Neuropsychological and cognitive studies of phonological reading*. Hillsdale, NJ: Lawrence Earlbaum.

Gonzalez-Rothi, L. J., Roeltgen, D. P., Kovistra, C. A. (1987). Isolated lexical agraphia in a right-handed patient with a posterior lesion of the right cerebral hemisphere. *Brain and Language* 30, 181–190.

Goodglass, H. (1981). Aphasia-related disorders. In M. T. Sarno (Ed.), *Aquired aphasia*. New York: Academic Press.

Gordon, H. W. (1980). Cognitive asymmetry in dyslexic families. *Neuropsychologia* 18, 645–656.

Grafman, J., Passafiume, D., Faglioni, P., & Boller, F. (1982). Calculation disturbances in adults with focal hemispheric damage. *Cortex* 18, 37–50.

Greenblatt, S. (1973). Alexia without agraphia or hemianopia: Anatomical analysis of an autopsied case. *Brain* 396, 307–316.

Greenblatt, S. (1976). Subangular alexia without agraphia or hemianopia. *Brain and Language* 3, 229–245.

Greenblatt, S. H. (1983). Localization of lesions in alexia. In A. Kertesz (Ed.), *Localization in neuropsychology*. New York: Academic Press.

Hatfield, F. M., & Patterson, K. E. (1984). Interpretation of spelling disorders in aphasia: Impact of recent developments in cognitive psychology. In F. C. Rose (Ed.), *Advances in neurology, Volume 42: Progress in aphasiology*. New York: Raven Press.

Heilman, K. M., & Gonzalez-Rothi, L. (1985). Apraxia. In K. M. Heilman and E. Valenstein (Eds.), *Clinical neuropsychology: 2nd edition*. New York: Oxford University Press.

Heilman K. M., Rothi L., Campanella D., & Wolfson S. (1979). Wernicke's and global aphasia without alexia. *Archives of Neurology* 36, 129–133.

Henderson, V. W. (1986). Anatomy of posterior pathways in reading: A reassessment. *Brain and Language* 29, 119–133.

Henderson, V. W., Alexander, M. P., & Naeser, M. A. (1982). Right thalamic injury impaired visuospatial perception, and alexia. *Neurology* 32, 235–240.

Henderson, V. W., Friedman, R. B., Teng, E. L., & Weiner, J. M. (1985). Left hemisphere pathways in reading: Inferences from pure alexia without hemianopia. *Neurology* 35, 962–967.

Horner, J., & Massey, E. W. (1986). Dynamic spelling alexia. *Journal of Neurology, Neurosurgery, and Psychiatry* 49, 455–457.

Hutchinson, B. B. (1983). Finger localization and reading ability groups of children ages three through twelve. *Brain and Language* 20, 143–154.

Hynd, G. W., & Cohen, M. (1983). *Dyslexia: Neuropsychological theory, research, and clinical differentiation.* New York: Grune & Stratton.

Hynd, G. W., Hynd, C. R., Sullivan, H. G., & Kingsbury, T. B. (1987). Regional cerebral blood flow (RCBF) in developmental dyslexia: Activation during reading in a surface and deep dyslexic. *Journal of Learning Disabilities* 20, 294–300.

Johnson, D. J. (1987). *Adults with learning disabilities: Clinical studies.* Orlando, Fl.: Grune & Stratton.

Kaplan, E., & Goodglass, H. (1981). Aphasia-related disorders. In M. T. Sarno (Ed.). *Acquired aphasia.* New York: Academic Press.

Kavale, K. A., & Forness, S. R. (1987). The far side of heterogeneity: A critical analyis of empirical subtyping research in learning disabilities. *Journal of Learning Disabilities* 20 (6), 374–382.

Kay, J., & Patterson, K. E. (1985). Routes to meaning in surface dyslexia. In K. E. Patterson, J. C. Marshall, & M. Coltheart (Eds.), *Surface dyslexia: Neuropsychological and cognitive studies of phonological reading.* Hillsdale, NJ: Lawrence Erlbaum.

Kertesz, A. (1984). Recovery from aphasia. In F. C. Rose (Ed.), *Advances in neurology, Volume 42: Progress in aphasiology.* New York: Raven Press.

Kinsbourne, M., & Warrington, E. K. (1962). A variety of reading disabilities associated with right hemisphere lesions. *Journal of Neurology, Neurosurgery, and Psychiatry* 25, 339–344.

Kirshner, H. S., & Webb, W. G. (1982). Alexia and agraphia in Wernicke's aphasia. *Journal of Neurology, Neurosurgery, and Psychiatry* 45, 719–724.

Laine, T., & Marttila, R. J. (1981). Note—Pure agraphia: A case study. *Neuropsychologia* 19, 311–316.

Leischner, A. (1983). Side differences in writing to dictation of aphasics with agraphia: A graphic disconnection syndrome. *Brain and Language* 18, 1–19.

Levin, H. S., & Spiers, P. A. (1985). Acalculia. In K. M. Heilman & E. Valenstein (Eds.), *Clinical neuropsychology: 2nd Edition.* New York: Oxford University Press.

Levine, D. N., Hier, D. V., & Calvanio, R. (1981). Acquired learning disability for reading after left temporal lobe damage in childhood. *Neurology* 31, 257–264.

Lezak, M. D. (1983). *Neuropsychological assessment: 2nd edition.* New York: Oxford University Press.

Lyon, G. R. (1985). Educational validation studies of learning disability subtypes. In B. P. Rourke (Ed.), *Neuropsychology of learning disabilities: Essentials of subtype analysis.* New York: Guilford Press.

Lyon, R., Rietta, S., Watson, B., Porch, B., & Rhodes J. (1981). Selected linguistic and perceptual abilities of empirically derived subgroups of learning disabled readers. *Journal of School Psychology* 19, 152–166.

Lyon, R., Stewart, N., & Freedman, D. (1982). Neuropsychological characteristics of empirically derived subgroups of learning disabled readers. *Journal of Clinical Neuropsychology* 4, 343–365.

Lyon, R., & Watson, B. (1981). Empirically derived subgroups of learning disabled readers: Diagnostic characteristics. *Journal of Learning Disabilities*, 14, 256–261.

Mann, V. A. (1986). Why some children encounter reading problems: The contribution of difficulties with language processing and phonological sophistication to early reading disability. In J. Torgeson & B. Wong (Eds.), *Psychological and educational perspectives on learning disabilities.* New York: Academic Press.

Margolin, D. J. (1984). The neuropsychology of writing and spelling: Semantic, phonological, motor, and perceptual processes. *The Quarterly Journal of Experimental Psychology* 36A, 459–489.

Margolin, D. J., & Binder, L. (1984). Multiple component agraphia in a patient with atypical cerebral dominance: An error analysis. *Brain and Language* 22, 26–40.

Margolin, D. J., & Wing, A. M. (1983). Agraphia and micrographia: Clinical manifestations of motor programming and performance disorders. *Acta Psychologia* 54, 263–283.

Marks, R. L., & De Vito, T. (1987). Alexia without agraphia and associated disorders: Importance of recognition in the rehabilitation setting. *Archives of Physical Medicine and Rehabilitation* 68, 1491–1495.

Marshall, J. C., & Newcombe, F. (1973). Patterns of paralexia: A psycholinguistic approach. *Journal of Psycholinguistic Research* 2, 175–199.

Marshall, J. C., & Newcombe, F. (1980). The conceptual status of deep dyslexia: An historical perspective. In M. Coltheart, K. Patterson, & J. Marshall (Eds.), *Deep dyslexia.* London:

Routledge & Kegan Paul.

Mattis, S. (1978). Dyslexia syndromes: A working hypothesis that works. In A. Benton & D. Pearl (Eds.), *Dyslexia: An appraisal of current knowledge*. New York: Oxford University Press.

Mattis, S., French, J. H., & Rapin, I. (1975). Dyslexia in children and young adults: Three independent neuropsychological syndromes. *Developmental Medicine and Child Neurology* 17, 150–163.

Mazzochi, F., & Vignolo, L. A. (1979). Localization of lesions in aphasia: Clinical-CT scan correlates in stroke patients. *Cortex* 15, 627–654.

McCloskey, M., Caramazza, A., & Basili A. (1985). Cognitive mechanisims in number processing and calculation: Evidence from dyscalculia. *Brain and Cognition* 4, 171–196.

Miceli, G., Caltagirone, C., Gainotti, G., Masullo, C., Silveri, M. C., & Villa, G. (1981). Influence of age, sex, literacy and pathologic lesion on incidence, severity and type of aphasia. *Acta-Neurologica-Scandinavia* 64, 370–382.

Momose, T., Yoshikawa, K., Bandish, M., Iwata, M., & Iio, M. (1986). MRI of callosal disconnection due to cerebral infarction. *Radiation Medicine* 4, 8–11.

Newcombe, F., & Marshall, J. C. (1985). Reading and writing by letter sounds. In K. E. Patterson, J. C. Marshall, & M. Coltheart (Eds.), *Surface dyslexia*. London: Erlbaum.

Newcombe, F., Marshall, J. C., Carrivick, P. J., & Hirons, R. W. (1974). Recovery curves in acquired dyslexia. *Journal of the Neurological Sciences* 24, 127–133.

Nicole, S., Nardi, P., & Fortuna, A. (1982). Alexia without agraphia: A case studied by means of computed axial tomography. *European Neurology* 21, 361–365.

Nolan, K. A., & Caramazza, A. (1982). Modality independent impairments in word processing in a deep dyslexic patient. *Brain and Language* 16, 237–264.

Nolan, K. A., & Caramazza, A. (1983). An analysis of writing in a case of deep dyslexia. *Brain and Language* 20, 305–328.

Patterson, K. E. (1985). From orthography to phonology: An attempt at an old interpretation. In K. E. Patterson, M. Coltheart, & J. C. Marshall (Eds.). *Surface dyslexia*. Hillsdale, NJ: Lawrence Earlbaum.

Patterson, K. E., Marshall, J. C., & Coltheart, M. (Eds.). (1985). *Surface dyslexia: Neuropsychological and cognitive studies of phonological reading*. Hillsdale, NJ: Lawrence Erlbaum.

Pontius, A. A. (1983). Finger misrepresentation and dyscalculia in an ecological context: Toward an ecological (cultural) evolutionary neuro-psychiatry. *Perceptual and Motor Skills* 57, 1191–1208.

Prior, M., & McCorriston, M. (1983). Acquired and developmental spelling dyslexia. *Brain and Language* 20, 263–285.

Prior, M., & McCorriston, M. (1985). Surface dyslexia: A regression effect? *Brain and Language* 25, 52–71.

Rapscak, S. Z., Gonzalez-Rothi, L. J., & Heilman K. M. (1987). Phonological alexia with optic and tactile anomia: A neuropsychological and anatomical study. *Brain and Language* 31, 109–121.

Rebert, C. S., Wexler, B. N., & Sproul, A. (1978). EEG asymmetry in educationnally handicapped children. *Electroencephalography and Clinical Neurophysiology* 45(4), 436–442.

Regard, M., Landis, T., & Hess, K. (1985). Preserved stenography reading in a patient with pure alexia: A model for dissociated reading processes. *Archives of Neurology* 42, 400–402.

Roeltgen, D. (1985). Agraphia. In K. M. Heilman & E. Valenstein (Eds.), *Clinical neuropsychology: 2nd edition*. New York: Oxford University Press.

Roeltgen, D. P. (1987). Loss of deep dyslexic reading ability from a second left-hemispheric lesion. *Archives of Neurology* 44, 346–348.

Roeltgen, D. P., Gonzalez-Rothi, L., & Heilman K. M. (1986). Linguistic semantic agraphia: A dissociation of lexical spelling system from semantics. *Brain and Language* 27, 257–280.

Roeltgen, D. P., & Heilman, K. M. (1983). Apractic agraphia in a patient with normal praxis. *Brain and Language* 18, 35–46.

Roeltgen, D. P., & Heilman, K. M. (1984). Lexical agraphia: Further support for the two-system hypothesis of linguistic agraphia. *Brain* 107, 811–827.

Roeltgen, D. P., Sevush, S., & Heilman, K. M. (1983). Phonological agraphia: Writing by the lexical-sematic route. *Neurology* 33, 755–765.

Roeltgen, D. P., Sevush, S., & Heilman, K. M. (1983). Pure Gerstmann's syndrome from a focal lesion. *Archives of Neurology* 40, 46–47.

Rosati, G., & DeBastiani, P. (1979). Pure agraphia: A discrete form of aphasia. *Journal of Neurology, Neurosurgery, and Psychiatry* 42, 266–269.

Rosati, G., DeBastiani, P., Aiello, I., & Agnetti, V. (1984). Alexia without agraphia: A study of a case of verbal alexia without accompanying colour-naming defect. *Journal of Neurology* 231, 20–25.

Rourke, B. P. (1981). Neuropsychological assessment of children with learning disabilities. In S. B. Filskov & T. J. Boll (Eds.), *Handbook of clinical neuropsychology*. New York: Wiley-Interscience.

Rourke, B. (1983). Reading and spelling disabilities: A developmental neuropsychological perspective. In U. Kirk (Ed.), *Neuropsychology of language, reading, and spelling*. New York: Academic Press.

Rudel, R. G. (1985). Hemispheric asymmetry and learning disability: Left-right or in-between. In C. T. Best (Ed.), *Hemispheric function and collaboration in the child*. New York: Academic Press.

Saffran, E. M. (1985). Lexicalization and reading performance in surface dyslexia. In K. E. Patterson, J. C. Marshall, & M. Coltheart (Eds.), *Surface dyslexia*. Hillsdale, NJ: Lawrence Earlbaum.

Sartori, G., Barry, C., & Job, R. (1984). Phonological dyselxia: A review. In R. N. Malatesha & H. A. Whitaker (Eds.), *Dyslexia: A global issue*. The Hague: Martinus Nijhoff.

Shallice, T. (1981). Phonological agraphia and the lexical route in writing. *Brain* 104, 413–429.

Siirtola, M., Narva, E. V., & Siirtola, T. (1977). On the occurrence and prognosis of aphasia in patients with cerebral infarction. *Scandinavian Journal of the Society of Medicine* (Supp) 14, 128–133.

Stark, R. E., & Tallal, P. (1979). Analysis of stop consonant production errors in developmentally dysphasic children. *Journal of the Acoustic Society of America* 66, 1703–1712.

Stark R., & Tallal, P. (1981). Selection of children with specific language deficits. *Journal of Speech and Hearing Disorders* 46, 114–122.

Strang, J. D., & Rourke, B. (1985). Arithmetic disability subtypes: The neuropsychological significance of specific arithmetic impairment in childhood. In B. P. Rourke (Ed.), *Neuropsychology of learning disabilities: Essentials of subtype analysis*. New York: Guilford.

Strub, R. L., & Geschwind, N. (1983). Localization in Gerstmann syndrome. In A. Kertesz (Ed.), *Localization in neuropsychology*. New York: Academic Press.

Tallal, P., & Stark, R. (1981). Acoustic analysis of speech discrimination abilities of normally developing and language impaired children. *Journal of the Acoustical Society of America* 69, 568–574.

Tallal, P., & Stark, R. (1983). Perceptual prerequisites for language development. In U. Kirk (Ed.), *Neuropsychology of language, reading and spelling*. New York: Academic Press.

Tandirag, O., & Kirshner, H. S. (1985). Aphasia and agraphia in lesions of the posterior internal capsule and putamen. *Neurology* 35, 1797–1801.

Velluntino, F. R. (1979). *Dyslexia: Theory and research*. Cambridge, MA: MIT Press.

Vignolo, L. A. (1983). *Modality-specific disorders of written language*. New York: Academic Press.

Vincent, C., Sandorsky, C. H., Saunders, R. L., & Reeves, A. G. (1977). Alexia without agraphia, hemianopia, or color naming defect: A disconnection syndrome. *Neurology* 27, 689–691.

Wagner, R. K. (1986). Phonological processing abilities and reading: Implications for disabled readers. *Journal of Learning Disabilities* 19, 623–630.

Wagner, W., & Gardner, H. (1979). A study of spelling in aphasia. *Brain and Language* 7, 363–374.

Wiegel-Crump, C. A., & Dennis, M. (1986). Development of word-finding. *Brain and Language* 27, 1–23.

Wolf, M., & Goodglass, H. (1986). Dyslexia, dysnomia and lexical retrieval: A longitudinal investigation. *Brain and Language* 28, 154–168.

4. COGNITION AND WATCHING TELEVISION

JOHN J. BURNS AND DANIEL R. ANDERSON

INTRODUCTION

Television viewing has been popularly hypothesized to shorten attention spans, increase frantic behavior, and cause brain damage. A review of the scientific literature reveals no support for these claims. In fact, contrary to popular conceptions, it appears that television viewing is a cognitively active behavior, sharing many characteristics of other leisure-time activities such as reading. Although there is some evidence of subtle cognitive effects, such findings require further study to verify the link and the direction of causality. In the same vein, though different patterns of EEG have been reported when comparing television viewing with other activities, these findings indicate only that television viewing differs in some respects from other activities. Like the research on cognitive effects, nothing in this research supports the commonly hypothesized devastating effects of television viewing.

Television causes brain damage. It also turns children into zombies, mesmerized by the medium. At the same time, it shortens attention spans and produces hyperactivity. Claims such as these have abounded since the introduction of television and are widely believed. In this chapter we will evaluate the evidence with respect to cognitive processes while watching television, what is known about the physiology of TV viewing, and the cognitive effects of TV viewing.

There has been no shortage of "experts" willing to make claims about the negative impact of TV viewing. In fact, a host of claims regarding the detrimental effects on cognitive processes have been made. Schorr (1983) and Moody (1980), for example, cited Edgar Gording to the effect that because television viewing reduces eye movements in young children, they do not get requisite eye movement practice and subsequently suffer retarded reading development. No evidence was offered in support of this claim.

In the same vein are claims made regarding the relationship between TV viewing and attentional development. Winn (1985), for example, accused "Sesame Street" (as well as other programs) of contributing to increased "frantic behavior" and inattentiveness observed in today's children. Winn argued that the magazine-style format and rapid pace of "Sesame Street" are to blame for this phenomenon. Swerdlow (1981) echoed these sentiments in considering the adverse effects of TV on classroom behavior. He noted that teachers increasingly complained about students' passivity, shortened attention spans, and lack of creativity. These characteristics, according to Swerdlow, were "attributable, at least in part, to TV viewing" (Swerdlow, 1981, p. 52). Finally, Halpern (1975) suggested that too much television viewing may result in clinically diagnosed hyperactivity in children.

Parallel claims have been made regarding the adverse physiological effects of TV viewing. In one of the most extreme, Emery and Emery (1974) contended that television viewing may result in cortical brain damage, especially in children. Only slightly less extreme is the claim of television-induced epilepsy (Moody, 1980).

Taken together, these claims, if warranted, paint a disturbing picture of the television viewing experience—especially with respect to children. A recent extensive review of the research literature, however, lends little support: Television viewing does not have the dire cognitive consequences that are so widely feared (Anderson & Collins, 1988). In the remainder of this chapter we will briefly summarize what is known about the cognitive processes and physiology of television viewing as well as the cognitive effects of TV viewing. We will conclude that there is at present little scientific basis for alarm concerning the influence of television per se.

TELEVISION VIEWING: FACTS AND MYTHS

To understand what can be definitively said about the cognitive effects of TV viewing, it is necessary to understand the general nature of the television viewing experience. In the sections that follow, we will first summarize the research describing TV viewing behavior and the cognitive processes involved. We will then turn to a consideration of research on cognitive and physiological effects in order to separate fact from myth.

Attention to Television

When using the term *attention*, most researchers refer to cognitive engagement and hence something that is not directly observable. A handful of studies have used visual fixation (location on screen toward which eyes are directed) as a measure of attention, but the most commonly used measure has been visual orientation toward the screen ("looking"). Listening, as well as intensity of attention, must be inferred from performance on recognition and recall tests, performance on secondary tasks, self-rating, and electrophysiological recordings.

Although popular belief contends that adult and child viewing is characterized by extended and high levels of visual attention, our research reveals that viewers typically look at and away from the TV screen between 100 and 200 times an hour (e.g., Anderson & Field, in press; Anderson & Smith, 1984). Moreover, examination of both looks at and looks away from the TV reveals that the vast majority are of relatively short duration (less than 5 seconds) and that viewers look at the TV only about two thirds of the time they are in the room (Anderson et al., 1986). Looks as long as 10 minutes do take place, but these are not representative of average look lengths for either children or adults. Moreover, viewers may be engaged in any number of concurrent activities such as play, housework, dressing, or eating while "watching" TV. Many of these activities can and do take place in front of the TV, but they can also necessitate leaving the room at different points. Indeed, television viewing is often part of passing through the room. Remarkably, viewers only spend an average of 7 to 10 minutes in the room before leaving (Anderson, 1987). These observations help to illustrate the surprisingly active nature of TV viewing, in both children and adults.

Determinants of attention to TV

A popular belief is that television captures and maintains attention by virtue of visual noncontent features such as movement and scene change. These features, however, have been found to have a relatively small influence on looking at TV (see Anderson & Lorch, 1983, for a review). Other factors are far more influential. Lorch, Anderson, and Levin (1979), for example, found that for children, availability of toys halved time spent looking at the TV. Anderson and colleagues (1981b) found that coviewing children have a large influence on one another's attention. These findings reflect the importance of the environment in which television viewing takes place.

Several studies found evidence of a strong relationship between comprehensibility of television content and attention. Anderson, Lorch, Field, and Sanders (1981a) noted that preschoolers' visual attention was higher during dialogue with immediate (here and now) referents than during dialogue with nonimmediate (displaced in time or space) referents. Anderson et al. (1981a) argued that dialogue with immediate referents is more comprehensible and that comprehensibility is essential for maintaining the attention of young children. In an experiment that supported this argument, Anderson et al. (1981a) found that visual attention was greater during normal segments of "Sesame Street" than for segments in which comprehensibility had been distorted by using backward speech or foreign language soundtracks.

With respect to listening, our research indicates that children are less likely to listen to television if they are not looking. Several studies (e.g., Field & Anderson, 1985; Lorch, Anderson, & Levin, 1979) found that auditory information was much less likely to be recalled if the child was not looking at the time the information was presented. Lorch et al. (1979) suggested, however, that listening guides looking at TV. They argued that children learn to monitor the audio for nonsemantic cues indicating important or interesting content. Children's voices, for example, are highly effective in eliciting looking because the content is likely "for kids" and thus comprehensible and interesting. Men's voices, on the other hand, are generally associated with content that is not interesting to young children and so serve to suppress looking. Not only have these effects been found in several studies (see Anderson & Lorch, 1983, for a review), but the effects are not found in children under 2.5 years of age, supporting the idea that deployment of attention to TV is a learned behavior. Children appear to develop an efficient strategy for monitoring both the audio and visual tracks of the television, thus enabling them to time-share TV viewing with other activities such as toy play.

Intensity of attention

Another commonly articulated belief about television viewing is that viewers enter an almost hypnotic state. This state is seen as essentially mindless, empty of cognition (Emery & Emery, 1976; Moody, 1980; Winn, 1985, 1987; Mander, 1978). The research on intensity of attention, however, offers evidence in sharp contrast to this popular view. This is not to say that viewers are exceptionally cognitively active during TV viewing. In fact, viewing is often chosen as a relaxing activity and usually rates as less demanding than other leisure activities (e.g., Csikszentmihalyi & Kubey, 1982).

Recall that looks at television tend to be quite brief, although some may be 10 minutes or more in length. In our research, we have noticed that the longer a look at the TV continues, the greater the probability is that it will be maintained (Anderson et al., 1979). This phenomenon, which we called attentional inertia, has been observed in both children and adults.

Anderson and Lorch (1983), in investigating attentional inertia, found that, for children, the longer a look is maintained prior to a content boundary, the longer it will be maintained after that content boundary. They concluded that attentional inertia drives looks across content boundaries. We have since replicated this finding with adults viewing prime-time TV. The longer a viewer maintains attention prior to a commercial, for example, the more likely he or she is to watch the commercial. Superficially, it might seem that the viewer is "mindlessly" watching TV. Anderson, Choi, and Lorch (1987), however, found that the longer a child maintained a look at TV, the less distractible he or she became. In addition, when distracted from long looks (looks greater than or equal to 15 seconds), head turns to a distractor were significantly slower than when distracted from short looks (looks less than 15 seconds). These findings are indicative of increased engagement with the TV and are supported by other work. In this research (Lorch & Castle, 1986), it was shown that children were slower to respond to a secondary reaction time task the longer they maintained attention to the TV.

Following up on this work, in our most recent research we discovered that for adults, recognition memory for material seen on TV was better if they had maintained visual attention for at least 15 seconds prior to viewing the material (Burns, 1988). Finally, we found that in many respects, free play with toys shows characteristics of attentional inertia during TV viewing (Choi, 1988).

Taken together, this research suggests that viewers increasingly become attentionally engaged with the medium over the time course of a look. This engagement reduces distractibility and increases information acquisition. Other research (e.g., Meadowcroft & Reeves, 1985) indicates that viewers appropriately become more engaged during material central for comprehension and less engaged during peripherally relevant content. Overall, intensity of attention to television appears unexceptional and likely shared many characteristics in common with other leisure time, more obviously cognitively active behaviors (e.g., toy play, reading).

Individual differences

While there is a marked similarity between the viewing behavior of children and adults, there are some differences across these as well as other groups. A number of different studies have found a great increase in looking at TV from infancy to 5 years of age. Anderson et al. (1986) verified this increase in observations of home viewing; they also reported that looking at TV leveled off at between 60 and 70% during the school-age years and declined somewhat in adulthood. Several studies (reviewed by Anderson and Collins, 1988) found significant correlations (about +.25) between looking at TV and IQ in children. More pronounced differences were reported by Grieve and Williamson (1977) when comparing viewing mentally retarded individuals to typical age cohorts. Grieve and Williamson found that mentally retarded individuals looked less at the TV than did the typical children. The two groups performed equally on visually presented comprehension test items, but the mentally retarded individuals' performance was worse than typical individuals on information presented audiovisually and on information presented on the audio track alone.

Examining one very important childhood pathology, Lorch and colleagues (1987) found that boys diagnosed with attention deficit disorder (ADD) performed somewhat less well than matched controls on comprehension tests following presentation of a television program. This reduction in comprehension was likely due to dramatically reduced visual attention by the ADD group. Although they looked at the TV as frequently as the controls, their looks averaged half the duration.

From the work already discussed, we can say that television viewing develops over time with exposure to the medium. Smith, Anderson, and Fischer (1985) showed that 4-year-olds engage in inferential activity appropriate to decoding cinematic montage. As they mature children become quite proficient at this activity, and by the time individuals reach later childhood television viewing is engaged in with ease, with comprehension approaching adult levels (Collins, 1982).

In contrast to popular characterizations of television viewing, American children and adults look at and away from the TV frequently. Listening, especially for children, is strongly related to looking. It is also clear that although viewers may choose to engage in television viewing as a relaxing pastime, it is not an exceptionally passive activity characterized by little or no cognitive activity. The "couch potato" characterization is amusing but receives little support from systematic research. As this brief review illustrates, many of the commonly articulated beliefs about the passive nature of television viewing are not supported by the research in this field. Attention to television involves a complex, active interplay between viewer interests and knowledge as well as the viewing environment and medium-specific variables. With this general description of television viewing as a backdrop, we can turn to an examination of cognitive and electrophysiological research on TV viewing.

TV and Brain Wave Activity

The existence of a relationship between electroencephalographic measurements and TV viewing was demonstrated as early as 1971. In one such study, Shagass et al. (1971) set out to determine if psychiatric patients could be differentiated from normal subjects based on examination of EEG recordings made while watching TV. Although this hypothesis was not supported, the researchers did find that alpha was suppressed during TV viewing.

While the bulk of research in the area of brain wave activity has correlated alpha with TV viewing, there has been some research using event-related potentials. Research in the area of event-related potentials generally indicates that the evoked potential demonstrates enhanced amplitude in response to attended stimuli and diminished amplitude to probe stimuli during distraction.

Using this procedure, Schafer (1978) inserted brief (33 millisecond) visual flicker probes in television programs of differing interest to subjects. Schafer found that evoked potentials were significantly reduced in response to the probes during programming of particular interest.

Using a different type of probe, Shagass et al. (1971) stimulated the median nerve at the wrist during TV viewing and did not find consistent evoked potential responses. In addition, while Shagass et al. (1971) did find that EEG amplitude was reduced during TV viewing, evoked response variations were not correlated with changes in EEG amplitude. Beyond this research, evoked potentials have not seen extensive application in the study of physiological correlates of attention to TV.

TV compared to other cognitive tasks

Early comparisons between EEG while watching TV and EEG while reading were based on the popular as well as academic belief that TV viewing is passive. Based on William James' conceptualization of dual attention systems (voluntary and involuntary attention), Krugman (1971) posited that whereas reading involved a series of successive efforts to attend (demanded voluntary attention), TV viewing involved little or no voluntary effort. Using an EEG measure from the occipital area, Krugman found a preponderance of slow waves (alpha, delta, and theta frequencies) whereas the corresponding characteristic response for EEG during reading involved little slow wave activity and considerable high-frequency or beta activity. He interpreted these findings as supporting the idea that the two media are processed differently, consistent with James' idea of two attentional systems.

Krugman's widely publicized findings were based on EEG recordings from one subject who was told to first look at several magazine ads, then to watch three commercials. The subject spent 15 minutes looking through the magazines before viewing the commercials, which were repeated several times. Though his findings are interesting, the use of a single subject limits their generalizability. In addition, Krugman concluded that it was not possible to determine which medium, print or television, better facilitated learning.

Attempting to expand on his conceptualization of television viewing as a passive activity, Krugman (1977) argued that motionless or focused eyes are typical of eye movement during television viewing whereas active or scanning eyes typify reading. Krugman further hypothesized that reading was primarily a left hemisphere dominant function since it involved gross eye movement and high involvement and that television viewing was primarily a right hemisphere function demanding focused attention and low involvement.

These hypotheses were expanded and examined in detail by Weinstein, Appel, and Weinstein (1980). The authors hypothesized that looking at magazine ads would generate more overall beta wave activity, as well as more left hemisphere beta wave activity, than would looking at television ads. They further hypothesized that advertising that generated more beta wave activity would also generate higher levels of brand recall. Based on data from 30 women, they found support for their hypothesis that magazine ads generated more beta wave activity, but support for their hypothesis that magazine ads would generate more left brain beta wave activity and greater brand recall was less impressive. Weinstein et al. nevertheless concluded that there were significant relationships in the direction they predicted.

While Weinstein and colleagues provide justification for acceptance of the hypothesis that magazine ads produce more beta, subsequent interpretations and manipulations of the data used in assessing their remaining hypotheses are open to question. For example, they based their conclusions on data from 18 of the original 30 subjects, those 18 subjects selected in order to maximize differences between conditions. In addition, the authors contended that since beta waves are indicative of increased attention, the magazine ads were more closely attended to than the television ads. It is also relevant to note that although there was some effort made to control for content differences in the two media by matching print ads with their corresponding TV ads, this manipulation does not eliminate the possibility that content differences accounted for their findings. A difference in task difficulty as a function of content may explain why subjects exhibited proportionately more beta wave activity when looking at magazine ads than when looking at TV ads.

The idea that television viewing may require less effortful processing than reading was directly examined by Featherman and colleagues (1979). They speculated that since the majority of people view TV to relax, this activity would involve a reduction in the frequency of saccades. They also hypothesized that, when compared with reading, television viewing would result in reduced levels of cortical activation in the occipital region. Decreased cortical activation was operationalized as increased alpha along with decreased beta and theta activity. In an effort to minimize the environmental differences between the two activities, Featherman et al. (1979) displayed reading material on a television screen.

Featherman et al. (1979) found a significant decrease in both theta and beta activity during television viewing when compared to reading. However, while television did produce a higher level of alpha than reading, this difference was not significant. With regard to saccades, these authors found that the frequency was somewhat reduced during television viewing when compared to reading. They pointed out, however, that these results may be confounded because content differences within TV viewing sessions and between media conditions were not controlled. These latter results are, in many respects, similar to those obtained by Krugman (1971) and Weinstein et al. (1980).

Walker (1980) had a group of university students engage in a variety of more or less demanding cognitive tasks, including resting with eyes closed, counting backwards, reading, and viewing television. Walker recorded EEG during these activities, giving special attention to levels of beta and alpha. His results indicated that reading and television viewing were associated with the highest levels of beta and the lowest levels of alpha. Comparisons between reading and television viewing revealed that although reading was characterized by slightly higher levels of beta and slightly lower levels of alpha, these differences were not statistically significant. The general pattern of results from these studies are slight, often nonsignificant, differences between the media.

In a similar vein, Radlick (1980) used EEG recordings in an attempt to determine if television viewing could be characterized as different in terms of processing demands when compared to reading and resting. To assess the possible effects of within-activity complexity, however, Radlick included four television stimuli varying in terms of content complexity as well as visual and auditory complexity. Radlick's results indicated that while reading produced more depth of processing, mental effort, and left hemisphere activation than the less complex television segments, the more complex television segments produced greater depth of processing, mental effort, and left hemisphere activation than reading. This result indicates that content complexity is the determining factor in the EEG studies comparing media. In most of the studies content was not controlled. Like Krugman (1971) and Weinstein et al. (1980), Radlick interpreted decreased alpha and increased beta as reflecting increased cognitive processing. Radlick also concluded that the rapid pace of visual or auditory television stimuli did not produce decreased attention or arousal.

The finding that television viewing and reading can differ in terms of characteristic patterns of brain wave activity is consistent throughout all of this work. Radlick's finding that, when content is systematically varied, these differences can be reversed suggests that these patterns are not medium specific. This is a key finding and illustrates a methodological shortcoming of much of the work previously discussed.

The patterns of brain wave activity may in fact support James's conceptualization of dual attentional systems. However, television may draw on an attentional system that is no less voluntary and active than the attentional system invoked when reading.

TV attributes, attention, and cognition
Like the research already discussed, initial research examining the relationship between EEG and learning and recall in the TV viewing context was based on the assumption that TV viewing was a low-involvement activity. Appel, Weinstein, and Weinstein (1979), for instance, hypothesized that TV viewing was a predominantly right brain activity but that recall of information presented on TV would show a strong relationship with left brain activity. Using 30-second commercials as stimuli, Appel and co-workers examined aggregate levels of alpha from 30 women to test their hypotheses. They found no support for their hypotheses that TV viewing was predominantly a right brain activity or that recall was positively correlated with left brain activity (as indicated by decreased levels of alpha). They did find that alpha was negatively correlated with immediate recall and concluded that EEG provided an indication of the possible effectiveness of TV commercials.

Mulholland (1968, 1974) argued that television becomes a conditioned stimulus for decreased brain activity. Examining EEG during TV viewing by children, Mulholland used alpha activity as feedback to the television: As long as subjects maintained lower levels of alpha, the television stayed on. The results indicated that the children had a great deal of difficulty keeping the TV on for any length of time, and Mulholland concluded that children learn to be inattentive when watching TV.

Mulholland's results are interesting, but his interpretation does not seem warranted. It may well have been the case that the children were devoting enough attention to comprehend the content. If so, their failure to keep the TV on represents nothing more than an inability to perform an unusual task in a highly atypical viewing situation. At most, Mulholland's research suggests only that TV viewing with unspecified content can differ in terms of alpha from other unspecified activities.

Perhaps the most sophisticated use of EEG in the field of television research has been in the study of moment-to-moment attention to television. A group at the University of Wisconsin at Madison have attempted to provide a detailed analysis of the relationship between ongoing cognitive processing and stimulus properties of TV. Based on the well-established fact that alpha has proven to be a reliable indicator of attention, this group has sought to more carefully examine the relationship between cognition and properties of the concurrent television message.

Using commercials as stimuli, Rothschild, Thorson, Reeves, Hirsch, and Goldstein (1986a) replicated earlier research that demonstrated a significant inverse relationship between alpha and subsequent paper-and-pencil measures of learning and recall. In simple terms, those commercials that resulted in high levels of learning were associated with lower alpha. Rothschild and colleagues found evidence of this relationship only when examining aggregate data, although it held for 30-minute as well as 2-week delay conditions.

Citing research on event-related potentials that indicates a maximum response about 300 milliseconds after the onset of the stimulus, Rothschild et al. (1986b) decided to examine the relationship between "epochs" of alpha and concurrent commercial activity. An epoch was defined as a period of commercial time that began with a sharp drop in alpha (indicating an increase in attention to the TV) and ended with the next sharp drop in alpha. Carrying out this analysis at the aggregate level, Rothschild et al. (1986b) identified 57 such epochs across 9 commercials. They found that 69% of all epochs started within half a second of an easily identifiable visual cue in the stimulus commercial.

Predicated on these findings, Rothschild et al. offer two intriguing conceptualizations of the relationship between attention and stimulus attributes. They first suggest that the initiation of an epoch represents an involuntary response of the attentional system to some change in the visual field (dominated by the commercial stimulus). They then suggest that the length of the epoch, or the length of time alpha is suppressed, represents the length of time in which effortful attention is brought to bear on the stimulus.

The work of Rothschild et al. (1986b) suggests the presence of an attentional system that responds to stimuli at two (at least) different levels. Such a system bears some resemblance to James's early conceptualization in that it involves involuntary attention as well as voluntary attention. Research by the same group has examined, in more detail, aspects of the television stimulus that invoke involuntary attention.

Working with the same data set as Rothschild et al. (1986b), Reeves et al. (1985) examined the relationship between alpha and two types of visual change:

scene changes (edits) and movement (e.g., a hand moving or a product rolling across the screen). Reeves et al. cited an extensive literature in visual perception that argues that perception of visual movement occurs innately. Based on this, they hypothesized that movement remains an important determinant of attention when translated to the TV screen.

To test this hypothesis, Reeves and co-workers (1985) correlated alpha with concurrent edits and movement and found that these features of the stimulus predicted significant variation in alpha. This finding extends the Rothschild et al. conceptualization that certain properties of the stimulus invoke involuntary attention, and Reeves et al. (1985) concluded that attention to TV, not surprisingly, shares a processing mechanism with attention to nontelevision stimuli.

TV Viewing and Cognitive Effects

We have already noted the many popular beliefs about the negative cognitive effects of TV viewing. These beliefs have focused on children as especially vulnerable. A commonly invoked mechanism is the displacement of "more important" activities such as reading or homework by TV viewing. Anderson and Collins (1988) argued that the displacement hypothesis cannot be accepted until it is demonstrated that displacement actually takes place and that the displaced activity is more valuable than TV viewing.

Research on displacement is difficult to conduct for two reasons. First and perhaps more obvious is that, given the degree to which television has penetrated our society, it is difficult to carry out controlled comparisons. Second, correlational studies in which time spent with television is compared with time spent with other activities are difficult to interpret. For example, if viewers spend 4 hours an evening viewing television, it does not necessarily follow that if their viewing is decreased by 2 hours, they will engage in other more cognitively important activities.

With respect to research examining behavior before and after the arrival of TV, in their review Anderson and Collins (1988) reported that TV primarily replaced consumption of other entertainment media (especially radio and comic books). Attendance at outdoor activities also declined. They concluded that the research did not offer clear-cut support for the displacement hypothesis, insofar as the displaced activities have not been shown to be more cognitively valuable than TV viewing.

Although somewhat less obvious, another possible effect of television viewing is its impact on a viewer's knowledge base. With children as well as adults spending anywhere from 10 to 25 hours per week watching TV (depending on the sample and the measuring procedure), it is clear that they are being exposed to a tremendous amount of information. The question is what are the effects of this exposure on knowledge? Here again, the bulk of the research on this issue involves children. Although there is generally a negative correlation between exposure to TV and vocabulary (Morgan & Gross, 1982), before and after studies (studies of the initial arrival of television) reveal increases in vocabulary or else no effect. The evidence is that brighter children simply choose to watch less TV (e.g., Williams, 1986), clearly confounding causal interpretations.

Perhaps the most common criticism of TV with respect to children is that it shortens attention span and produces heightened activity levels. Unfortunately, only a small number of studies have examined these claims, and close inspection reveals serious methodological problems in some studies and mixed findings in others.

Typical of the flawed work is a study reported by Halpern (1975). Halpern described 2-year-olds referred to a mental health center for problems with hyperactivity. Citing evidence of compulsive repetition of numbers and letters as well as behavior akin to "wound-up robots" (p. 68), Halpern suggested that this behavior was "directly traceable" to "Sesame Street." He argued that the rapid pacing and repetition of "Sesame Street" led to the behaviors he observed. Halpern provided no details on numbers of children involved nor did he indicate whether nonhyperactive 2-year-olds also recited numbers and letters from "Sesame Street." In addition to these shortcomings Halpern himself pointed out that he could not later replicate these observations. Despite these flaws and the study's clear lack of scientific value, this paper is consistently cited in popular books and magazine articles.

Substantive research examining the relationship between TV viewing and perseverance has relied on both correlational and experimental designs. Using a correlational approach, Anderson, Levin, and Lorch (1977) found no relationship among 5-year-olds between total amount of TV viewing (reported by parents) and tests of perseverance and impulsivity. In contrast, Anderson and McGuire (1978) reported a small positive correlation between TV viewing and impulsivity in Canadian third and fourth graders. However, the problem of establishing a causal direction was not addressed, and once again it is not clear whether TV viewing causes impulsivity or whether children with higher levels of impulsivity simply watch more TV.

Experimental studies have shown the same sort of mixed findings. Salomon (1979), for example, had one group of second graders watch "Sesame Street" over 8 days while a control group watched adventure and nature films for the same period. Subsequent testing revealed that the children who had watched "Sesame Street" performed better on some tests of attention and perception but also showed less perseverance on a tedious task than the comparison children. These findings are difficult to interpret however, as it is unclear whether "Sesame Street" or the adventure and nature films or both produced the group differences.

In contrast, Gadberry (1980) found that 6-year-olds who were restricted over a 6-week period to lower levels of commercial TV were less impulsive than a control group whose viewing was not restricted. The restricted group primarily watched educational programs such as "Sesame Street" and "Mister Rogers' Neighborhood," while the unrestricted group tended to watch action-oriented shows. The difference in viewing diet may have produced the difference in impulsivity as much as reduction in viewing per se.

It is difficult to determine cause and effect relationships, but the research is suggestive of a relationship between TV viewing and impulsivity as well as perseverance. When the full pattern of results is considered, it appears that viewing educational TV programs (e.g., "Sesame Street," "Mister Rogers' Neighborhood") is associated with enhanced attentional skills and that viewing violent action and adventure programming is associated with increased impulsiveness and reduced perseverance (see Anderson & Collins, 1988, for a detailed review).

CONCLUSIONS AND FUTURE DIRECTIONS

As this chapter demonstrates, television viewing does not appear to be the destructive force suggested by writers in the popular press. It does not mesmerize viewers by the use of hypnotic formal features, nor does it apparently lead to brain damage (there are no such reports in the scientific literature). In fact, scientific research indicates that TV viewing likely shares many characteristics of other leisure-time activities such as reading. Attentional patterns during toy play, for example, have aspects in common with TV viewing. Although most TV viewing may not be as cognitively demanding as most reading, TV viewing certainly demands active cognitive processing. Differences from reading may be due more to typical content than form. We are not suggesting that TV viewing does not merit further study, but rather than it should not be seen as something in a totally different class from any other leisure activity.

For many, the most surprising finding regarding typical TV viewing is the fact that it takes place in such a busy environment. Viewers come and go, and while in the room with the TV they may be engaged in any number of concurrent activities. These findings serve to remind us of the importance of considering ecological validity when evaluating investigations of TV viewing.

The study of physiological correlates of TV viewing is still in its infancy, yet several important advances have been made. Like the cognitive effects research, EEG investigation has helped to dispel some commonly held conceptions of television viewing. Despite the evidence of different patterns of EEG when comparing television viewing to other cognitive activities such as reading, this difference does not necessarily mean television is cognitively less demanding than reading. The fact that only one study effectively varied content differences across media points to a major deficit in much of the research comparing TV viewing to other activities. In fact, the most important finding may simply be that different kinds of content have different cognitive demands. Although a review of the scientific research reveals lack of support for hypothesized devastating cognitive effects of TV viewing, there may well be more subtle effects. For example, there does appear to be a relationship between viewing of action adventure programming and impulsivity as well as perseverance. As we have indicated, however, the nature of this relationship has not been thoroughly explored, and as such this is one area deserving of additional study.

There has not been any research suggesting that TV causes brain damage. In fact, it is unlikely that TV causes anything quite so dramatic. While there are possible cognitive effects of TV viewing, it is likely that these are mediated by a variety of factors other than TV viewing itself. In any event, detailed explanation of these effects awaits future research. Perhaps the most newsworthy finding in all this research is that TV viewing is not unlike other leisure-time activities both in terms of cognitive demands and cognitive processes involved. Although the mode of presentation is strikingly different when compared to reading, for example, it appears that TV viewing is similar in many other respects. The most important influences of television are probably not cognitive per se but instead depend on the content viewed. Educational content appears to educate in the manner intended (Bryant, Alexander, & Brown, 1983), and entertainment content may educate in unintended manners. Such unintended effects may include increasing aggressive behavior and influencing constructs of social reality (Pearl, Bouthilet, and Lazar, 1982). The effects appear to be more a property of the message than the medium.

NOTE

This chapter was supported in part by a research grant from the National Institute of Health.

REFERENCES

Anderson, D. (1987). *Analysis of lengths of TV viewing sessions.* Paper presented at the annual meeting of the Association for Consumer Research, Boston.

Anderson, D., Alwitt, L., Lorch, E. & Levin, S. (1979). Watching children watch television. In G. Hale & M. Lewis (Eds.), *Attention and cognitive development* (pp. 331–361). New York: Plenum Press.

Anderson, D., Choi, H., & Lorch, E. (1987). Attentional inertia reduces distractibility during young children's television viewing. *Child Development* 58, 798–806.

Anderson, D., & Collins, P. (1988). *The impact on children's education: Television's influence on cognitive development.* Washington D.C.: U.S. Department of Education.

Anderson, D., & Field, D. (In press). Online and offline assessment of the television audience. In J. Bryant & D. Zillmann (Eds.), *Responding to the screen: Reception and reaction processes.* Hillsdale, NJ: Earlbaum.

Anderson, D., Levin, S., & Lorch, E. (1977). The effects of TV program pacing on the behavior of preschool children. *AV Communication Review* 25, 159–166.

Anderson, D., & Lorch, E. (1983). Looking at television: Action or reaction?. In J. Bryant & D. Anderson (Eds.), *Children's understanding of television: Research on attention and comprehension* (pp. 1–34). New York: Academic Press.

Anderson, D., Lorch, E., Field, D., Collins, P., & Nathan, J. (1986). Television viewing at home: Age trends in visual attention and time with television. *Child Development* 57, 1024–1033.

Anderson, D., Lorch, E., Field, D., & Sanders, J. (1981a). The effects of TV program comprehensibility on preschool children's visual attention to television. *Child Development* 52, 151–157.

Anderson, D., Lorch, E., Smith, R., Bradford, R., & Levin, S. (1981b). Effects of peer presence on preschool children's television viewing behavior. *Developmental Psychology* 17, 446–453.

Anderson, D., & McGuire, T. (1978). The effect of TV viewing on the educational performance of elementary school children. *The Alberta Journal of Educational Research* 24, 156–163.

Anderson, D., & Smith, R. (1984). Young children's TV viewing: The problem of cognitive continuity. In F. Morrison, C. Lord, & D. Keating (Eds.), *Advances in applied developmental psychology* (Vol. 1, pp. 115–163). New York: Academic Press.

Appel, V., Weinstein, S., & Weinstein, C. (1979). Brain activity and recall of TV. *Journal of Advertising Research* 19, 7–15.

Bryant, J., Alexander, A., & Brown, D. (1983). Learning from educational television programs. In M. J. Howe (Ed), *Learning from television: Psychological and educational research* (pp. 1–30). London: Academic Press.

Burns, J. (1988). *The relationship between attentional inertia and recognition memory*. Unpublished Masters Thesis, University of Massachusetts, Amherst.

Choi, H. (1988). *Attentional patterns in five year olds' toy play: Test of attentional inertia in toy play*. Unpublished Doctoral Dissertation, University of Massachusetts, Amherst.

Collins, W. (1982). Cognitive processing aspects of television viewing. In D. Pearl & L. Bouthilet (Eds.), *Television and behavior: Ten years of scientific progress and implications for the eighties* (Vol. 2, pp. 9–23). Rockville, MD: National Institute of Mental Health.

Csikszentmihalyi, M., & Kubey, R. (1982). Television and the rest of life: A systematic comparison of subjective experience. In D. Whitney & E. Wartella (Eds.), *Mass communication review yearbook* (Vol. 3, pp. 317–328). Beverly Hills, CA: Sage.

Emery, F., & Emery, M. (1974). *A choice of futures: To enlighten or inform*. Canberra, Australia: Australian National University.

Emery, F., & Emery, M. (1976). *A choice of futures*. Leiden: Martinus Nijhoff Social Sciences Division.

Featherman, G., Frieser, D., Greenspun, D., Harris, B., Schulman, D., & Crown, P. (1979). *Electroencephalographic and electrooculographic correlates of television viewing*. Final Technical Report: National Science Foundation Student-Oriented Studies (Grant No. SPI78–03698). Hampshire College: Amherst, MA.

Field, D., & Anderson, D. (1985). Instruction and modality effects on children's television attention and comprehension. *Journal of Educational Psychology* 77, 91–100.

Gadberry, S. (1980). Effects of restricting first graders' TV viewing on leisure time use, IQ change, and cognitive style. *Journal of Applied Developmental Psychology* 1, 45–47.

Grieve, R., & Williamson, K. (1977). Aspects of auditory and visual attention to narrative material in normal and mentally handicapped children. *Journal of Child Psychology and Psychiatry* 18, 251–262.

Halpern, W. (1975). Turned-on toddlers. *Journal of Communication* 25, 66–70.

James, W. (1890). *The principles of psychology*. New York: Holt.

Krugman, H. (1971). Brain wave measures of media involvement. *Journal of Advertising Research* 11, 3–9.

Krugman, H. (1977). Memory without recall, exposure without perception. *Journal of Advertising Research* 17, 7–12.

Lorch, E., Anderson, D., & Levin, S. (1979). The relationship of visual attention to children's comprehension of television. *Child Development* 50, 722–727.

Lorch, E., & Castle, V. (1986). *Preschool children's attention to television: Visual attention and probe response times*. Unpublished manuscript, University of Kentucky, Lexington.

Lorch, E., Milich, R., Welsh, R., Yocum, M., Bluhm, C., & Klein, M. (1987). *A comparison of the television viewing and comprehension of attention deficit disorders and normal boys*. Paper presented at the meeting of the Society for Research in Child Development, Baltimore, MD.

Mander, J. (1978). *Four arguments for the elimination of television*. New York: William Morrow.

Meadowcroft, J., & Reeves, B. (1985). *The development of schema-based strategies for attending to television stories*. Paper presented at the Speech Communication Association Convention, Denver.

Moody, K. (1980). *Growing up on television: The TV effect*. New York: Times Books.

Morgan, M., & Gross, L. (1982). Television and educational achievement and aspiration. In D. Pearl, L. Bouthilet, & J. Lazar (Eds.), *Television and behavior* (Vol. 2): Technical reviews (pp. 78–90). Washington D.C.: Department of Health and Human Services.

Mulholland, T. (1968). Feedback electroencephalography. *Activitas Nervosa Superior* (Prague), 10, 410–438.

Mulholland, T. (1974). Training visual attention. *Academic Therapy* 10, 5–17.

Pearl, D., Bouthilet, L., & Lazar, J. (1982). *Television and behavior: Ten years of scientific progress and implications for the eighties.* Washington D.C.: Department of Health and Human Services.

Radlick, M.S. (1980). *The processing demands of television: Neurophysiological correlates of television viewing.* Unpublished doctoral dissertation, Rensselaer Polytechnic Institute, Troy, NY.

Reeves, B., Thorson, E., Rothschild, M., McDonald, D., Hirsch, J., & Goldstein, M. (1985). Attention to television: Intrastimulus effects of movement and scene change on alpha variations over time. *International Journal of Neuroscience* 27, 241–255.

Rothschild, M., Thorson, E., Reeves, B., Hirsch, J., & Goldstein, R. (1986a). EEG activity and the processing of television commercials. Communication and scene change on alpha variations over time. *International Journal of Neuroscience* 27, 241–255.

Rothschild, M., Thorson, E., Reeves, B., Hirsch, J., & Goldstein, R. (1986b). EEG activity and the processing of television commercials. *Communication Research* 13, 182–220.

Salomon, G. (1979). *Interaction of media, cognition and learning.* San Francisco: Jossey-Bass.

Schafer, E. (1978). Brain responses while viewing television reflect program interest. *International Journal of Neuroscience* 8, 71–77.

Schorr, L. (1983). Environmental deterrents: Poverty, affluence, violence and television. In M. Levine, W. Carey, A. Crocker, & R. Gross (Eds.), *Developmental-behavioral pediatrics* (pp. 293–312). Boston: W. B. Saunders.

Shagass, C., Overton, D., Bartolucci, G., & Straumanis, J. (1971). Effect of attention modification by television viewing on somatosensory evoked responses and recovery functions. *Journal of Nervous and Mental Disease* 152, 53–62.

Smith, R., Anderson, D., & Fischer, C. (1985). Young children's comprehension of montage. *Child Development* 56, 962–971.

Swerdlow, J. (1981). What is television doing to real people?. *Today's Education* 70, 50–57.

Walker, J. (1980). Changes in EEG rhythms during television viewing: Preliminary comparisons with reading and other tasks. *Perceptual and Motor Skills* 51, 255–261.

Williams, T. (1986). *The impact of television: A natural experiment in three communities.* Orlando: Academic Press.

Winn, M. (1985). *The plug-in-drug.* New York: Viking Press.

Winn, M. (1987). *Unplugging the plug-in-drug.* New York: Viking Press.

5. EPILEPSY IN CHILDREN AND ADULTS

RICHARD C. DELANEY AND MARY L. PREVEY

INTRODUCTION

Epilepsy has been a focus of interest, research, and speculation for clinicians of many disciplines, perhaps more so than any other medical disorder. Features of seizure disorders and our lack of understanding of their mechanisms have led to numerous misperceptions and myths but have also provided the impetus for investigations in an area that has been alluded to as the border between neurophysiology and behavior (e.g., Gowers, 1881). The purpose of this chapter is to review the neuropsychology of seizure disorders and to consider the impact of epilepsy on daily living. Developmental factors are discussed where possible because, although an individual of any age may have seizures, different issues present themselves depending on the age of the patient. The presentation is divided into four sections reviewing neurological, neurobehavioral, psychiatric, and psychosocial aspects of epilepsy. Neuropsychology has been most concerned with understanding brain–behavior relationships associated with seizure disorders and how epilepsy is related to other more general problems in living and adjustment. In this presentation, neurological and psychiatric considerations will be somewhat deemphasized. Although it is not possible in a single chapter to provide an exhaustive review of all the relevant research, our goal is to provide an overview that does justice to the main issues of this area. In areas provided less coverage, we hope to direct the reader to appropriate sources.

EPILEPSY AND NEUROLOGICAL FACTORS

Definition, Description, and Treatment

Epilepsy is a term used to refer to a number of disorders of the central nervous system that cause recurrent seizures. Seizures involve the sudden, occasional, excessive, and disorderly discharge of grey matter. This characterization owes much to Jackson (1870, cited in Taylor, 1958), from whom the modern age of study and understanding of the epilepsies derives. The prevalence of epilepsy has been variously estimated to be between about .5% (Hauser & Kurland, 1975) and 2% (Epilepsy Foundation of America, 1975), though some research has suggested that these figures underestimate prevalence due to the failure of many cases to come to medical attention (Zielinski, 1986). Thus epilepsy is a disorder that affects a significant proportion of the population. Neither a unitary phenomena nor a specific disease is implied by the general definition of epilepsy, and several classification schema have been proposed for both the epilepsies (each as a broadly described syndrome) and epileptic seizures. An outline of the International Classification (revised, Dreifuss, 1981) is presented in table 5–1. Working from that framework, a brief description of seizure manifestations and their treatments can be provided.

Partial seizures may be defined as seizures involving a limited portion of the cerebrum. They can be subdivided into simple (elementary) partial or complex partial, the latter referring to the occurrence of an associated alteration in consciousness. Simple partial seizures reflect the involvement of a very delimited region of one cerebral hemisphere, for example, with only sensory or motor symptoms. In such cases sensation, such as localized tingling or flashing lights, or a specific movement—for example, involving the eyes, posture, or the rhythmic contraction/relaxation of muscle groups—may represent the seizure and be associated with localized spiking or sharp discharges on the EEG. There are also instances of simple partial seizures involving phonation, olfactory, or gustatory sensation, aphasia, amnesia, cognition, emotion, or dizziness as specific expressions, though conscious awareness is

Table 5–1. An abbreviated classification of seizures

Partial seizures
  Simple partial (motor, sensory, autonomic, or psychic)
  Complex partial (with or without automatisms)
  Simple or complex partial that generalize to tonic–clonic

Generalized seizures
  Absence (petit mal)
  Myoclonic
  Clonic
  Tonic
  Tonic–Clonic (grand mal)
  Atonic

Unclassified

---

unaffected. Partial complex seizures, on the other hand, more typically involve larger regions of the brain, particularly temporal lobe or deep frontal lobe regions that have limbic structure involvement, and they are more frequently bilateral in expression when documented by the EEG. There is an impairment in consciousness and the seizure can include behavioral automatisms and psychic symptoms, hence the older, descriptive term of a psychomotor seizure. The partial complex seizure may be preceded by a simple partial component, sometimes referred to as the aura.

Generalized seizures are those with widespread involvement of both cerebral hemispheres either initially, as in primary generalized epilepsy, or quickly following a more focal (or partial) manifestation, as in secondary generalized epilepsy. A generalized seizure may be convulsive—e.g., the tonic-clonic seizures often referred to as grand mal—or nonconvulsive—e.g., the absence seizures that are frequently labeled petit mal. There is nearly always an impairment or loss of consciousness with generalized seizures. A tonic-clonic (grand mal) seizure consists of an initial increase in muscle tone with posturing, forcible emission of air and subsequent apnea, and frequently incontinence (tonic phase, typically 10–15 seconds), followed by the bilateral and symmetrical jerking of the extremities, pronounced salivation and sweating, and grimacing (clonic phase, typically 1–2 minutes). In a generalized tonic, clonic, or tonic-clonic seizure the effects on consciousness are obvious and there are often postictal features as well (grogginess or confusion). In contrast, absence seizures may be very brief and include no pre- or postictal symptoms, which contributes to their being overlooked initially in schoolchildren. Characteristic EEG patterns are usually obtained with the several varieties of convulsive and nonconvulsive seizure.

A further dichotomy of the epilepsies is that they may be "symptomatic"—that is, related to a specific etiology (tumor, trauma, abscess, infection, etc.)—or "idiopathic" (where there is no other known cause). The presence of identifiable brain damage associated with seizures has been a relevant parameter in studies involving neuropsychological findings, as will be discussed later. Primary generalized epilepsy, especially that expressed by absence seizures, has been considered to have a significant genetic component. However, the concept of a seizure threshold, varying among individuals and involving a complex, multifactor genetic basis, could apply to the expression of many types of seizure disorders.

In the treatment of symptomatic epilepsy there may be a need to attack an underlying cause in addition to pharmacologic therapy, the first line treatment of the seizures themselves. There are several major classes of anticonvulsant medications with differential efficacy depending upon seizure type. They include phenytoin, phenobarbitol, and carbamazepine for tonic-clonic, partial complex, and simple partial seizures; for absence seizures ethosuximide and benzodiazepines are frequently employed. Valproic acid is the most important recently approved medication, and it appear to have wide applicability, particularly for absence seizures, primary generalized tonic-clonic seizures, and myoclonic seizures. These and other anticonvulsants can provide good to excellent seizure control in the vast majority of epileptic patients. However, to varying degrees there may be a cost to the patient in terms of side effects, frequently including interference with cognitive and functional abilities. In situations where anticonvulsants are ineffective, and a well-defined region of epileptogenic activity can be accessed without serious neurologic consequence, the patient may be considered for surgical therapy such as temporal lobectomy. Again, possible cost to the patient in terms of changes in pattern of neuro-behavioral abilities must be weighed against the benefit of effective seizure control. The possible effects of treatment on behavior will be addressed in a subsequent section.

Finally, it is noted that age is an important variable in terms of the types and incidences of the epilepsies. For example, there is an overall high incidence in the first year of life that drops off until around age 30–40, with a subsequent rise after 50. Absence seizures most typically begin between the ages of 5 and 10 and often cease spontaneously when the individuals reach their teens or 20s. This has been a very simplified overview of seizure expressions and medical treatments; the interested reader is encouraged to consult additional sources, such as Browne and Feldman (1983) or Adams and Victor (1985) for an excellent description of the various types, etiologies, treatments, and prognoses for the epilepsies.

Environmental and Psychological Aspects of Seizures and Their Treatment

Seizures can obviously have an impact on an individual's opportunities in life, and the far-ranging psychosocial consequences of epilepsy will be discussed further in a later section. However, there are also certain factors in daily living that can impact on the expression of seizures themselves. Topics considered under this heading include (1) reflex epilepsy, (2) the relationship of drug and psychological factors to seizures, and (3) behavioral interventions as treatments.

Reflex epilepsy

Seizures frequently occur in patients without warning or obvious trigger, but in some cases (perhaps 5% of seizure patients; Servit et al., 1963) a specific environmental or behavioral stimulus can induce seizures in a reliable fashion. For example, photic stimulation at 15 to 20 flashes per second has been used as a diagnostic procedure to induce EEG abnormalities or seizures (Newmark & Penry, 1979). Other visual triggers that have been described include observation of patterns or colors and watching television (Bickford & Klass, 1962). Seizures have been associated in some individuals with listening to music, sometimes of a relatively specific type (Joynt et al., 1962) and specific somato-sensory stimulation. In addition, seizures in certain individuals have been reported to result from a variety of complex activities including toothbrushing

(Holmes et al., 1982), dressing (Cirignotta et al., 1982), or eating (Forster, 1971) or from aspects of communication such as reading or writing (Daly & Forster, 1975). Forster (1977) provided an excellent review of this topic. Reflex epilepsy can affect an individual's everyday life and influence how a person might choose to spend time, though interestingly there are reports of purposeful self-induction of seizures. The existence of specifiable stimulus triggers for certain seizure patients has also been useful in research toward understanding epilepsy. In addition, since the seizure trigger may not be under the ready control of the patient and may be both unpredictable and unavoidable in daily living, behavioral interventions have been employed, as described later.

Drug and psychological factors
Other facets of everyday life may also have special significance for individuals with epilepsy. For example, several drugs have known interaction with epileptic seizures, including alcohol (Mattson, 1983; Chan, 1985), several medications and antibiotics, and possibly oral contraceptives (Kutt, 1984). Seizure frequency may increase during periods of high estrogen in menarche and decrease when progesterone dominates (Mattson & Cramer, 1985).

   Some patients have seizures only out of sleep, though sleep deprivation has been shown to be related to increased seizure frequency and expression of EEG abnormalities (Mattson, Pratt, & Claverly, 1975). Other aspects of stressful experience, including emotional state (Glass & Mattson, 1973) and life events, both major and minor (Temkin & Davis, 1984), have been linked to an increase in seizures. The mechanisms by which stress can contribute to seizures are poorly understood, but many stressful aspects of life may be involved in a cyclic interaction with the expression of seizures, with each factor influencing the other in a manner detrimental to the patient.

Behavioral interventions as treatment
Because certain environmental or behavioral stimuli can evoke seizures in some patients and there is a relationship between seizures and the experience of stress, psychological/behavioral treatments are sometimes used in conjunction with anticonvulsant therapy. Biofeedback-based approaches have been employed as a direct method of treating seizures or "normalizing" the EEG, though the results appear equivocal in terms of outcome. Sterman and his colleagues were among the first to investigate such an approach and described beneficial effects of seizure suppression with sensorimotor EEG-feedback training (Sterman & Friar, 1971). However, reviews of subsequent research have raised questions regarding the specificity of the treatment, the size and meaningfulness of effects, and methodological issues in the studies (Feldman, Ricks, & Orren, 1983). A number of investigators have attempted to treat reflex epilepsy by applying the principles of behavioral therapy, principally through methods of avoidance conditioning or those similar to systematic desensitization (Forster, 1977). This approach has not invariably been success-

ful, but there are some indications of beneficial results in reducing seizures or raising the threshold of response to the stimulus. Finally, efforts to employ relaxation or cognitive behavioral therapy to reduce the possibilities of stress or psychosocial difficulties contributing to seizures have met with little success to date in controlled studies (Snyder, 1983; Tan & Bruni, 1986). For the most part these efforts represent clinically applied research, and behavioral approaches are at best adjunctive to pharmacological treatment. There has been little consideration to date of age as a factor in success or failure, and most of the work accomplished, with the exception of reflex epilepsy treatment, has been with adults.

EPILEPSY AND NEUROPSYCHOLOGICAL ASPECTS

Intelligence and Adaptive Abilities

The remaining sections of this chapter will consider primarily interictal behavior and abilities, that is, functioning that occurs apart from actual seizure occurrences rather than during a seizure. Historically, the most prominant methodology employed has been the investigation of the intellectual capacities of seizure patients in comparison to nonepileptic samples. Because most of the early studies utilized institutionalized subjects, an early but erroneous conception of epilepsy was that it is invariably associated with mental inferiority or progressive deterioration, despite the few studies that argued to the contrary (e.g., Paskind, 1932). Collins (1951), selecting seizure patients from a private practice sample, found generally above average functioning with no evidence of deterioration in the epileptic group. Winfield (1951) demonstrated the heterogeneity of the epileptic population by separating his sample into symptomatic and idiopathic (cryptogenic) subgroups. Results suggested that it might be the presence of identifiable brain damage that decreases cognitive abilities and test scores rather than seizures per se, since the symptomatic group performed significantly worse. In 1953 Folsom reviewed the literature and concluded that there is no cognitive deficit characteristic of all epilepsies and that it is important to correlate specific types of dysfunction with specific types of seizure phenomena.

Research across the next two decades continued to demonstrate that test scores of seizure patients are skewed toward the lower end of the distribution, particularly in child samples; but that epilepsy itself precludes neither normality nor genius as reflected by intelligence measures. Outpatients continued to outperform inpatient samples, and those with identifiable brain damage underlying the seizures typically obtained lower scores (Angers, 1963; Rodin, 1968; Needham et al., 1969). However, additional factors of importance were also identified during this period, as neuropsychological test batteries were employed to further define behavioral abilities in patients with epilepsy. These factors include the age of the individual when recurring seizures started, how long the patient had experienced seizures, the frequency of the seizures, the types of electroencephalographic abnormalities, and the effects of treatment. If an epileptic disorder can be linked to a pattern of deficits, then these epilepsy-related factors should reflect the association. By far the most frequently employed neuropsychological battery used to investigate the effects of epilepsy and epilepsy-related variables has been that developed by Halstead and Reitan (e.g., Reitan & Davison, 1974).

Klove and White (1963) were able to relate the degree of EEG abnormality in patients to their performance on neuropsychological tests. This relationship was particularly evident for the Halstead-Reitan Impairment Index, which was found to be more sensitive than intelligence test data in categorizing patients. Questions similar to those that had been investigated through the use of intelligence tests were also addressed with the Halstead-Reitan Battery, with generally parallel results. A series of studies at the University of Wisconsin demonstrated that the severity of neuropsychological impairment could be associated with the presence of identifiable brain damage, the presence of major motor seizures, and an earlier age at onset (Klove & Matthews, 1966, 1969; Matthews & Klove, 1967).

Tartar (1972) provided a review of research that corroborated many of the conclusions of Folsom (1953) and summarized studies considering various epilepsy-related factors. Major seizures (grand mal or tonic-clonic type generalized seizures) were associated with greater deficit than minor seizures (petit mal or absence). Patients with temporal lobe or "psychomotor" seizures and mixed seizure types were also shown to be at risk for impairments in functioning. Frequency of seizures, as could be documented, was not consistently associated with dysfunction, but both duration of epilepsy and earlier age at onset were found to be associated with less proficient cognition. There were indications that, aside from petit mal epilepsy, functioning might be negatively correlated with lifetime number of seizures. Thus it could be concluded that it is more deleterious to have identifiable cerebral damage, to begin having seizures younger, to have seizures longer, and to have a more pronounced type or multiple types of seizures.

It has been logical to assume that higher seizure frequency would be associated with lowered performance, but this has been difficult to demonstrate. To some degree this may be because it is very difficult to ascertain seizure frequency with reasonable accuracy, since patients or even those close to them are often not aware of minor seizures. It is also probable that research would need to consider the type or severity of the seizure, since a brief absence is not likely to produce disruption comparable to a generalized tonic-clonic seizure. Nevertheless, Seidenberg and co-workers (1981) compared individuals on a test-retest paradigm with the WAIS, noting "practice effects" only in adult seizure patients who had reported decreases in recent seizure frequency. These results suggested a frequency effect on cognitive functioning that is consistent with research with the Halstead-Reitan Battery (e.g., Dikmen & Matthews, 1977).

The level and pattern of psychological abilities as expressed by patients with varying seizure types continues to be of interest. Giordani et al. (1985) recently reported a comparison of subgroups with primary generalized epilepsy, partial epilepsy, and partial epilepsy with secondary generalization on the WISC-R/WAIS-R instruments. Their findings, largely consistent with the prior research, suggested that generalized epilepsy (primary or secondary) is correlated with worse performance. However, results were significant for specific subtests (primarily those related to attention or visual-spatial skill) rather than for the global IQ index. This study was methodologically sophisticated, utilizing a modern system of diagnosis and classification of the epilepsies and in controlling for age, socioeconomic status, education, duration, onset, frequency, anticonvulsant types, and seizure type as important factors. However, including small groups of absence patients with the tonic-clonic patients in the primary generalized group and simple partial with complex partial may have diluted the results by obscuring group differences.

An issue of considerable importance that has just begun to be addressed is the effect of a seizure disorder on the developing central nervous system. For example, a younger age at onset, particularly during early development (0–5 years of age), has been associated with worsened performance even apart from disease duration (Dikmen, Matthews, & Harley, 1975; Dikmen & Matthews, 1977). This finding has been further substantiated with children for both partial and generalized seizure disorders (O'Leary et al., 1981, 1983). Recently, Farwell et al. (1985) employed a neuropsychological battery adjusted for children to study the behavioral abilities of those from 6 to 16. Their findings underscored the relationships previously noted between duration, age at onset, and seizure frequency. This investigation also related the presence of seizures to scholastic progress, indicating that children with seizures have significant problems and require special placement or repetition of a grade much more frequently than controls. Several other investigators have noted the serious disadvantage faced by children with epilepsy in learning situations (Stores, 1981; Rutter, Graham, & Yule, 1970).

The effects of seizures often appear more marked for children than for adults. Certainly, a young child with seizures might show delays in neuro-behavioral as well as psychological development that would be magnified by standard test procedures that expect growth and higher performance with increasing age. Several investigators (e.g., O'Leary et al., 1983) have pointed out that the often cited advantage of incurring CNS damage in youth (with time and plasticity on the side of recovery) rather than late in life does not hold for seizure disorders. The lack of "recovery" from the effects of a seizure disorder may reflect one of the essential differences between static and discharging lesions and could be understood in terms of the disruptive effects of seizures upon presumed neural reorganization. There is also the possibility that the deleterious effects of the treatments play a role in maintaining or exacerbating deficits. The results of a recent longitudinal study by Rodin, Schmaltz, and Twitty (1986) speak to these issues. For children whose epilepsy had improved but who remained on anticonvulsant medication, stability or slight rise in WAIS-R IQ was indicated in a 5-year (or greater) retest. Children whose epilepsy had remained uncontrolled showed a modest decline that actually appeared to reflect slowed growth. Phenobarbitol, not phenytoin, was associated with deficit. However, an important question that has not been adequately investigated is whether critical periods can be defined developmentally in which the onset or occurrence of a seizure disorder, particularly a disorder with poor or marginal control, can be associated with specific types of behavioral problems.

The recognition that seizures result in problems that may differ somewhat from those presented by static brain lesions led to refinements in the neuropsychological battery, with additions and deletions based on empirical findings with seizure patients (Dodrill, 1978). Using this battery, Dodrill and Wilkus (1978) were able to corroborate the findings of Klove and White (1963) on the relationship between behavioral functioning and EEG abnormalities, but suggested that generalized slowing rather than epileptiform activity per se may be more closely related to observed neuropsychological deficit. There has been additional work developing batteries of neuropsychological tests specifically to define possible anticonvulsant effects (e.g., Lewis & Rennick, 1979; Thompson & Trimble, 1982, 1983).

In summary, it may be said that batteries of tests, either those of psychometric intelligence or those specifically designed to assess neurobehavioral abilities, have broadly addressed a number of important issues. The significance of observations regarding epilepsy related factors (age at onset, duration of illness, seizure frequency, EEG abnormalities, and the presence of identifiable damage) should be emphasized. However, in part because of the ways in which subject groups have been defined in most of these studies, specific patterns of impairment in relation to brain function or the nature of the observed deficits have not been adequately elucidated by these approaches. For example, patients with partial complex seizures may have cerebral dysfunction that is localized (for example, either in temporal or frontal brain regions) or may have both specific and general damage. Where secondary generalized seizures are the defining characteristic of the group, the possibility of a heterogeneous sample in terms of neural dysfunction is even more likely. Employing a battery aimed at assessing multiple and overlapping functional systems, an approach initially grounded in the diagnosis of abnormalities rather than their explication, identifies the presence of relative group impairment without necessarily taking us further in understanding specific brain–behavior relationships. Research aimed at those relationships has been stimulated by theories of brain organization rather than issues of epilepsy per se.

Epilepsy and Specific Deficits: Learning and Memory Impairment

Numerous studies have described specific types of dysfunction associated with certain varieties of seizure disorders. Lennox and Lennox (1960) suggested that an attention/distractibility factor might be particularly relevant in seizure patients. Mirsky and his associates (Mirsky et al., 1960; Fedio and Mirsky, 1969) demonstrated the importance of attention- and vigilance-related problems for adults or children with generalized seizures, especially childhood absence seizures. Dennerll (1964) demonstrated that left and right hemisphere laterality of seizure focus could be associated with verbal and nonverbal cognitive defects, respectively, similar to nondischarging lesion laterality effects. This finding, however, was not uniformly confirmed (Blakemore et al., 1966; Klove & Fitzhugh, 1962). Visual-motor deficits (Blundell, 1966; Crawford, 1967), perceptual (Webb & Berman, 1973), motoric (Sillanpaa, 1975), and mental speed/reaction time (Bruhn & Parsons, 1977) are among the functions found to be affected by various presentations of seizure disorders.

To some degree, this type of research has been directed by considerations of how specific types of functions may be correlated with particular brain regions and, therefore, the effects of more localized brain disturbances. The greatest impetus to this line of inquiry has been the work of Milner and her co-workers with focal seizure patients, especially following surgical resection. Milner and her associates documented the material-specific memory disorder present in lateralized temporal lobe seizure patients. Patients undergoing left temporal lobectomy were shown to have primarily verbal memory difficulties, whereas those undergoing right temporal lobectomy were shown to have primarily nonverbal memory problems (Milner, 1958, 1970; Milner & Teuber, 1968; Kimura, 1963). Inconsistent findings emerged in subsequent research with nonsurgical epilepsy patients (Glowinski, 1973; Scott et al., 1967; Stevens et al., 1972). However, studies selecting well-defined, focal patient samples, using sensitive tasks and controlling across groups for essential variables such as age, education, age at onset, and duration, have been able to extend Milner's initial findings to samples without surgical interventions or large, atrophic lesions in adults (Delaney et al., 1980) and children (Fedio & Mirsky, 1969). These studies also indicated a specificity such that patients with frontal seizure foci or with primary generalized epilepsy do not show similar memory deficiencies. The existence of material-specific memory difficulties in lateralized temporal lobe seizure patients has been corroborated (e.g., Ladavas et al., 1979; Berent et al., 1980; Mungas et al., 1985), though others who used techniques with only immediate recall or recognition memory testing on delay have failed to demonstrate such effects (Loiseau et al., 1983). Although memory deficits are probably not independent of cognitive and attentional problems identified in less specifically defined seizure populations, the results of these studies suggest that attention and general intellect cannot account for either the specificity or relative severity of the problem.

However, the nature of the learning/memory defect has yet to be fully explicated. Milner (1975) has considered that a problem in the consolidation of material from short-term to long-term memory is the essential feature, but others have implicated either retrieval or storage capacity (Drachman & Arbit, 1966). While there are several etiologies for the occurrence of a dense anterograde memory disorder (e.g., Squire & Cohen, 1984), it has been well established that bilateral hippocampal damage, through trauma or disease, can result in an amnestic syndrome. Researchers must explore the relationship between the memory deficit observed in temporal lobe seizure patients, most of whom likely have deep temporal pathology involving such limbic structures as the hippocampal complex and amygdala (e.g., Margerison & Corsellis, 1966; Falconer, 1974), and the more pronounced memory disorder of the amnestic syndrome.

Nevertheless, Mayeux and co-workers (1980) suggested that the memory deficit in focal left temporal lobe seizure patients might be a function of a subtle language dysfunction or dysnomia and that the relationship between information retrieval and word finding in these patients deserves more research. Recently, Delaney, Prevey, and Mattson (1986) provided evidence that both left and right temporal focal seizure patients show deficiencies in short-term phonemic memory paradigms that are not easily explained by a subtle language defect. Furthermore, the types of errors made by seizure patients (primarily perseverative intrusions) differed from those that dominated normal control performances (primarily omissions), suggesting an effect of proactive interference rather than dysnomia in the seizure sample. This pattern of errors on short-term memory tasks is similar to that observed with Korsakoff amnestics and Alzheimer's disease patients who have well-documented lesions in diencephalic and basal frontal regions that have important limbic system connections (Butters, 1985). Of course, as Mungas et al. (1985) suggested, it is possible that an impairment in phonemic processing contributes to both a subtle language deficit and a memory deficit with these patients. One could also speculate regarding the underlying relationship between the functions of memory retrieval and word finding.

In addition, a consideration of metacognitive and learning strategies has shown a complex relationship between memory dysfunction and such factors as self-monitoring, the implementation of learning strategies, and the individual's awareness of difficulties (Prevey, Delaney, & Mattson, 1988a, b). Focal seizure patients may perform poorly on memory tasks due to a deficit related to information processing abilities (short-term encoding, consolidation, retrieval) and problems in executive control factors that minimize the use of appropriate strategies or interfere with making the behavioral adjustments necessary to succeed. The research with these factors is preliminary in nature, but their findings carry significant implications for rehabilitation and training with patients having learning and memory deficits.

Impact of Treatment on Behavioral Abilities

So far we have reviewed research on the behavioral effects believed attributable either to the epileptic disorder or to the underlying cerebral damage. However, epilepsy is certainly a disorder whose treatment carries with it a cost in terms of side effects, some of which have been shown to be of behavioral significance. There remains considerable question regarding the severity and breadth of behavioral effects of anticonvulsant medication. Several careful reviews considering both methodological issues and clinical findings appear to emphasize either the relatively minimal effects expected of current therapy (Dodrill, 1981) or, conversely, the likelihood of impairment attributable to medication in demanding daily activities (Trimble, 1985).

Nevertheless, there is a growing and general consensus with respect to several issues. For example, most researchers believe that anticonvulsant effects are reflected by impairment on tasks involving high degrees of concentration, motor speed/steadiness, or a rapid rate of mental processing (Matthews & Harley, 1975; Thompson & Trimble, 1982; Dodrill & Troupin, 1977). Considerable evidence exists that effects are dose or level related and that reducing drug levels or using monotherapy is advantageous where possible (Thompson & Trimble, 1983; Mattson et al., 1985; Matthews & Harley, 1975).

It is also increasingly recognized that some anticonvulsants have greater detrimental effects (e.g., barbiturates; Giordani et al., 1983), whereas others are associated with lesser attributable dysfunction (e.g., carbamazepine; Andrewes et al., 1986; or valproic acid; Aman et al., 1987). Some research has implicated phenytoin as producing significant problems in concentration, mental or motor speed, and memory (Thompson & Trimble, 1982; Andrewes et al., 1986), but others minimize its effects when well within therapeutic ranges (Dikmen et al., 1984). The fact that the two drugs least implicated for producing behavioral side effects have been the more recently developed may reflect progress in treatment specificity or the need for additional research that may reveal occult effects. Indeed, MacPhee et al. (1986) recently presented evidence of psychomotor impairment in normal volunteers with one dose of carbamazepine in comparison to placebo. However, this approach has been criticized as likely to maximize the likelihood of finding effects (with any active agent), particularly in short-term testing (Dodrill, 1981).

Although the treatment rationale for adults and children with epilepsy is similar, there are differences in approach that relate to adverse reactions that occur more frequently in children as well as to differences in frequency of seizure types. For example, ethosuximide is a common therapy for the generalized absence seizures of childhood, though it has occasional side effects that relate to sleep disorders. There is an increasing recognition that phenobarbitol and primidone can contribute to a syndrome of hyperactivity and behavior disturbance in children; thus other medications may be preferentially employed. Anticonvulsant treatment with children represents a particularly thorny problem, in that multiple drug treatment and pushing drugs toward toxic levels in an effort to achieve total seizure control has been more closely associated with decreased functioning than have measures of actual seizure control (Bourgeois et al., 1983).

It is certainly difficult to separate the effects of seizures, underlying cerebral damage or metabolic disturbance, and chemical treatments. However, in a unique and important opportunity, Smith et al. (1986) reported on preliminary results of a large VA Cooperative Study (Mattson et al., 1985) and described deficits relating to motor speed, cognition, attention, and mood status in seizure patients *prior* to anticonvulsant treatment. The patients were recently diagnosed, noninstitutionalized individuals without such complications as alcoholism, chronic psychiatric disturbance, or progressive neurological disease. The authors found that while the intelligence of the sample was not skewed to below average, a number of deficits were documented in comparison to age/education matched control subjects in such areas as motor speed, concentration, mental agility, and mood. Following the administration of anticonvulsants (principally carbamazepine, phenytoin, and phenobarbitol), the seizure patients showed no significant declines but had less of a practice effect on 30-day retest than control subjects. These results suggest that difficulties on tasks designed to assess behavioral toxicity are present prior to treatment and that the effects of a single well-monitored anticonvulsant may be more subtle than pronounced once the patient has adjusted to use.

In her review of experience with surgical treatment of focal epilepsy, Milner (1975) suggested that surgical excision of a discharging lesion tended to result in a mild worsening of function subserved primarily by that brain region, but with some amelioration of deficits associated with areas at a distance from the epileptogenic source. Although little preoperative/postoperative data were presented, subsequent research has tended to support Milner's observation. For example, following left temporal lobectomy, the verbal memory impairment is seen to worsen immediately postoperatively and not to regain preoperative levels, whereas nondominant temporal lobe surgery yields verbal memory improvement beyond preoperative levels (Novelly et al., 1984). The converse was noted for visual memory. These studies, as well as those of Wannamaker and Matthews (1976), suggest that there is a greater cost in overall cognitive functioning with a dominant than a nondominant temporal lobe resection. Research has noted a significant correlation between the reduction in seizure frequency postoperatively and improved intellectual functioning, and similar findings are reported in such psychosocial areas as occupational status (Augustine et al., 1984). In addition, Lieb et al. (1982) noted that patients most likely to show a postlobectomy drop in intellect were those with poor seizure relief, a lack of pathology in the resected specimen, and residual EEG abnormalities. Poor seizure relief was also correlated with lower preoperative intellect. Thus the results to date indicate that surgical considerations need to include psychological and neuropsychological factors as well as the evidence for otherwise intractable, circumscribed epileptogenic tissue (e.g., Browne & Feldman, 1983). With optimal procedures, selected cases can achieve results that are notably beneficial in terms of long-term seizure relief and greatly reduced anticonvulsant treatment without marked cost in terms of behavioral skills.

Overview of Findings and Prognosis

The deficits that have been documented in connection with various types of epilepsy are of a far-reaching variety and are apparently associated somewhat more closely with the underlying cerebral pathology than with the seizures themselves (with the possible exception of vigilance failures in patients with frequent absence seizures). However, the fact that the cerebral pathology either at a structural or subcellular level provides the substrate for abnormal and excessive discharge has several consequences. First, of course, are the seizures themselves varying in severity and frequency and with their attendant interference with immediate activity. Second, there is the opportunity for the interictal disruption of otherwise normal neuronal activity through the transmission of abnormal, though subclinical, discharge more broadly, both within and between hemispheres. Finally, there is the necessity for anticonvulsant therapy that is responsible for at least mild, but in some cases more marked, exacerbation of attentional, perceptual-motor, and cognitive dysfunction. These factors combine to produce a significant disadvantage for the individual with seizures, one that can obviously interfere with learning as expressed in development, in scholastic progress, or in work adjustment. The implications have now begun to be explored in a less clinical and more empirical fashion. It is important to note that many patients with epilepsy can lead normal lives and adapt to or overcome the subtle deficits that can best be documented through research methodologies. In working with patients having epilepsy, clinicians and educators need to maintain an individualized approach rather than one based on a group identification such as "epileptic," since there is no specific deficit or pattern across patients and the problems that are present encompass a wide range of severity.

It is clear that deficits do occur in conjunction with seizure disorders, but what is the prognosis for patients with epilepsy? The concept of a necessary significant deterioration in the presence of epilepsy has been disputed for years (e.g., Rodin, 1968). However, there is increasingly strong evidence that when deterioration occurs (apart from an identified progressive brain disease), seizure severity can be an important predictor. The concept of the severity of the seizure disorder needs to include at least seizure type and frequency (e.g., Mattson et al., 1985), and some consideration of duration of illness is probably also important to differentiate effects. The likelihood that seizures themselves have the effect of producing actual neuronal damage has been suggested by neuropathological studies (Markiewicz & Dymecki, 1969; Scheibel et al., 1974). The issues in this area were carefully reviewed by Lesser et al. (1986), who underscore that cognitive deterioration is not "expected" but occurs in conjunction with underlying pathophysiological abnormalities that may be responsible for the seizure severity factor as well.

EPILEPSY AND PSYCHIATRIC DISTURBANCE

Perhaps more than any other neurological disorder, epilepsy has been linked to the presence of psychiatric disturbances. Relationships have been suggested to exist between epilepsy and such disorders as hysteria (e.g., Roy, 1977), depersonalization (e.g., Kenna & Sedman, 1965), depression (e.g., Robertson & Trimble, 1983), and various characterological problems (such as aggression/ violence, disorders of sexuality, and criminality; e.g., Pincus, 1980; Blumer, 1975). Evidence has also been presented that epilepsy might contribute to psychosis, particularly a schizophreniclike condition. It was further proposed that differences might exist in the type of psychotic manifestation, depending on the side of lesion (e.g., Flor-Henry, 1969), though subsequent research has not consistently supported that contention (Jensen & Larsen, 1979). Some investigators have indicated that the psychosis that can be associated with seizure disorders may take considerable time to develop (Slater & Beard, 1963). In this regard it is of interest that the literature on behavior disorders in children with epilepsy presents a wide variety of possible abnormalities, but psychosis is not well represented. A recent review identified studies that would categorize the behavior abnormalities in children under four major headings: (1) anxious/withdrawn/dependent, (2) inattentive, (3) hyperactive/impulsive, and (4) aggressive/antisocial (Curley, 1986).

There has also been a long-running debate regarding whether there exists a specifiable "epileptic personality" (e.g., Delay et al., 1958). Personality traits such as explosive impulsivity, affective viscosity, and egocentricity have been proposed as common across seizure patients. However, their existence as pervasive traits has been questioned, and when such features are present it is not clear whether these traits are the direct result of heredity, of seizures, of the underlying pathology as expressions of "organicity," of a reaction to painful social situations, of a subclinical epileptiform discharge, of medication, or perhaps of psychodynamic processes.

Although these are important issues both for clinicians and for those trying to understand the central nervous system, their investigation from a scientific perspective has proven difficult indeed. Thus contradictory findings emerge in the research, and controversy predominates. The literature on these and related topics is extensive, and one can draw quite different conclusions from overviews that have been presented; while some would emphasize the primacy of neurophysiological mechanisms, others view the development of psycho-pathology and behavioral abnormalities in a more complex light (see, for example, Geschwind, 1977, 1979; Blumer, 1984; Reynolds & Trimble, 1981; Hermann & Whitman, 1984; Whitman & Hermann, 1986).

With regard to psychopathology, temporal lobe epilepsy and partial complex seizures have been the focus of the most interest by investigators and been accorded a central position in the etiology of many of the behavioral disturbances cited here. Over the past decade in particular, the concept of the epileptic personality has been refined somewhat and focused into a consideration of the contribution of abnormalities within the temporal lobes. Gastaut, Morin, and Lesevre (1955) described a pattern that they believed represented a relatively direct result of the neuropathology within the temporal lobe and limbic system. The pattern of hypometamorphosis (viscosity/verbosity in conversation and writing), hyperemotionality, and hyposexuality has been thought to represent a partial inverse of the pattern observed (primarily in animals) following bilateral temporal lobe ablation, that is, the Kluver-Bucy syndrome. Waxman and Geschwind (1975) pointed to the occurrence of behavior changes in patients with temporal lobe epilepsy involving alterations in sexual behavior, religiosity, and compulsive writing, which they felt could be attributed etiologically to interictal temporal lobe spiking. More recently, researchers have attempted to verify the presence of these personality traits as a syndrome related to abnormal neuronal activity within the temporal lobes, a "temporal-limbic hyperconnection" (Bear & Fedio, 1977). Although the results of that initial effort were felt by many to be both promising and exciting (Geschwind, 1977), subsequent replication efforts have certainly not provided unequivocal support (Hermann & Riel, 1981; Bear, 1982; Tucker et al., 1987).

Nevertheless, consistent data suggest that the incidence of psychopathology is increased in samples with epilepsy as compared to healthy samples and that an increase in the likelihood of psychosis may be especially prominent. There is also a body of research that argues that behavior disorders in children are more prevalent in conjunction with epilepsy than with other chronic medical disorders (Rutter et al., 1970). Behavioral abnormalities may be especially serious and common in patients suffering from multiple types of seizures (Hermann et al., 1982). The factors responsible for these findings merit further consideration. In a careful and thorough review Hermann and Whitman (1984) presented a synopsis of this complicated area, including a methodological analysis of the research carried out to date. Among the problems identified in their review is a tendency of investigators to neglect variables that could well contribute to the presence or development of psychopathology in patients with seizures. Interestingly, researchers frequently have found these variables to be important in the area of general psychopathology, such as socioeconomic status, psychosocial parameters, and developmental/family factors. Additional variables that have a secondary relationship to the epileptic disorder, including neuropsychological status and treatment effects, were also underscored. This perspective led the authors to consider a conceptual model for various types of psychopathology associated with epilepsy that would include "brain-related," "nonbrain-related", and treatment-related variables, perhaps contributing in different degrees to different types of psychological problems. Considering the variability of either the presence or type of psychopathology in both general seizure populations or subgroups such as temporal lobe epilepsy, this approach has an intuitive appeal. Thus the most promising and exciting investigations of psychiatric complications of epilepsy are likely to be those that consider the etiology of the behavioral and emotional problems from a multivariate perspective, including social and psychological factors as well as the neurophysiological. It continues to be important for those working with patients having epilepsy to use an individualized approach rather than one based on group membership.

EPILEPSY AND PSYCHOSOCIAL FACTORS

In considering the psychosocial effects of epilepsy we move to those factors that most obviously involve everyday life functioning. Included are such central issues as educational and vocational experiences, financial stress, interpersonal functioning (including marriage and family interactions), and medical management/physician–patient rapport. As noted by Dodrill (1986b) in his excellent review of the psychosocial consequences of seizures, epilepsy "is a disorder that lends itself to the study of the interrelationships between brain disorders and psychosocial problems." This can be attributed to many factors and their interactions.

In the first section of this chapter we reviewed some of the seizure manifestations themselves as well as effects of their treatment, each of which can interfere markedly with affective behaviors in nearly any situation. In the subsequent sections we considered deficits in behavioral abilities and problems in emotional adjustment and personality, complex factors that are clearly capable of contributing to difficulties in educational, vocational, or interpersonal situations. It should be evident at this point that there is a wide degree of variation among patients with epilepsy in the range and severity of problems faced. For patients with incomplete seizure control, the unpredictability of seizures often leads to additional, externally imposed limitations intended for their safety and the safety of others. These limitations can preclude activities that are taken for granted in our society such as driving or certain sports activities. Although these concerns are practical and appropriate for some, they can be unfortunately limiting to others. It is also the case that unnecessary psychosocial problems occur whose source may involve the patients, their families or guardians, or those with whom they interact (educators, employers, and social agencies).

Considering first the patients themselves, factors such as fear of public censure, loss of self-esteem, social isolation, and despair of a normal life have been noted to contribute to poor psychosocial adjustment (Fraser & Smith, 1982). Hermann and Whitman (1986) reviewed the literature documenting how a patient's fear of seizures, expectation of discrimination, and lack of perceived control over life events can lead to depression, anxiety, withdrawal, and limited coping. The sense that a diagnosis of epilepsy includes a social stigmatization motivates some patients to hide their illness or even to avoid treatment. Noncompliance with medication regimens is a further complication that can stem from patient misperceptions about their illness, though simply imparting information does not solve the problem of erratic medication usage (Peterson et al., 1982; Pryse-Phillips, 1982). In adolescence non-compliance can also be associated with a restriction of independence, a lack of family harmony, or lowered self-esteem (Freidman et al., 1986). One might be led to think that these difficulties with adjustment and everyday life might dissipate if only the epilepsy could vanish. It is a measure of the complexities of "having epilepsy" that a cure, as through surgery, does not invariably lead to an improvement in psychosocial functioning. Several authors discussed the difficult time individuals may have in living without seizures following effective surgical treatment, since epilepsy had become an integral part of their identification (Ferguson & Rayport, 1965; Horowitz & Cohen, 1968).

Factors external to the patients most importantly include their immediate family. This is particularly relevant in considering the child and adolescent with epilepsy. Evidence has been presented that family functioning is vulnerable to disruption when a child has a seizure disorder and that the child's mother may often behave in an overprotective manner or in a fashion that reduces optimal communication and family cohesion as well as the child's self-concept (e.g., Ferrari et al., 1983). Appropriate caution versus overprotectiveness is discussed by O'Donohoe (1983) among others, who notes that an ambience of overconcern limits a child's development and experience of normality. A model suggesting that parental overprotectiveness is related to the unpredictability of seizures and the consequent feeling of incompetence or lack of control was presented by Ziegler (1981). Matthews et al. (1982) showed that epileptic children are more likely than either diabetic children or healthy peers to attribute control over events in their lives to external sources, even occurrences that represent successes. From a clinical perspective, Ziegler (1982) discussed the child with epilepsy in terms of additional issues related to school, social relationships, and treatment.

Another external factor affecting the patient with epilepsy is the public perception of epilepsy and its victims. Surveys have pointed to numerous misperceptions and prejudices regarding epilepsy. For example, many people tend to associate epilepsy with insanity or would prefer that individuals with seizures were kept from the labor market (e.g., Gutteling et al., 1986). The effects such attitudes might have on teachers, potential employers, or those individuals who might otherwise be available as friends or social supports are obvious. It is important to note that all of these factors, both internal and external to the patient, interact and in many cases are likely to intensify each other's effects. For example, the fact that some deal with epilepsy patients through prejudice contributes to patients' desire to hide their illness or to withdraw, lessening the opportunity for more rewarding experiences.

The difficulties experienced by patients in adjusting to the practicalities of having epilepsy and with developing as optimal a life-style as possible around a seizure disorder have been well recognized by clinicians. However, prior to 1980 relatively few studies objectively evaluated psychosocial problems. In an effort to provide a method for rating the severity and pattern of psychosocial stressors in a patient's life, Dodrill et al. (1980) developed the Washington Psychosocial Seizure Inventory (WPSI). Designed in a manner similar to the prototypical personality inventory (MMPI), this measure allows for a quantification of relevant factors including family background, emotional adjustment, interpersonal adjustment, vocational adjustment, financial status, adjustment to seizures, medicine and medical management, and an overall index of psychosocial functioning. The scale has proven to have reasonable reliability, validity, and utility and has been useful in research as well as in a more limited manner in clinical situations. For example, it has been possible to characterize the similarities and differences in psychosocial problems across regions and even among countries (Dodrill et al., 1984a, b). A comparison of patterns and "two-point" configurations allows a consideration of individual differences and could raise hypotheses for intervention (Dodrill, 1986b).

CONCLUSIONS AND NEW DIRECTIONS

This chapter has provided an overview of the major behavioral facets of epilepsy and, in a limited manner, implied areas of overlap and interaction between these areas. Seizures are stressful and life stress increases the likelihood of seizure occurrence; treatment can improve everyday life but can interfere with specific functions; behavioral deficits contribute to psychosocial limitations that may well contribute to depression or psychiatric disturbances. Although there is unquestionably a need for continued careful research in each of the areas reviewed, one of the more exciting directions currently underway is more direct consideration of the interplay among the biological, psychological, and social variables.

Examples of these types of studies are increasingly common. For example, Hermann (1982) compared groups of epileptic children defined as having good or poor neuropsychological functioning, though otherwise closely matched, on measures of aggression, overall behavioral pathology, and social competence. A greater degree of psychopathology and aggression was found in the group with greater neuropsychological impairment. Dodrill (1986a) considered intellectual, neuropsychological, emotional, and social functioning in patients with generalized tonic-clonic epilepsy. High-frequency seizures and the occurrence of status epilepticus were associated with decreased functioning in all areas, with emotional and psychosocial dysfunction most prominent in the former and abilities most reduced in the latter. Dodrill has also begun looking at relationships between scales measuring emotional, psychosocial, and neuropsychological factors in samples of seizure patients (Dodrill, 1986b). As noted, Hermann and Whitman (1984) proposed a multietiologic model for the development of psychopathology associated with seizure disorders that would include neurophysiological, psychosocial, and treatment-related parameters. This model was further elaborated recently (Whitman & Hermann, 1986).

As a final example, a recent study has made more explicit use of the biopsychosocial model of Engel (1980) in attempting to understand the increased presence of behavior problems in children with seizures as compared to healthy children or others with chronic illness (Curley et al., 1987). Using a hierarchical multiple regression analysis, this research documented that three variables—(1) general neuropsychological functioning, (2) overall seizure severity, and (3) parental disagreement about child rearing—contribute to the presence of significant behavior disturbance in epileptic boys, while measures of overall marital satisfaction and overprotectiveness did not. It is the recognition of the multivariate determination of complex behaviors that should direct both interventions and future research in this area.

REFERENCES

Adams, R. D., & Victor, M. (1985). *Principles of neurology* (3rd ed.). New York: McGraw-Hill.

Aman, M. G., Werry, J., Paxton, J., & Turbott, S. (1987). Effect of sodium valproate on psychomotor performance in children as a function of dose, fluctuations in concentration, and diagnosis. *Epilepsia* 28, 115–124.

Andrewes, D. G., Bullen, J. G., Tomlinson, L., Elwes, R. D. C., & Reynolds, E. H. A. (1986). Comparative study of the cognitive effects of phenytoin and carbamazepine in new referrals with epilepsy. *Epilepsia* 27, 128–134.

Angers, W. (1963). Patterns of abilities and capacities in the epileptic. *Journal of Genetic Psychology* 103, 59–66.

Augustine, E. A., Novelly, R. A., Mattson, R. H., Glaser, G. H., Williamson, P. D., Spencer, D. D., & Spencer, S. S. (1984). Occupational adjustment following neurosurgical treatment of epilepsy. *Annals of Neurology* 15, 68–72.

Bear, D. M. (1982). Interictal behavior in hospitalized temporal lobe epileptics: Relationship to idiopathic psychiatric syndromes. *Journal of Neurology, Neurosurgery, and Psychiatry* 45, 481–488.

Bear, D. M. & Fedio, P. (1977). Quantitative analysis of interictal behavior in temporal lobe epilepsy. *Archives of Neurology* 34, 454–467.

Berent, S., Giordani, B., Boll, T. (1980). Hemispheric site of epileptogenic focus: Cognitive, perceptual and psychomotor implications for children and adults. In R. Cange, R. Angeleri, & K. Penry (Eds.), *Advances in epileptology: The XI Epilepsy International Symposium*, New York: Raven Press.

Bickford, R. G., & Klass, D. W. (1962). Stimulus factors in the mechanism of television-induced seizures. *Transactions of the American Neurological Association* 89, 136.

Blakemore, C., Ettlinger, G., & Falconer, M. (1966). Cognitive abilities in relation to frequency of seizures and neuropathology of the temporal lobes in man. *Journal of Neurology, Neurosurgery, and Psychiatry* 29, 268–72.

Blumer, D. (1975). Temporal lobe epilepsy and its psychiatric significance. In F. Benson & D. Blumer (Eds.), *Psychiatric aspects of neurologic disease*. New York: Grune & Stratton.

Blumer, D. (1984). Psychiatric complications in epilespy. In H. Sands (Ed.), *Epilepsy: A handbook for the mental health professional*. New York: Brunner/Mazel.

Blundell, E. (1966). Parietal lobe dysfunction in subnormal patients. *Journal of Mental Deficiency Research* 10, 141–52.

Bourgeois, B., Prensky, A., Palkes, H., Talent, B., & Busch, S. (1983). Intelligence in epilepsy: A prospective study in children. *Annals of Neurology* 14, 438–444.

Browne, T. R. (1983). Epilepsy, sexual function, and pregnancy. In T. R. Brown & R. G. Feldman, *Epilepsy diagnosis and management*. Boston: Little, Brown.

Browne, T. R. & Feldman, R. G. (1983). *Epilepsy diagnosis and management*. Boston: Little, Brown.

Bruhn, P., & Parsons, O. (1977). Reaction time variability in epileptic and brain damaged patients. *Cortex* 13, 373–384.

Butters, N. (1985). Alcoholic Korsakoff syndrome: Some unresolved issues concerning etiology, neuropathology, and cognitive deficits. *Journal of Clinical and Experimental Neuropsychology* 7,

181–210.

Chan, A. (1985). Alcoholism and epilepsy. *Epilepsia* 26, 323–33.

Cirignotta, F., Montagna, P., Lugaresi, E., & Gervasio, L. (1982). Seizures provoked by dressing. *Archives of Neurology* (letter), 39, 785–786.

Collins, L. (1951). Epileptic intelligence. *Journal of Consulting Psychology* 15, 392–329.

Crawford, J. P. (1967). Cerebral localization of psychological functions. *British Medical Journal* 4, 483.

Curley, A. D. (1986). *Behavior problems in children with seizures and parental influences*. Unpublished doctoral dissertation, State University of New York at Stony Brook.

Curley, A. D., Delaney, R. C., Mattson, R. H., Holmes G. L., & O'Leary, K. D. (1987). Determinants of behavioral disturbance in boys with seizures. Paper presented at the Annual Meeting of the American Psychological Association, New York.

Daly, R. F. & Forster, F. M. (1975). Inheritance of reading epilepsy. *Neurology* 25, 1051–1054.

Delaney, R. C., Mattson, R. H., Rosen, A., & Novelly, R. A. (1980). Memory function in focal epilepsy: A comparison of unilateral temporal lobe and frontal lobe samples. *Cortex* 16, 103–117.

Delaney, R. C., Prevey, M. L., & Mattson, R. H. (1986). Short term retention with lateralized temporal lobe epilepsy. *Cortex* 22, 591–600.

Delay, J., Pichot, P., Lemperiere, T., & Perse, J. (1985). In A. Benton (Ed.), *The Rorschach and the epileptic personality*. New York: Logos Press.

Dennerll, R. (1964). Cognitive deficits and lateral brain dysfunction in temporal lobe epilepsy. *Epilepsia* 5, 177–191.

Dikmen, S., Matthews, C., & Harley, J. P. (1975). The effect of early versus late onset of major-motor epilepsy upon cognitive-intellectual performance. *Epilepsia* 16, 73–81.

Dikmen, S., & Matthews, C. (1977). The effect of major-motor seizure frequency upon cognitive-intellectual functions in adults. *Epilepsia* 18, 21–30.

Dikmen, S., Temkin, N., Weiler, M., & Wyler, A. (1984). Behavioral effects of anticonvulsant prophylaxis: No effect of artifact. *Epilepsia* 25, 741–746.

Dodrill, C. B. (1978). A neuropsychological battery for epilepsy. *Epilepsia* 19, 611–623.

Dodrill, C. B. (1981). The neuropsychology of epilepsy. In S. Filskov and T. Boll (Eds.), *Handbook of clinical neuropsychology*. New York: Wiley-Interscience.

Dodrill, C. B. (1986a). Correlates of generalized tonic-clonic seizures with intellectual, neuropsychological, emotional, and social function in patients with epilepsy. *Epilepsia* 27, 399–411.

Dodrill, C. B. (1986b). Psychosocial consequences of epilepsy. In S. Filskov & T. Boll (Eds.), *Handbook of clinical neuropsychology (Vol. 2)*. New York: Wiley-Interscience.

Dodrill, C. B., Batzel, L. W., Queisser, H. R., & Temkin, N. (1980). An objective method for the assessment of psychological and social problems among epileptics. *Epilepsia* 21, 123–135.

Dodrill, C. B., Beier, R., Kasparick, M., Tacke, I., Tacke, U., & Tan, S. (1984a). Psychosocial problems in adults with epilepsy: Comparison of findings from four countries. *Epilepsia* 25, 176–183.

Dodrill, C. B., Breyer, D. N., Diamond, M. B., Dubinsky, B. L., & Geary, B. B. (1984b). Psychosocial problems among adults with epilepsy. *Epilepsia* 25, 168–175.

Dodrill, C. B., & Troupin, A. S. (1977). Psychotropic effects of carbamazepine in epilepsy: A double blind comparison with phenytoin. *Neurology* 33, 1023–1028.

Dodrill, C. B. & Wilkus, R. (1978). Neuropsychological correlates of the EEG in epileptics III. Generalized non-epileptiform abnormalities. *Epilepsia* 19, 453–462.

Drachman, D., & Arbit, J. (1966). Memory and the hippocampal complex. *Archives of Neurology* 10, 232–248.

Dreifuss, F. E. (1981). Proposal for revised clinical and electroencephalographic classification of epileptic seizures. *Epilepsia* 22, 489.

Engel, G. L. (1980). The clinical application of the biopsychosocial model. *American Journal of Psychiatry* 137, 535–544.

Epilepsy Foundation of America. (1975). *Basic statistics on the epilepsies*. Philadelphia: F. A. Davis.

Falconer, M. (1974). Mesial temporal sclerosis as a common cause of epilepsy: Etiology, treatment, and prevention. *Lancet* 2, 767–770.

Farwell, J., Dodrill, C., & Batzel, L. (1985). Neuropsychological abilities of children with epilepsy. *Epilepsia* 26, 395–400.

Fedio, P., & Mirsky, A. (1969). Selective intellectual deficits in children with temporal lobe and centrencephalic epilepsy. *Neuropsychologia* 3, 287–300.

Feldman, R. G., Ricks, N. L., & Orren, M. (1983). Behavioral methods of seizure control. In T. R. Brown & R. G. Feldman (Eds.), *Epilepsy diagnosis and management.* Boston: Little, Brown.

Ferguson, S. M., & Rayport, M. (1965). The adjustment to living without epilepsy. *Journal of Nervous and Mental Disease* 140, 26–37.

Ferrari, M., Matthews, W. S., & Barabas, G. (1983). The family and the child with epilepsy. *Family Processes* 22, 53–59.

Flor-Henry, P. (1969). Psychosis and temporal lobe epilepsy: A controlled investigation. *Epilepsia* 10, 363–395.

Folsom, A. (1953). Psychological testing in epilepsy. *Epilepsia* 2, 15–22.

Forster, F. M. (1971). Epilepsy associated with eating. *Transactions of the American Neurological Association* 96, 106–107.

Forster, F. M. (1977). *Reflex epilepsy, behavioral therapy, and conditional reflexes.* Springfield, IL: Charles C Thomas.

Fraser, R. T. & Smith, W. R. (1982). Adjustment to daily living. In H. Sands *Epilepsy: A handbook for the mental health professional.* New York: Brunner/Mazel.

Friedman, I. M., Litt, I. F., King, D. R., Henson, R., Holtzman, D., Halverson, D., & Kraemer, H. C. (1986). Compliance with anticonvulsant therapy by epileptic youth. *Journal of Adolescent Health Care* 7, 12–17.

Gastaut, H. (1970). Clinical and electroencephalographic classification of epileptic seizures. *Epilepsia* 11, 102.

Gastaut, H., Morin, G., & Lesevre, N. (1955). Etude de compotement des epileptiques psychomoteurs dans l'intervalle, de leurs crises; les troubles de l'activite globale et de la sociabilite. *Annales Medico-Psychologiques* 112, 657–696.

Geschwind, N. (1977). Behavioral change in temporal lobe epilepsy. *Archives of Neurology* 34, 453.

Geschwind, N. (1979). Behavioral changes in temporal lobe epilepsy. *Psychological Medicine* 9, 217–219.

Giordani, B., Berent, S., Sackellares, J. C., Rourke, D., Seidenberg, M., O'Leary, D., Dreifuss, F., Boll, T. (1985). Intelligence test performance of patients with partial and generalized seizures. *Epilepsia* 26, 37–42.

Giordani, B., Sackellares, J. C., Miller, S. M., Berent, S., Sutula, T., Seidenberg, M., Boll, T. J., O'Leary, D., & Dreifuss, F. (1983). Improvement in neuropsychological performance in patients with refractory seizures following intensive diagnostic and therapeutic intervention. *Neurology* 33, 489–493.

Glass, D., & Mattson, R. H. (1973). Psychopathology and emotional precipitants of seizures in temporal lobe epilepsy. *Proceedings of the 81st Annual Convention of the American Psychological Association* 8, 425–426.

Glowinski, H. (1973). Cognition in temporal lobe epilepsy. *Journal of Nervous and Mental Disease* 157, 129–137.

Gowers, W. R. (1881). *Epilepsy and other chronic convulsive disorders.* London: Churchill.

Gutteling, J. M., Seydel, E. R., & Wiegman, O. (1986). Previous experience with epilepsy and effectiveness of information to change public perception of epilepsy. *Epilepsia* 27, 739–745.

Hauser, W., & Kurland, L. (1975). The epidemiology of epilepsy in Rochester Minnesota, 1935–1967. *Epilepsia* 16, 1.

Hermann, B. P. (1982). Neuropsychological functioning and psychopathology in children with epilepsy. *Epilepsia* 23, 545–554.

Hermann, B. P., Dikmen, S., & Wilensky, A. J. (1982). Increased psychopathology associated with multiple seizure types: Fact or Artifact? *Epilepsia* 23, 587–596.

Hermann, B. P., & Riel, P. (1981). Interictal personality and behavioral traits in temporal lobe and generalized epilepsy. *Cortex* 17, 125–128.

Hermann, B. P., & Whitman, S. (1984). Behavioral and personality correlates of epilepsy: A review, methodological critique, and conceptual model. *Psychological Bulletin* 95, 451–497.

Hermann, B. P., & Whitman, S. (1986). Psychopathology in epilepsy: A multietiologic model. In S. Whitman, & B. Hermann (Eds.), *Psychopathology in epilepsy: Social dimensions.* New York: Oxford University Press.

Holmes, G. L., Blair, S., Eisenberg, E., Scheebaum, R., Margraf, J., & Zimmerman, A. (1982). Toothbrushing induced epilepsy. *Epilepsia* 23, 657–661.

Horowitz, M. J., & Cohen, F. M. (1968). Temporal lobe epilepsy: Effect of lobectomy on psychosocial functioning. *Epilepsia* 9, 23–41.

Hutt, S. J., & Fairweather, H. (1971). Some effects of performance variables upon generalized spike-wave activity. *Brain* 94, 321–326.

Jackson, J. H. (1958). *Selected writings of J. H. Jackson* (Vol. 1), J. Taylor (Ed.), London: Staples Press.

Jensen, I., & Larsen, J. K. (1979). Psychosis is drug resistant temporal lobe epilepsy. *Journal of Neurology, Neurosurgery, and Psychiatry* 42, 948–954.

Joynt, J., Green, D., & Green, R. (1962). Musicogenic epilepsy caused only by a discrete frequency band of church bells. *Brain* 85, 77.

Kenna, J. C., & Sedman, G. (1965). Depersonalization in temporal lobe epilepsy and the organic psychoses. *British Journal of Psychiatry* 111, 293–299.

Kimura, D. (1963). Right temporal lobe damage. *Archives of Neurology* 8, 264–271.

Klove, H., & Fitzhugh, K. (1962). The relationship of differential EEG patterns to the distribution of Wechsler-Bellevue scores in a chronic epileptic population. *Journal of Clinical Psychology* 18, 334–337.

Klove, H., & Matthews, C. (1966). Psychometeric and adaptive abilities in differential etiology. *Epilepsia* 7, 330–338.

Klove, H., & Matthews, C. (1969). Neuropsychological evaluation of the epileptic patient. *Wisconsin Medical Journal* 68, 296–301.

Klove, H., & White, P. (1963). Relationship of the degree of EEG abnormality to the distribution of Wechsler-Bellevue scores. *Neurology* 13, 423–430.

Kutt, H., (1984). Interactions between anticonvulsants and other commonly prescribed drugs. *Epilepsia* 25 (Suppl.), S118–S131.

Ladavas, E., Umilta, C., & Provinciali, L. (1979). Hemispheric cognitive performance in epileptic patients. *Epilepsia* 20, 493–502.

Lechtenberg, R. (1984). *Epilepsy and the family*. Cambridge, MA: Harvard University Press.

Lennox, W. G., & Lennox, M. A. (1960). *Epilepsy and related disorders*. New York: Little, Brown.

Lesser, R., Luders, H., Wyllie, E., Dinner, D., & Morris III, H. H. (1986). Mental deterioration in epilepsy. *Epilepsia* 27, S105–S123.

Lewis, R., & Rennick, P. (1979). *Manual for a repeated cognitive-perceptual-motor battery*, Grosse Point, MI: Axon.

Lieb, J., Rausch, R., Engel, J., Brown, W., & Crandall, P. (1982). Changes in intelligence following temporal lobectomy: Relationship to EEG activity, seizure relief, and pathology. *Epilepsia* 23, 1–13.

Loiseau, P., Strube, E., Broustet, D., Battellochi, S., Gomeni, C., & Moselli, P. (1983). Learning impairment in epileptic patients. *Epilepsia* 24, 183–192.

MacPhee, G., Goldie, C., Roulston, D., Potter, L., Agnew, E., & Laidlaw, M. (1986). Effect of carbamazepine on psychomotor performance in naive subjects. *European Journal of Clinical Pharmacology* 30, 37–42.

Margerison, J., & Corsellis, J. (1966). Epilepsy and the temporal lobes. *Brain* 89, 499–530.

Markiewicz, D., & Dymecki, J. (1969). Neuropathological changes in epilepsy with behavior and intellectual disorders. *Polish Medical Journal* 8, 181–192.

Matthews, C., & Harley, J. P. (1975). Cognitive and motor-sensory performances in toxic and non-toxic epileptic subjects. *Neurology* 25, 184–188.

Matthews, C., & Klove, H. (1967). Differential psychological performances in major-motor, psychomotor, and mixed seizure classifications of known and unknown etiology. *Epilepsia* 8, 117–128.

Matthews, W. S., Barabas, G., & Ferrari, M. (1982). Emotional concommitants of childhood epilepsy. *Epilepsia* 23, 671–681.

Mattson, R. H. (1983). Seizures associated with alcohol use and alcohol withdrawal. In T. R. Brown & R. G. Feldman (Eds.), *Epilepsy diagnosis and management*. Boston: Little, Brown.

Mattson, R. H., & Cramer, J. A. (1985). Epilepsy, sex hormones, and antiepileptic drugs. *Epilepsia* 26 (Suppl. 1), S40–S51.

Mattson, R. H., Cramer, J. A., Collins, J., Smith, D., Delgado-Escueta, A., Browne, T., Williamson, P., Treiman, D., McNamara, J., McCutcheon, C., Homan, R., Crill, W., Lubozynski, M., Rosenthal, N. P., & Mayersdorf, A. (1985). Comparison of carbamazepine, phenobarbitol, phenytoin, and primidone in partial and secondarily generalized tonic-clonic seizures. *New England Journal of Medicine* 313, 145–151.

Mattson, R. H., Pratt, K. L., & Claverly, J. R. (1975). Electroencephalograms of epileptics following sleep deprivation. *Archives of Neurology* 25, 361.

Mayeux, R., Brandt, J., Rosen, J., & Benson, D. F. (1980). Interictal memory and language impairment in temporal lobe epilepsy. *Neurology* 30, 120–125.

Merlis, J. K. (1970). Proposal for an international classification of the epilepsies. *Epilepsia* 11, 114–119.

Milner, B. (1958). Psychological deficits produced by temporal lobe excision. *Research Publications of the Association of Nervous and Mental Disease* 36, 244–257.

Milner, B. (1970). Memory and the medial temporal regions of the brain. In K. Pribram and D. Broadbent (Eds.), *Biology of memory*. New York: Academic Press.

Milner, B. (1975). Psychological aspects of focal epilepsy and its neurosurgical management. In D. Purpura (Ed.), *Advances in neurology* (Vol. 8). New York: Raven Press.

Milner, B., & Teuber, H. L. (1968). Alteration of perception and memory in man: Reflections and methods. In L. Weiskrantz (Ed.). *Analysis of behavioral change*. New York: Harper & Row.

Mirsky, A., Primac, D., Marsan, C., Rosvold, H., & Stevens, J. (1960). A comparison of the psychological test performance of patients with focal and non-focal epilepsy. *Experimental Neurology* 2, 79–85.

Mungas, D., Ehlers, C., Walton, N., & McCutchen, C. (1985). Verbal learning differences in epileptic patients with left and right temporal lobe foci. *Epilepsia* 26, 340–345.

Needham, W., Dustman, R., Bray, P., & Beck, E. (1969). Intelligence and EEG studies in families with idiopathic epilepsy. *JAMA* 207, 1497–1501.

Newmark, M. E., & Penry, J. K. (1979). *Photosensitivity and epilepsy: A review*. New York: Raven Press.

Novelly, R. A., Augustine, E., Mattson, R. H., Glaser, G., Williamson, P., Spencer, D., & Spencer, S. (1984). Selective memory improvement and impairment in temporal lobe epilepsy. *Annals of Neurology* 15, 64–67.

O'Donohoe, N. V. (1983). What should a child with epilepsy be allowed to do? *Archives of Disease in Childhood* 58, 934–937.

O'Leary, D., Lovell, M., Sackellares, J. C., Berent, S., Giordani, B., Seidenberg, M., & Boll, T. (1983). Effects of age of onset of partial and generalized seizures on neuropsychological performance in children. *Journal of Nervous and Mental Disease* 171, 624–629.

O'Leary, D., Seidenberg, M., Berent, S., & Boll, T. (1981). Effects of age of onset of tonic-clonic seizures on neuropsychological performance in children. *Epilepsia* 22, 197–204.

Paskind, H. (1932). Extramural patients with epilepsy with special reference to the frequent absence of deterioration. *Archives of Neurology and Psychiatry* 28, 370–385.

Peterson, G. M., McLean, S., & Millingen, K. S. (1982). Determinants of patients compliance with anticonvulsant therapy. *Epilepsia* 23, 607–613.

Pincus, J. (1980). Can violence be a manifestation of epilepsy? *Neurology* 30, 304–307.

Prevey, M. L., Delaney, R. C., & Mattson, R. H. (1988a). Gist recall in temporal lobe seizure patients: A study of adaptive memory skills. *Cortex* 24, 301–312.

Prevey, M. L., Delaney, R. C., & Mattson, R. H. (1988b). Metamemory in temporal lobe epilepsy: Self-monitoring of memory functions. *Brain and Cognition* 7, 298–311.

Pryse-Phillips, W., Jardine, F., & Bursey, F. (1982). Compliance with drug therapy by epileptic patients. *Epilepsia* 23, 269–274.

Reitan, R., & Davison, L. A. (1974). *Clinical neuropsychology: Current status and applications*. New York: Wiley and Sons.

Reynolds, E., & Trimble, M. (Eds.). (1981). *Epilepsy and psychiatry*. Edinburgh: Churchill Livingstone.

Robertson, M., & Trimble, M. R. (1983). Depressive illness in patients with epilepsy: A review. *Epilepsia* 24 (Supp. 2), S109–S116.

Rodin, E. A. (1968). *Prognosis of patients with epilepsy*. Springfield, IL: Charles & Thomas.

Rodin, E., Schmaltz, S., & Twitty, G. (1986). Intellectual functions of patients with childhood onset epilepsy. *Developmental Medicine and Child Neurology* 28, 25–33.

Roy, A. (1977). Cerebral disease and hysteria. *Comprehensive Psychiatry* 18, 607–609.

Rutter, M., Graham, P., & Yule, W. (1970). *A neuropsychiatric study in childhood. Clinics in developmental medicine Numbers 35/36*. London: S.I.M.P. and Philadelphia: Lippincott.

Scheibel, M., Crandall, P., & Scheibel, A. (1974). The hippocampal-dentate complex in temporal lobe epilepsy. *Epilepsia* 15, 55–80.

Scott, D., Moffat, A., Matthews, C., & Ettlinger, G. (1967). Effect of epileptic discharges on learning and memory in patients. *Epilepsia* 8, 188–194.

Seidenberg, M., O'Leary, D., Berent, J., & Boll, T. (1981). Changes in seizure frequency and test-retest scores on the WAIS. *Epilepsia* 22, 75–83.

Servit, Z., Machek, J., & Stercova, A. (1963). Reflex influences in the pathogenesis of epilepsy. In *Reflex mechanisms in the genesis of epilepsy*. Amsterdam: Elsevier.

Sillanpaa, M. (1975). Significance of motor handicap in the prognosis of childhood epilepsy. *Developmental Medicine and Child Neurology* 17, 52–57.

Slater, E., & Beard, E. W. (1963). Schizophrenia-like psychoses of epilepsy. *British Journal of Psychiatry* 109, 95–105.

Smith, D., Craft, B., Colins, J., Mattson, R. H., Cramer, J. A., & the VA Cooperative Study Group 118. (1986). Behavioral characteristics of epileptic patients compared to control subjects. *Epilepsia* 27, 760–768.

Snyder, M. (1983). Effect of relaxation on psychosocial functioning in persons with epilepsy. *Journal of Neurological Nursing* 15, 250–254.

Squire, L., & Cohen, N. (1984). Human memory and amnesia. In G. Lynch, J. L. McGaugh, & N. Weinberger (Eds.), *Neurobiology of learning and memory*. New York: Guilford Press.

Sterman, M. B., & Friar, L. (1971). Suppression of seizures in an epileptic following sensorimotor EEG feedback training. *Electroencephalography and Clinical Neurophysiology* 33, 89.

Stevens, J., Milstein, V., & Goldstein, S. (1972). Psychometric test performance in relation to the psychopathology of epilepsy. *Archives of General Psychiatry* 26, 532–538.

Stores, G. (1981). Problems in learning and behavior in children with epilepsy. In E. H. Reynolds & M. R. Trimble (Eds.), *Epilepsy and psychiatry*. Edinburgh: Churchill Livingstone.

Tan, Siang-Yang, and Bruni, J. (1986). Cognitive-behavior therapy with adult patients with epilepsy: A controlled outcome study. *Epilepsia* 27, 225–233.

Tartar, R. (1972). Intellectual and adaptive functioning in epilepsy. *Diseases of the Nervous System* 33, 763–770.

Temkin, N., & Davis, G. (1984). Stress as a risk factor for seizures among adults with epilepsy. *Epilepsia* 25, 450–456.

Thompson, P., & Trimble, M. (1982). Anticonvulsant drugs and cognitive functions. *Epilepsia* 23, 531–544.

Thompson, P., & Trimble, M. (1983). Anticonvulsant serum levels: Relationship to impairments of cognitive functioning. *Journal of Neurology, Neurosurgery, and Psychiatry* 46, 227–233.

Trimble, M., & Thompson, P. (1986). Neuropsychological aspects of epilepsy. In I. Grant & K. Adams (Eds.), *Neuropsychological assessment of neuropsychiatric disorders*. New York: Oxford University Press.

Tucker, D., Novelly, R. A., & Walker, P. J. (1987). Hyperreligiosity in temporal lobe epilepsy: Redefining the relationship. *Journal of Nervous and Mental Disease* 175, 181–184.

Wannamaker, B. B., & Matthews, C. (1976). Prognostic implications of neuropsychological test performance for surgical treatment of epilepsy. *Journal of Nervous and Mental Disease* 163, 29–34.

Waxman, S. G., & Geschwind, N. (1975). The interictal behavior syndrome of temporal lobe epilepsy. *Archives of General Psychiatry* 32, 1580–1588.

Webb, T., & Berman, P. (1973). Stereoscopic form disappearance in temporal lobe dysfunction. *Cortex* 9, 239–245.

Whitman, S., & Hermann, B. (Eds.). (1986). *Psychopathology in epilepsy: Social dimensions*. New York: Oxford University Press.

Winfield, D. (1951). Intellectual performance in cryptogenic epileptics, symptomatic epileptics, and post-traumatic encephalopaths. *Journal of Abnormal and Social Psychology* 46, 336–343.

Ziegler, R. G. (1981). Impairments of control and competence in epileptic children and their families. *Epilepsia* 22, 339–346.

Ziegler, R. G. (1982). The child with epilepsy. In H. Sands (Ed.), *Epilepsy: A handbook for the mental health professional*. New York: Brunner/Mazel.

Zielinski, J. J. (1986). Selected psychiatric and psychosocial aspects of epilepsy as seen by an epidemiologist. In S. Whitman & B. Hermann (Eds.), *Psychopathology in epilepsy*. New York: Oxford University Press.

6. ASSESSMENT OF EVERYDAY FUNCTIONING IN NORMAL AND MALIGNANT MEMORY DISORDERED ELDERLY

HOLLY A. TUOKKO AND DAVID J. CROCKETT

INTRODUCTION

Previous means of assessing everyday functioning may be either too limited or too broadly defined to be useful in a research context. This study describes the development of a questionnaire to obtain comprehensive information regarding collaborative informants' perceptions of the elderly patient's ability to function within everyday situations and a rating scale to provide objective estimates of impairment necessary to establish diagnoses in dementia. The existence of nonlinear relationships between rated levels of impairment and problems reported by collaborative informants suggested the possibility of multiple threshold points in the course of dementia. Multidisciplinary professionals often identified problems at a higher rate than the collaborative informants. This suggests that the collaborative informant may have either been unaware of these problems or was facilitating the impaired elderly's ability to adapt to everyday life. Neuropsychological examination indicated that measures of memory functioning were most sensitive to emerging problems in adapting to everyday functioning. Measures of expressive and receptive language functioning indicated the importance for language in determining the patients' ability to either cope with everyday life or make their needs known. These results suggested the utility of questionnaire and rating data for predicting levels of functional impairment and everyday problems in elderly samples.

Table 6–1. DSM-3 criteria for determing dementia

A. A loss of intellectual abilities of sufficient severity to interfere with social or occupational functioning
B. Memory impairment
C. At least one of the following:
    (1) impairment of abstract thinking, as manifested by concrete interpretation of proverbs, inability to find similarities and differences between related words, difficulty in defining words and concepts, and other similar tasks
    (2) impaired judgement
    (3) other disturbance of higher cognitive function, such as aphasia (disorder of language due to brain dysfunction), apraxia (inability to carry out motor activities despite intact comprehension and motor function), agnosia (failure to recognize or identify objects despite intact sensory function), "constructional difficulty" (e.g., inability to copy three-dimensional figures, assemble blocks, or arrange sticks in specific designs)
    (4) personality change (i.e., alteration or accentuation of premorbid traits)
D. State of consciousness not clouded (i.e., does not meet the criteria for delirium or intoxication, although these may be superimposed)
E. Either (1) or (2):
    (1) evidence from the history, physical examination, or laboratory tests of a specific organic factor that is judged to be etiologically related to the disturbance
    (2) in the absence of such evidence, an organic factor necessary for the development of the syndrome can be presumed if conditions other than organic mental disorders have been reasonably excluded and if the behavioral change represents cognitive impairment in a variety of areas

---

Source: Adapted from American Psychiatric Association, *Diagnostic and Statistical Manual of Mental Disorders, Third edition* (pp. 11–12), 1980.

Definitions of Dementia

Dementia is a nonspecific diagnosis referring to an overall decline in mental capacity that affects the individual's ability to cope with everyday life. It has been estimated to affect approximately 10 to 15% of the population over the age of 65 years; Alzheimer's disease, one type of dementia, alone accounts for 50% of all cases of dementia (Plum, 1979; Schneck et al., 1982; Wells, 1982). Criteria for diagnosing the presence of dementia have been developed that specify the nature of cognitive and behavioral changes involved, and many subclassifications of dementia have been suggested.

The DSM-3 (APA, 1980) criteria for diagnosing dementia are included in table 6–1. These criteria, as in most of the criteria for disorders classified by DSM-3, were developed within a group decision-making context. As such, they are essentially atheoretical but represent the clinical wisdom of professionals coming into contact with patients having this disorder. In a similar fashion, the Ninth Revision of the International Classification of Diseases (WHO, 1978) defines dementia as being organic, psychotic conditions of "chronic or progressive nature, which if untreated are usually irreversible and terminal." Organic psychotic conditions are referred to as "syndromes in which there is impairment of orientation, memory, comprehension, calculation, learning capacity, and judgment. These are essential features but there may also be: shallowness or lability of affect; more persistent disturbance of mood; lowering of ethical standards; and exaggeration or emergence of personality traits and diminished capacity for independent decision" (WHO, 1978).

In both DSM-3 and ICD-9, further criteria are applied for differentiating between types of dementing disorders. Etiological considerations serve to differentiate some forms of dementia considered possibly reversible with the provision of prompt and appropriate treatment. Specific characteristics such as onset, course, and presence of concomitant symptomology are also applied to differentiate among forms of dementia. For example, subsequent to the diagnosis of dementia, a DSM-3 diagnosis of Primary Degenerative Dementia (PDD: 290.XX) may be made if, as essential features, the dementia is of an insidious onset and gradual progressive course for which all other specified causes have been excluded by history, physical examination, and laboratory tests. Phenomenological subtypes within the diagnostic category of PDD include distinction between age of onset and clinical presentation with delirium, delusions, depression, or uncomplicated.

Criteria for the DSM-3 diagnosis of PDD parallel the research criteria established by the NINCDS-ADRDA Work Group for Alzheimer's Type Dementia. (McKhann et al. 1984). These research criteria are presented in table 6–2. These criteria initially specify that the decline of memory and other cognitive functioning must be present when compared to the patient's previous level of functioning as determined by a history of decline in performance and by abnormalities noted from clinical examination and neuropsychological tests. When delirium, drowsiness, stupor, coma, or other clinical abnormalities prevent adequate evaluation of mental status, a diagnosis of dementia *cannot be made*. Although the application of these criteria have enhanced our ability to compare research work done across groups, it has done little to clarify standards for evaluating functioning in everyday life.

The identification of Alzheimer's type dementia involves the application of exclusionary criteria only after a diagnosis of dementia has been made. It is apparent from these various definitions that cognitive and behavioral deterioration is the hallmark of dementia during life and deficits in activities of daily living would be expected, as a matter of course. Various approaches have been taken to assessment and description of a patient's cognitive and behavioral status in order to establish the presence of dementia and document deterioration over time. Many examination procedures have been employed in order to provide a brief, yet limited investigation of the diverse range of cognitive abilities subsumed under the rubric of "mental status." Unfortunately, there has been a tendency to confuse the concept "mental status," which often includes a much more diverse range of cognitive skills than could be possibly represented in a 30-item test, with the name of an instrument designed to provide a *brief* screening tool to be used in a clinical situation. It should be apparent that a patient's mental status is not equivalent to any single test score. Although these brief "mental status" examinations are easy to administer and

Table 6–2. Criteria for clinical diagnosis of Alzheimer's disease from the NINCDS-ADRDA report

I. The criteria for the clinical diagnosis of PROBABLE Alzheimer's disease include:
  – dementia established by clinical examination and documented by the Mini-Mental Test (Folstein et al., 1975), Blessed Dementia Scale (Blessed et al., 1968), or some similar examination, and confirmed by neuropsychological tests
  – deficits in two or more areas of cognition
  – progressive worsening of memory and other cognitive functions
  – no disturbance of consciousness
  – onset between ages 40 and 90, most often after age 65
  – absence of systemic disorders or other brain diseases that in and of themselves could account for the progressive deficits in memory and cognition
II. The diagnosis of PROBABLE Alzheimer's disease is supported by:
  – progressive deterioration of specific cognitive functions such as language (aphasia), motor skills (apraxia), and perception (agnosia)
  – impaired activities of daily living and altered patterns of behavior
  – family history of similar disorders, particularly if confirmed neuropathologically
  – laboratory results of:
    – normal lumbar puncture as evaluated by standard techniques
    – normal pattern or nonspecific changes in EEG, such as increased slow-wave activity
    – evidence of cerebral atrophy on CT with progression documented by serial observation
III. Other clinical features consistent with the diagnosis of PROBABLE Alzheimer's disease, after exclusion of causes of dementia other than Alzheimer's disease, include:
  – plateaus in the course of progression of the illness
  – associated symptoms of depression; insomnia; incontinence; delusions; illusions; hallucinations; catastrophic verbal, emotional, or physical outbursts; sexual disorders; and weight loss
  – other neurological abnormalities in some patients, especially with more advanced disease, and including motor signs such as increased muscle tone, myoclonus, or gait disorder
  – seizures in advanced disease
  – CT normal for age
IV. Features that make the diagnosis of PROBABLE Alzheimer's disease uncertain or unlikely include:
  – sudden, apoplectic onset
  – focal neurologic findings such as hemiparesis, sensory loss, visual field deficits, and incoordination early in the course of the illness
  – seizures or gait disturbances at the onset or very early in the course of the illness
V. Clinical diagnosis of POSSIBLE Alzhiemer's disease:
  – may be made on the basis of the dementia syndrome, in the absence of the neurologic, psychiatric, or systemic disorders sufficient to cause dementia, and in the presence of variations in the onset, in the presentation, or in the clinical course
  – may be made in the presence of a second systemic or brain disorder sufficient to produce dementia, which is not considered to be the cause of the dementia
  – should be used in research studies when a single, gradually progressive severe cognitive deficit is identified in the absence of other identifiable cause
VI. Criteria for diagnosis of DEFINITE Alzheimer's disease are:
  – the clinical criteria for probable Alzheimer's disease
  – histopathologic evidence obtained from a biopsy or autopsy
VII. Classification of Alzheimer's disease for research purposes should specify features that may differentiate subtypes of the disorder, such as:
  – familial occurrence
  – onset before age of 65
  – presence of trisomy-21
  – coexistence of other relevant conditions such as Parkinson's disease

Source: Adapted from McKhann et al., 1984.

may provide some information regarding the upper and lower range of a patient's status, their sensitivity is limited for the purpose of detecting mild deficits or documenting changes over the entire course of the disease. Moreover, these abbreviated measures do not correlate well with other measures of daily living (Winograd, 1984).

Extensive assesssment of cognitive and behavioral functioning via quantitative neuropsychological testing (NPT) procedures may be particularly useful for disclosing subtle abnormalities in mentally impaired patients and for characterizing the exact type of disabilities they exhibit. For example, memory loss is essential for establishing a diagnosis of dementia, but the specific details regarding the type or types of memory disorders are not mandated by the diagnostic systems and require further clarification (Miller, 1971; Tuokko & Crockett, 1987). As apparent from the definitions of dementia and the criteria for specific types of dementia (e.g., PDD), wide variations may exist in terms of the presence of other cognitive impairments such as receptive/expressive language deficits, deficits in visual-spatial, and verbal-abstract problem solving skills. Clarifying the unique aspects of an individual's functioning within and across areas of cognitive ability is an ongoing process (Martin et al., 1986) and will potentially contribute even more to our comprehensive understanding of the capacity of impaired elderly patients for engaging in independent living.

As an alternative to objective measures of performance, some rating scales have been developed for the purpose of characterizing the level of residual independent functioning in patients with dementia. Berger (1980) described a unidimensional scale to determine the level of severity of dementia based on how much personal assistance the patient requires. More recent attempts at developing scales have focused on characterizing the stages of dementia across various domains of functioning. The Global Deterioration Scale (GDS), by Reisberg and co-workers (1982), is another example of a unidimensional scale describing clusters of symptoms associated with the development of PDD. For each stage of PDD, the clinical characteristics are defined with particular emphasis on memory functioning, although alterations in social skills, self-care functioning, problem solving, comprehension, and personality-emotional changes are included as well. In contrast, the Clinical Dementia Rating (CDR), by Hughes et al. (1982), is a multidimensional scale for assessing the various components of cognitive and behavioral functioning, including memory, orientation, judgment and problem-solving, community affairs, and home/hobbies. These areas are rated by the examiner on a 5-point scale from healthy to severely impaired. The memory scale is the primary criterion for determining the presence of dementia. The frequency of occurrence of other scores above, below, or equal to the memory scale is used to define the actual level of impairment exhibited by the patient. This allows for the possibility that the patients may deviate in their rate of decline across areas of functioning.

Both the GDS and CDR were developed for the purpose of assessing various stages of PDD, but only after the initial diagnosis of PDD was established. No attempt was made to take into account factors that may be important for consideration while the diagnosis is being established. Both the Dementia of the Alzheimer Type (DAT) Inventory (Cummings & Benson, 1986) and the Functional Rating Scale (FRS) (Tuokko et al., 1986) were designed to improve the accuracy in establishing the diagnosis of PDD. The FRS also facilitates the collection of important information regarding the patient's everyday functioning.

The DAT inventory assesses a total of ten parameters, five of which measure intellectual ability (memory, visuospatial, cognitive, personality, and language) and five that evaluate primarily motor functioning (speech, psychomotor speed, posture, gait, and movement). These domains were used in keeping with the original description of DAT (Alzheimer, 1977) as a progressive dementia with prominent features of aphasia, amnesia, and cognitive impairment but with relatively intact psychomotor functioning, except at the final stages of this disease. To emphasize this clinical pattern, the authors assigned a weight of 3 to each domain such that the highest score is associated with the most abnormal intellectual functioning and relatively preserved psychomotor functioning. In a retrospective study of patients with a diagnosis of DAT (Cummings & Benson, 1986), the DAT inventory was clinically useful for differentiating between patients with and without DAT.

The FRS was developed in an attempt to define the necessary components for establishing the diagnosis of dementia. The individual scales and their anchor points are contained in table 6–3. The areas of functioning are compatible with the criteria described by DSM-3 and ICD-9 as definitions of dementia. The ratings are to be made on the basis of medical history, clinical examination, laboratory assessment, and information from a collaborative informant. To establish the diagnosis of DAT, the criteria behavior must not only be exhibited but also be present in the form of an insidious onset and in the absence of any other systemic or brain diseases that might produce the cognitive deficits. Memory functioning is given a prominent role, in keeping with its status as a crucial variable in establishing a diagnosis of dementia. Language skills and affect are also rated since they may be extremely important in making diagnostic decisions and in planning follow-up care. The traditional components of social/community/occupation; homes/hobbies; personal care; and problem solving/reasoning are also included, in keeping with the accepted definitions of dementia. The FRS serves as a vehicle to facilitate input for members from multidisciplinary teams and to allow the monitoring of changes in patient functioning over time.

Everyday Functioning

In the broadest sense, the concept of everyday functioning may be equated with Lawton's (1983) construct of "behavioral competency." Investigators vary widely in their assumptions regarding the number and types of behavior

Table 6–3. Components and threshold points for functional rating scale

Variable	Healthy (1)	Questionable (2)	Mild (3)	Moderate (4)	Severe (5)
Memory	No deficit or inconsistent forgetfulness evident only on clinical interview	Variable symptoms reported by patient or relative; seemingly unrelated to level of functioning	Memory losses which interfere with daily living; more apparent for recent events	Moderate memory loss; only highly learned material retained, new material rapidly lost	Severe memory loss; unable to recall relevant aspects of current life, very sketchy recall of past life
Social/ community and occupational	Neither patient nor relatives aware of any deficit	Variable levels of functioning reported by patient or relatives; no objective evidence of deficits in employment or social situations	Patient or relative aware of decreased performance in demanding employment or social settings; appears normal to casual inspection	Patient or relative aware of ongoing deterioration; does not appear normal to objective observer; unable to perform job; little independent functioning outside home	Marked impairment of social functioning; no independent functioning outside home
Home and hobbies	No changes noted by patient or relative	Slightly decreased involvement in household tasks and hobbies	Engages in social activities in the home but definite impairment on some household tasks; some complicated hobbies and interests abandoned	Only simple chores/ hobbies preserved; most complicated hobbies/ interests abandoned	No independent involvement in home or hobbies

Table 6–3. (continued)

Variable	Healthy (1)	Questionable (2)	Mild (3)	Moderate (4)	Severe (5)
Personal care	Fully capable of self-care	Occasional problems with self-care reported by patient/relatives or observed	Needs prompting to complete tasks adequately (i.e. dressing, feeding, hygiene)	Requires supervision in dressing, feeding, hygiene and keeping track of personal effects	Needs constant supervision and assistance with feeding, dressing, or hygiene, etc.
Language skills	No disturbance of language reported by patient or relative	Subjective complaint of, or relative reports, language deficits; usually limited to word finding or naming	Patient or relative reports variable disturbances of such skills as articulation or naming; occasional language impairment evident during examination	Patient or relative reports consistent language disturbance, language disturbance evident on examination	Severe impairment of receptive and/or expressive language; production of unintelligible speech
Problem solving and reasoning	Solves everyday problems adequately	Variable impairment of problem solving, similarities, differences	Difficulty in handling complex problems	Marked impairment on complex problem solving tasks	Unable to solve problems at any level; trial and error behaviour often observed
Affect	No change in affect reported by patient or relative	Appropriate concern with respect to symptomatology	Infrequent changes in affect (e.g. irritability) reported by patient or relative; would appear normal to objective observer	Frequent changes in affect reported by patient or relative; noticeable to objective observer	Sustained alterations of affect; impaired contact with reality observed or reported
Orientation	Fully oriented	Occasional difficulties with time relationships	Marked difficulty with time relationships	Usually disoriented to time and often to place	Oriented only to person or not at all

Source: Adapted from Tuokko et al., 1986.

indicative of behavioral competency. Lawton summarized the most agreed upon domains as follows: physical health, physical self-maintenance skills, cognition, instrumental activities of daily living, time use, and social behavior. Each of these areas is crucial to the comprehensive assessment of the older individual's capacity to function independently in the community. Additional areas such as "nutritional status" and "presence of behavioral psychiatric symptoms" should be included in order to evaluate more fully everyday functioning in elderly samples (Lawton, 1983). Moreover, events external to these individuals such as availability of housing, neighborhood quality, economic resources, as well as the subjective evaluation of psychological well-being and subjective evaluation of external situations, may be predictive of behavioral competence in elderly individuals.

The Philadelphia Geriatric Center Multi-Level Assessment Instrument (MAI) was developed by Lawton and co-workers (1982) as an integrated assessment package to address most of these issues. Indices and subindices are provided for the following domains: physical health (self-rated health, reported condition, and health behavior); functional health (physical and instrumental activities of daily living); cognition (mental status and cognitive symptoms); time use; social behavior (family and friends); personal adjustment (morale and psychological symptoms); and perceived environmental quality (housing, neighborhood, and security).

Other comprehensive batteries include the Duke University Older American's Resource and Service Multi-Dimensional Functional Questionnaire (OARS) (Duke University Center, 1978), the Comprehensive Assessment and Referral Evaluation (CARE) (Gurland et al., 1977–1978), and the Self-Evaluation of Life Function (SELF) (Linn & Linn, 1984). The OARS allows ratings of the subject's well-being in the following domains: physical health, mental health (combining cognitive skills and psychological health), activities of daily living (physical and instrumental), social (both time use and inter-action with family and friends), and economic. The CARE consists of 1500 items covering a wide range of psychiatric, medical, and social problems of elderly adults. One of the major drawbacks of these extensive scales is the time demands they might make on frail, sometimes multiply handicapped, subjects. Reduced versions have been developed that focus on even more limited aspects of functioning.

Of these, the SHORT-CARE and CORE-CARE batteries are the most commonly encountered in the research literature. The SHORT-CARE (Gurland et al., 1984) consists of selected items from the indicator scales of depression/demoralization, dementia, subjective memory impairment, sleep disorders, somatic symptoms and disability, and additional items for arriving at an operational diagnosis of depression, dementia, and disability. The CORE-CARE (Golden, Teresi, & Gurland, 1984) provides an extensive view of each individual based on inquiries into medical, psychiatric, and social realms of functioning. The CORE-CARE contains information on many of the instrumental activities of daily living measured by the OARS or MAI batteries, but in greater detail. The SELF is a self-report scale that measures physical disability, symptoms of aging, self-esteem, social satisfaction, depression, and personal control. The major advantage of this measure is its brevity (i.e., 55 items), which lends itself to situations where assessment time is limited. However, the fact that this is solely a self-report instrument limits its usefulness in problematic settings as in the assessment of dementing or amnesic patients who may not be able to provide accurate information.

More circumscribed measures of functioning on everyday tasks have focused on limited areas such as "activities of daily living" (ADL) and "instrumental activities of daily living" (IADL). ADL instruments tend to focus on the diverse set of skills represented by the domain of physical self-maintenance skills such as toileting, dressing, eating habits, bathing, ambulation, and grooming. In contrast, IADL measures tend to assess more complex activities of daily life, such as shopping, use of transportation, cooking, house cleaning, laundry, use of telephone, medical compliance, financial management, and heavy house- and yardwork. Linn and Linn (1981) reported on the use of ADL instruments in community-dwelling elderly and indicated that very little disability was revealed in these groups and that their ratings were very stable over time. They concluded that these instruments were more appropriate to hospitalized patients, particularly those with physical illness alone or in combination with mental illness, but not much use in assessing benign elderly. IADL instruments tend not to be applicable to most institutionalized patients, as the institution often performs the function assessed by these items. Thus IADL measures focus on behaviors in which nonperformance is likely to signal a degree of impairment that would demand intervention by others primarily for the community dwelling segment of the elderly population.

Many ADL scales have been developed and published, but the reliability and validity of these scales remains unspecified. However, two specific indices may be useful to assess particular aspects of ADL: the Physical Self-Maintenance Scale (PSMS) (Lawton & Brody, 1969) and the Rapid Disability Rating Scale (RDRS-2) (Linn, 1967; Linn & Linn, 1982). The PSMS was designed to coordinate observations in various areas—toileting, eating, dressing, grooming, ambulation, and bathing—by having the care-giving staff provide rating of five levels of functioning ranging from "completely independent" to "dependent." Of particular interest is the RDRS-2, for it includes areas of physical functioning beyond the usual components of ADL scales. The ADL areas covered by the RDRS-2 include eating, walking, mobility, bathing, dressing, toileting, grooming, and adaptive tasks (managing money/possessions, telephoning, and buying newspapers, toilet articles, or snacks). Additional areas assessed include items reflecting Degrees of Disabilities (communication, hearing, sight, diet, in bed during day, incontinence, and medications) and Degree of Special Problems (mental confusion, uncooperativeness, and depression). Each item in the instrument is to be rated on a 4-point scale in terms of the amount of assistance or degree of disability evidenced by the subject.

The Instrumental Activities of Daily Living Scale (IADLS) (Lawton & Brody, 1969) rates subjects along scales ranging from 3 to 5 points. Each scale point was defined in order to reflect varying degrees of competency in the following areas: ability to use a telephone, shopping, food preparation, housekeeping, laundry, mode of transportation, responsibility for own medication, and ability to handle finances. The OARS incoporates the IADLS in its schedule of interviews as a separate composite scale, but the individual items making up the IADLS have not been analyzed or published as separate components (Lawton, 1983). The IADLS and its companion scale, the PSMS, have been used in the evaluation of individuals residing in or applying for admission to institutions of various types, as well as patients admitted to psychiatric screening wards and residents of institutions for whom returning to the community was under consideration (Linn & Linn, 1983). They reported that the correlation ($Rxy = 0.61$) between the two scales indicated a moderate degree of overlap between functioning on these two scales.

It has been postulated that cognitive facilities and daily living activities may deteriorate at different rates, particularly in the early stages of dementing disorders (Weintraub, Baratz, & Mesulam, 1982), but this assumption has yet to be evaluated in the research literature. Clinically, Weintraub et al. reported two case studies of elderly individuals in which there was marked discrepency between the extent of their cognitive deficits and the degree of impairment in daily living activities. Also, Vitaliano and colleagues (1984) examined the degree to which cognitive test scores could predict functional competency in patients with DAT. Their samples included 23 controls, 18 mildly impaired DATs, and 16 moderately impaired DAT patients. Attention and memory items, selected from Mini-Mental State Examination (Folstein, Folstein, & McHugh, 1975), and the Dementia Rating Scale (Coblentz et al., 1973; Mattis, 1976), were grouped into five classes of cognitive functioning: attention, calculation, recognition memory, recall, and orientation. The Record of Independent Living (Weintraub et al., 1982) was used to assess functional competency. This measure assessed basic activities of living as well as higher-level activities such as recreation, reading, and writing. It was possible to predict some aspects of functional competency in DAT patients from a knowledge of attention and memory scores. Lower levels of functional competence were associated with poor performance on relatively simple tests of recall and recognition.

By definition, disturbances in everyday functioning would be assumed in the presence of dementia, but the relationship between the instruments used in the assessment of dementia and measures of everyday functioning have not been thoroughly investigated. Even though the presence of impairment in social functioning is required to meet the criteria for diagnosis of dementia, very little is known about the forms these impairments may take or how they change as the disease progresses. Moreover, although the utility of neuropsychological instruments for predicting "everyday" life functioning has been investigated in a variety of other disorders of neurological patients, very little attention has been focused on the elderly and groups of demented patients.

This review of the criteria for establishing the diagnoses in dementing patients and the techniques for gathering such information indicates that there are some major gaps in our understanding of the relationship of everyday functioning to the dementing process. In the remainder of this chapter, we hope to provide some psychometric information regarding the utility of rating scales designed to assess everyday functioning in elderly samples. The reliability and discriminant validity of each of the measures from different data sources will be established in order to justify further analyses. In addition, we present a model for analyzing the relationship of data coming from significant others, professionals who have assessed the dementing patient, and objective test performance by the patient. This model will be based on the severity of impairment shown by the patient rather than a focal-feature model. Although other models may have been used, it is hoped that the subsequent analyses will indicate that the amount of improvement in our ability to predict everyday functioning based on these other, alternative models will be a minimal.

INSTRUMENTS

Before describing the variables used in this study, a few words are in order regarding the way in which they were selected. The challenge for professionals involved with assessing patients with Alzheimer's disease or related dementing disorders is to choose appropriate instruments. Although the assessment needs will vary depending on whether the inquiry involves diagnostic issues, care/management planning, in- or outpatients, and time constraints, it is imperative that a broad range of cognitive and behavioral measures be utilized in order to fully understand the nature of the disorder and how it impinges on everyday functioning.

To be included in this research, our assessment procedures had to satisfy a number of criteria. They had to be (1) related to the signs and symptoms associated with dementing disorders; (2) behaviorally defined with objective anchor points to describe the levels of functioning measured by them; (3) capable of being corroborated by either an examiner or a reliable informant; (4) capable of demonstrating adequate reliability and validity coefficients; and (5) samples of the data domains represented by observations from significant others, clinical investigations, and neuropsychological functioning. These criteria are interrelated in that objective measures will often demonstrate adequate reliability and validity, whereas representative measures of the domains of everyday functioning in the elderly will most often include aspects of patient functioning relevant to establishing diagnoses in the area of dementia.

On the other hand, selecting the variables on the basis of these requirements imposed on the design some significant limitations. For example, by confining ourselves to objective measures that are repeatable by reliable observers, we rule out employing a case study approach that might focus on the subjective experience in the elderly associated with their encountering either success or frustration in everyday life. By the same token, our insistence on measures that would demonstrate reliable differences among subjects implies that we would employ relatively large numbers of subjects and made an attempt to measure changes in the organic substrata associated with these changes in levels of everyday functioning impractical. It was felt that these limitations were acceptable in that elaborate microscopic studies of patients with very selective features may be more relevant to the development of models of brain–behavior relationships than the assessment of everyday functioning.

Present Functioning Questionnaire

The Present Functioning Questionnaire (PFQ) was constructed by reviewing the research literature associated with problems of everyday functioning in elderly (W. J. Koch, personal communication). Sixty items were developed to reflect the deficits reported in this population and were organized into five problem areas: personality, everyday functioning, language skills, memory, and self-care. Items were scored on a presence or absence basis, as presented

Table 6–4. Present Functioning Questionnaire (PFQ)

Variable	Presence/Absence
Personality	
Being irritable or angry	_____
Being misersable or depressed	_____
Being tense or panicky	_____
Being apathetic	_____
Being agitated or hyperactive	_____
Being anxious or afraid	_____
Stating that "things aren't real"	_____
Complaining of "upsetting thoughts"	_____
Being aggressive	_____
Being suspicious	_____
Being insensitive to others' feelings	_____
Showing inappropriate smiles or laughter	_____
Showing decreased hobby involvement	_____
Talking to imaginary others	_____
Exhibiting inappropriate sexual activities	_____
Everyday Tasks	
Problems performing household tasks	_____
Problems handling money	_____
Problems shopping	_____
Problems finding their way inside a house or building	_____
Problems finding their way around familiar streets	_____
Problems recognizing surroundings	_____
Problems recognizing the date or day of the week	_____
Problems recognizing the time of day	_____
Awaking at night and thinking it is day	_____
Problems reading (except as caused by poor vision)	_____
Problems performing job	_____
Problems driving a car (if could before)	_____

Table 6–4. (continued)

Variable	Presence/Absence
Language Skills	
Problems finding words to express him/herself	_____
Losing his/her vocabulary	_____
Problems pronouncing words	_____
Problems understanding others	_____
More frequently slurring words	_____
Problems clipping ends off words or sentences	_____
More frequently stuttering	_____
Problems finding names for common objects	_____
Problems forming any intelligible speech	_____
Memory Functions	
Problems remembering previous actions on the same day	_____
Problems remembering past life events	_____
Asking questions repeatedly (despite answers)	_____
Problems recognizing faces of old friends or family	_____
Problems recognizing names of old friends or family members	_____
Problems remembering newly introduced persons	_____
Problems leaving stove burners, water taps, and light switches turned on	_____
Problems maintaining a train of thought	_____
Problems remembering where he/she placed objects	_____
Problems concentrating	_____
Increasingly frustrated over problems remembering or thinking	_____
Increasingly defensive about problems remembering	_____
Problems remembering important personal dates	_____
Seemingly unaware of important current events	_____
Does not know own name	_____
Self-Care Functions	
Eating messily with spoon only	_____
Eating messily with spoon *and* with solid foods	_____
Has to be fed by someone else	_____
Problems dressing, e.g., occasional misplaced buttons	_____
Problems dressing, e.g., puts on clothes in wrong sequence	_____
Problems dressing, e.g., unable to dress self	_____
Problems with occasionally wetting bed	_____
Problems with frequently wetting bed	_____
Doubly incontinent	_____
Does not wash him/herself enough	_____
Must be bathed by someone else	_____
Grooming (combing of hair, etc.) inadequate	_____
Must be groomed by someone else	_____
Needs constant supervision in caring for self	_____

Source: Adapted from: W. J. Koch (personal communication).

in table 6–4. Once the scales were constructed, the test was administered in a structured interview format. Care was taken to pursue problem areas, even if initial inquiry resulted in denial of symptoms. When symptoms were reported within an area, they were used as further probes into other areas of everyday functioning that may be problematic but denied on previous inquiry. These probes would take the form of inquiring first whether the individual had noted a problem, and then whether he or she had noted any other problems in that

Table 6–5. Psychometric characteristics of the Present Functioning Questionnaire (PFQ)

No. of Items	Item–Total Correlation Range	Reliability Coefficient Alpha
Personality Total	.33–.49	.8106
Everyday Tasks Total	.36–.75	.8829
Language Skills Total	.33–.73	.8028
Memory Total	.41–.67	.8835
Self-Care Total	.42–.71	.9020

**Correlation Matrix for
Scales of the PFQ**

SCALE	PART–WHOLE CORRELATION	PTOT	ETOT	LSTOT	MEMTOT
Personality Total	.63				
Everyday Tasks Total	.84	.595			
Language Skills Total	.65	.386	.638		
Memory Total	.75	.640	.750	.568	
Self-Care Total	.60	.395	.664	.546	.433

Note: Reliability coefficient alpha = .865.

area. The source of information for this questionnaire was a collaborative informant, usually the patient's spouse or, more rarely, the patient's child. All interviewing of the collaborative informant was done separately from the patient.

To determine the reliability of this instrument, the psychometric characteristics of each PFQ subscale were computed, as shown in table 6–5. An examination of the item—total correlation matrices associated with each one of the subscales indicated that two items, item 15 of the Personality Subscale (i.e., "exhibits inappropriate sexual activities") and item 15 of the Memory Subscale (i.e., "does not know own name"), had inadequate reliability and thus were discarded. After these items were discarded, the range of the item— total correlations was sufficiently high to ensure adequate overall subscale reliability (i.e., .8028–.9020) and low enough to ensure a heterogeneous sample of the activities of everyday life was obtained. Table 6–5 also shows the correlation matrix for the PFQ subscales. The range of intercorrelations of these subscales (i.e., .38–.84) was high enough to imply a high degree of consistency of competency in everyday life yet low enough to indicate that substantially different areas of everyday functioning were being measured. The reliability coefficient (i.e., alpha = .865) was also sufficiently high to indicate that this measure was relatively stable.

Table 6–6 contains the means and standard deviations for the individual subscales of the PFQ for the normal elderly (NE), malignant memory disorder group (MMD), and the combined group. The normal elderly samples consisted of 70 volunteers recruited from senior citizens activity groups in the community. The subjects had a mean age of 70.2 years (range = 50–90; SD = 7.6).

Table 6–6. Means and standard deviation (SD) for normal elderly (NE) and malignant memory disorder (MMD) groups in the Present Functioning Questionnaire

Variable	NE	MMD	F value	NE & MMD
Personality Total				
Mean	1.40	5.43	104.39	4.63
SD	1.91	3.16		3.33
N	70	298		368
Everyday Tasks Total				
Mean	.17	5.19	153.31	4.29
SD	.589	3.40		3.69
N	70	298		368
Language Skills Total				
Mean	.16	2.79	93.10	2.34
SD	.65	2.28		2.37
N	70	298		368
Memory Total				
Mean	.80	8.17	311.36	6.77
SD	1.62	3.43		4.28
N	70	298		368
Self-Care Total				
Mean	.09	1.98	27.59	1.71
SD	.442	3.02		2.97
N	70	298		368
Present Functioning Total				
Mean	2.60	23.70	219.85	19.81
SD	3.68	11.83		13.60
N	70	298		368

Notes: 95% confidence interval for PTOT $\quad$ = (1.64 × 1.91) + 1.40 = 4.53.
$\quad\quad$ 95% confidence interval for ETOT $\quad$ = (1.64 × .59) + .17 = 1.14.
$\quad\quad$ 95% confidence interval for LSTOT $\quad$ = (1.64 × .65) + .16 = 1.22.
$\quad\quad$ 95% confidence interval for MEMTOT = (1.64 × 1.62) + .80 = 3.45.
$\quad\quad$ 95% confidence interval for SCTOT $\quad$ = (1.64 × .44) + .09 = .83.
$\quad\quad$ All F values (df = 1/352) significant ($p < .001$).

Twenty-eight (39.7%) of the subjects were male and 42 (60.3%) were female. Each subject was judged suitable for inclusion in the study on the basis of interview and medical questionnaire material. Only individuals who met the following criteria were included: (1) not receiving institutional care or services, (2) no present treatment for neurological or psychiatric disturbance, and (3) age 50 or older. The subjects in the NE group typically reported few problems. Out of the 63 possible problems, the NE group indicated the presence of, on average, less than three problems (PFQTOT mean = 2.86; SD = 3.84). From the observed rate of collaborative informant reported problems, it is apparent that this is a very benign normal elderly group. There existed consistent and statistically significant differences between the NE and MMD groups. These data indicate that the PFQ has an acceptable level of reliability and discriminant validity.

Despite the PFQ's demonstration of adequate reliability and discriminant validity, it was necessary to examine the influence of demographic variables on this questionnaire. When subjects who were within a continuing relationship, whether common-law or marriage, were compared to those who were currently without such a relationship (i.e., single, widowed, or separated), no significant multivariate or univariate relationships were found on the PFQ. On the other hand, age and self-reported level of education were more closely related to level of reported problems on the PFQ. For all subjects, age was related to the number of problems reported in the areas measured by PTOT ($R = .12$; $p < .009$), ETOT ($R = .15$; $p < .002$), MEMTOT ($R = .19$; $p < .001$), and SCTOT ($R = .128$; $p < .007$). Though consistent, the relationship was nonetheless small, typically accounting for less than 4% of the variance. Self-reported levels of education had the same small but significant relationship with PTOT ($R = -.21$; $p < .001$), ETOT ($R = -.17$; $p < .001$), LSTOT ($R = -.136$; $p < .005$), MEMTOT ($R = -.229$; $p < .001$), and SCTOT ($R = .093$; $p < .04$). Overall, it was felt that the existence of these small but reliable trends did not compromise the interpretation of our data.

The Functional Rating Scale

The Functional Rating Scale (FRS) (Tuokko et al., 1986) was developed to assist in establishing a diagnosis and monitoring patient changes in functioning over time. In developing this instrument a multidimensional approach was used. Eight areas of psychosocial functioning were rated along a 5-point scale: memory; social/occupational/community functioning; home and hobbies; problem solving; personal care; affect; language; and orientation. The areas and the rating scale are presented in table 6–3, and the means and standard deviations in table 6–7. The rating criteria for memory, social/occupational/community functioning, home and hobbies, problem solving, personal care, and orientation were devised to conform to the hierarchical structure of deficits associated with PDD (Hughes, 1982). Memory function was given a prominent role as were language skills and affect because they can be extremely important in making differential diagnostic decisions about management, planning, follow-up care and/or treatment. For example, language disorders are a common occurrence in some forms of dementia but not in others (e.g., dementias of the Alzheimer type and Huntington's disease, respectively) (Albert, 1987). Social/community/occupational, home and hobbies, personal care, and problem solving/reasoning components were also included because they are crucial to establishing the diagnosis of dementia (APA, 1980).

The interdisciplinary team members rated patients independently on the basis of information obtained from the referral source and from their own structured interviews. The multidisciplinary team included a neuropsychologist, a social worker, a psychiatrist, and a geriatrician/internist. Individual interviews with the patient and primary care giver, usually a spouse or close relative, were conducted by each team member. Each member of the assess-

Table 6–7. Means and standard deviation (SD) for malignant
memory disorder (MMD) groups on the Functional Rating Scale (FRS)

FRS Variables	Group 1 $n = 70$	Group 2 $n = 77$	Group 3 $n = 74$	Group 4 $n = 79$	F value df = 3/299
Memory					
Mean	2.09	2.99	3.59	4.68	275.92
SD	0.63	0.60	0.57	0.47	
Social					
Mean	2.16	3.09	3.71	4.48	263.11
SD	0.69	0.37	0.48	0.50	
Home					
Mean	1.91	2.90	3.70	4.47	201.88
SD	0.76	0.68	0.64	0.57	
Personal Care					
Mean	1.09	1.45	2.40	4.00	209.03
SD	0.28	0.62	0.94	1.04	
Language					
Mean	1.40	2.04	2.74	4.11	140.65
SD	0.62	0.95	0.86	0.92	
Problem Solving					
Mean	1.43	2.53	3.53	4.53	239.89
SD	0.55	1.02	0.69	0.60	
Affect					
Mean	2.80	3.19	3.44	4.10	20.19
SD	1.08	0.99	1.16	0.99	
Orientation					
Mean	1.24	2.19	3.16	4.58	296.94
SD	0.55	0.71	0.94	0.61	

Note: Since average ratings on the FRS were used to assign subjects to MMD groups, F value may be inflated. All F values beyond $p = .0001$. Group 1 (FRS ≤ 2.13); Group 2 (2.14 ≤ FRS ≤ 2.88); Group 3 (2.89 ≤ FRS ≤ 3.63); Group 4 (3.64 ≤ FRS).

ment team developed his or her own structured interview for assessing the patient's level of functioning. Subsequently, each patient underwent a neurological evaluation to assess the presence of significant neurological signs or symptoms for use in making a differential diagnosis when the condition of dementia had been established. However, no rating on the FRS was contributed by the neurologist.

The subjects for the interrater reliability study of the FRS were 52 consecutive referrals to the Clinic for Alzheimer Diseases and Related Disorders, University Hospital. There were 20 male and 32 female patients in the sample, with an average age of 70.0 years (range = 53 to 85; SD = 7.7). Manifest right handedness was reported by 96% of the group, and an average of 11.5 years of education (range = 6–19; SD = 2.9) was reported. Subjects for the study of the intervariable relationships were a group of 358 subjects resulting from combining the NE and MMD groups. There were 159 male and 199 female subjects with a mean age of 70.1 years (range = 40 to 88; SD = 8.4). A mean of 11.8 years of education was reported by this sample (range 0–21; SD = 3.4).

The interrater reliability for the FRS was determined by calculating Cronbach's Alpha (Cronbach, 1951) for each of the scales between the four raters. The intervariable relationships were examined using a principal component analysis (PCA). The four scores for each scale were summed across judges, producing one set of eight scores for each patient. All calculations were performed using SPSS-X (SPSS-X, 1983). The Pearson product–moment correlation matrix of the eight scales was then calculated. The PCA was performed and all factors with eigen values greater than 1.0 were retained. The retained factor matrix was rotated using varimax procedures.

Table 6–7 contains the results of a one-way analysis of variance comparison between groups of MMD subjects formed on the basis of the overall ratings of their functioning as measured by the FRS according to the method described by Tuokko et al. (1986). Group 1 had the lowest levels of observed problems in the eight areas (FRS < 2.13), group 2 (2.14 < FRS < 2.88) and group 3 (2.89 < FRS < 3.63) had an intermediate level of observed impairment, and group 4 (3.64 < FRS) had the greatest degree of impairment. All comparisons were highly significant, indicating the groups' ratings on the individual scales making up the FRS had non-overlapping distributions and were strongly related to overall estimates of their functioning. Since the average ratings in all eight scales of the FRS were used to assign the subjects to their groups, the F values for the individual scales may have been inflated. An additional comparison using a linear discriminant function analysis (LDFA) indicated that 89.8% of the subjects could be assigned to their correct group. This indicates the homogeneity of functioning in MMD subjects across the eight areas of everyday skills. The alpha coefficients for the FRS were: affect, .87; language, .92; social/community/occupational, .95; home and hobbies, .96; personal care, .96; problem solving, .96; orientation, .96; and memory, .97—indicating that the interrater reliability of these scales was very good. The PCA produced a single factor containing high loadings for all eight dimensions of the rating scale. This single factor accounted for approximately 77.5% of the variance. The loadings on this factor for the subscales for the FRS were: affect, .69; language, .84; social/community/occupation, .94; home and hobbies, .92; personal care, .86; problem solving, .91; orientation, .91; and memory, .94. These loadings suggest that patient ratings were typically similar across domains and reflect the presence of a generalized level of impairment.

Neuropsychological Test Battery

The neuropsychological test battery was constructed to measure a wide variety of skills and abilities that we felt would be necessary to enable the patient to function within a variety of everyday situations. All subjects were administered the Multifocus Assessment Scale for the frail elderly according to the manual for this test battery (MAS) (Coval et al., 1985). The MAS comprises eight subscales and is typically administered within a 45-minute time frame. The subscales consist of three rating subscales and five performance subscales. The rating subscales are completed by the examiner either during or shortly after interacting with the subject. Social Behavior Skills (MAS1) require the examiner to rate the presence/absence of basic behavioral skills necessary for sustaining social interactions. These items were adapted from the Minimal Social Behavior Scale by Lawton (1971). Receptive Language Skills—Oral Stimulus (MAS2) is comprised of eight verbally presented requests to perform

Table 6–8. Means ($\bar{X}$) and standard deviations (SD) for the normal elderly (NE) and malignant memory disorders (MMD) groups on the Multifocus Assessment Scale (MAS)

	GROUPS		
Variable	NE	MMD	F value
MAS1			
$\bar{X}$	11.0	10.64	6.77
SD	0.0	1.16	
N	71	298	
MAS2			
$\bar{X}$	7.54	6.61	13.61
SD	.81	2.08	
N	71	297	
MASVIS			
$\bar{X}$	8.83	7.06	27.35
SD	.45	2.85	
N	71	290	
MAS3			
$\bar{X}$	9.99	6.02	93.44
SD	.12	3.46	
N	297	297	
MAS4			
$\bar{X}$	9.97	7.06	63.67
SD	.17	3.07	
N	17	297	
MAS5			
$\bar{X}$	23.27	19.59	22.28
SD	4.62	6.13	
N	71	278	
MAS6			
$\bar{X}$	3.00	2.47	30.03
SD	0.00	.82	
N	71	294	
MAS7			
$\bar{X}$	9.87	8.97	25.24
SD	.34	1.51	
N	71	298	

simple commands (e.g., "touch your nose"). Receptive Language Skills—Visual Stimulus (MASVIS) consisted of nine visually presented requests to perform similar tasks (e.g., "point to the square"). Mental Status (MAS3) contained ten items assessing orientation to time, place, and person. These items were presented orally, and responses were checked against information available through the collateral informant in order to determine its accuracy (see table 6–8). Orientation (MAS4) consisted of ten items designed to measure the subject's awareness of his or her immediate environment (e.g., "where do you live?"). All questions were presented orally and verified against external sources. The Mood subscale (MAS5) was adapted from the Memorial University of Newfoundland's Scale of Happiness (MUNSH) (Kozma & Stones, 1980). Fourteen MUNSH items designed to assess the presence of general demoralization were used. Expressive Language Skills (MAS6) requires the examiner to rate the subject's ability to communicate verbally using three dimensions (e.g., "was the verbal behavior appropriate to the situation"). Finally, Accessibility and Sensory Abilities (MAS7) required the examiner to rate the capacity of the subject to attend to a conversation or instruction from care givers based on ten items. The reliability of the MAS has been studied (Coval et al., 1985), and alpha coefficients ranging from 0.92 to 0.99 have been reported. A PCA showed a high degree of homogeneity of scale content reflected by the presence of a single factor accounting for a majority of the variance associated with this scale. In addition, the MAS has been shown to differentiate among elderly samples on the basis of their ability to live independently in the community (Tuokko et al., 1987).

From the Wechsler Adult Intelligence Scale—Revised Form (WAIS-R; Weschler, 1981) the following subtests were administered according to the directions for administration and scoring: Information (WAIS-I), Digit Span (WAIS-DT), Similarities (WAIS-S), Vocabulary (WAIS-VOC), Block Design (WAIS-BD), Object Assembly (WAIS-OA), and Digit Symbol (WAIS-DS). The scores for these subtests were converted into Age Scale Scores (ASS) (see table 6–9). These variables were included in order to determine levels of intellectual skills necessary to support activities of everyday living. Although the WAIS-R is a well-established means of assessing cognitive functioning in the normal population, research on the subscales making up this battery of tests indicates that the subtests included in this study also make a valuable contribution to the differentiation of SDAT from other problems of cognitive functioning associated with elderly samples (Tuokko & Crockett, 1987; Brinkman & Braun, 1984; Fuld, 1984).

Expressive and receptive language functioning was assessed using several subtests drawn from the Neurosensory Center Comprehensive Examination for Aphasia (NCCEA). From this battery, the following subtests were administered and scored according to the manual provided for this test (Spreen & Benton, 1969): Word Fluency (WF); Tactual Naming—right hand (TAC-NAM-R); Tactual Naming—left hand (TAC-NAM-L); Visual Naming (Vis-

Table 6–9. Means ($\bar{X}$) and standard deviations (SD) for the normal elderly (NE) and malignant memory disorders (MMD) groups on the selected subtests from the WAIS-R★

| | GROUPS | | |
	NE	MMD	F value
Variable			
Information			
$\bar{X}$	13.38	7.40	124.39
SD	2.34	2.34	
N	71	285	
Digit Span			
$\bar{X}$	13.00	8.57	64.91
SD	2.95	4.39	
N	71	286	
Similarities			
$\bar{X}$	14.33	7.81	121.74
SD	2.56	4.81	
N	71	283	
Vocabulary			
$\bar{X}$	14.86	9.91	84.78
SD	2.00	3.91	
N	71	54	
Digit Symbol			
$\bar{X}$	15.01	6.76	192.93
SD	2.64	4.01	
N	69	58	
Block Design			
$\bar{X}$	13.30	7.61	89.18
SD	3.13	4.60	
N	70	166	
Object Assembly			
$\bar{X}$	12.66	7.67	77.78
SD	2.87	3.48	
N	71	55	

★ Age-corrected scaled scores.

Nam); and Visual Description of Use—Trays C and D (Desuse). These tests were included to provide measures of verbal fluency, haptic naming, and naming to visual presentation (see table 6–10). The NCCEA has been shown to have adequate reliability for the purpose of assessing language dysfunctioning as a consequence of acquired brain disorders (Spreen & Benton, 1969). It has also been shown to provide important information regarding the organization of residual language functioning among groups of language-impaired subjects (Crockett, 1977; Crockett et al., 1981).

Measures from the Halstead-Reitan Neuropsychological Test Battery were employed to assess psychomotor speed and strength of grip (Reitan & Davison, 1974). The Finger Tapping Test measures the patient's ability to tap his dominant or nondominant index finger. The first three 10-second trials are

Table 6–10. Means ($\bar{X}$) and standard deviations (SD) for the normal elderly (NE) and malignant memory disorders (MMD) groups on the Neuropsychological Test Battery

	GROUPS		
Variable	NE	MMD	F value
Word Fluency			
$\bar{X}$	38.61	19.94	93.37
SD	12.35	14.58	
N	71	278	
Tactile Naming, Right-hand			
$\bar{X}$	15.49	12.94	22.35
SD	1.25	4.64	
N	71	160	
Tactile Naming, Left-hand			
$\bar{X}$	14.80	11.82	24.20
SD	2.00	4.91	
N	71	150	
Visual Naming (A & B)			
$\bar{X}$	15.84	13.58	17.44
SD	.71	4.54	
N	71	155	
Description of Use (C & D)			
$\bar{X}$	15.92	13.97	15.34
SD	.26	4.08	
N	67	132	
Tactile Description of Use, Left hand			
$\bar{X}$	15.62	13.68	16.80
SD	1.02	3.89	
N	71	114	
Tactile Description of Use, Right Hand			
$\bar{X}$	15.00	12.76	15.97
SD	1.72	4.53	
N	71	104	
Description of Use (A & B)			
$\bar{X}$	15.97	14.59	11.74
SD	.23	3.40	
N	71	109	
Visual Naming (C & D)			
$\bar{X}$	15.90	13.98	17.01
SD	.53	3.78	
N	67	85	

administered to the dominant hand and the next three to the nondominant hand. Trials 7 and 8 are administered to the dominant hand and the final two trials to the nondominant hand. The average of the five trials with the dominant hand (TAP-DOM) and nondominant hand (TAP-ND) are shown in table 6–11. The Dynamometer test measures the subject's strength of grip.

Table 6–11. Means ($\bar{X}$) and standard deviations (SD) for the normal elderly (NE) and malignant memory disorders (MMD) groups on psychomotor and memory variables

	GROUPS		
Variable	NE	MMD	F value
Tapping, Right Hand			
$\bar{X}$	46.76	36.54	27.28
SD	9.11	15.84	
N	71	287	
Tapping, Left Hand			
$\bar{X}$	41.33	34.48	15.19
SD	8.39	14.20	
N	71	287	
Dynamometer, Right Hand			
$\bar{X}$	31.09	26.99	6.18
SD	12.60	12.41	
N	71	290	
Dynamometer, Left Hand			
$\bar{X}$	28.10	24.74	5.05
SD	11.32	11.29	
N	71	288	
Buschke			
Total Free Recall			
$\bar{X}$	69.18	33.28	178.15
SD	21.20	21.20	
N	68	149	
Total Recall			
$\bar{X}$	83.73	69.67	40.00
SD	.97	18.25	
N	68	149	

The subject is asked to squeeze a measuring device as "hard as you can." This procedure was administered to the dominant and nondominant hand on an alternating basis for two trials. The score is the average strength of grip measured in kilograms over the two trials for the dominant (DYN-DOM) and nondominant hand (DYN-ND). The Dynamometer Test and Finger Tapping Tests have been shown to measure important components of neuropsychological performance (Reitan & Davison, 1974). The effects of age and the ability of patients with the degenerative disorders have also been studied (Bigler, Steinman, & Newton, 1981).

To differentiate between rates of acquisition and retrieval, each subject was administered a version of the Buschke's Cued Recall Test of Memory (Buschke, 1984). Subjects were presented a random display of 12 pictures of common objects and directed to engage in a visual search to find the object that represented a semantic category (e.g., part of the body, furniture). A distraction task was employed between the initial presentation and the first recall (i.e., counting backward from 100 by 1 for 60 seconds). On each of the six recall trials, the subject engaged in free recall of the items. Following each free recall trial, semantic cues were provided for items not previously recalled under the free recall condition (i.e., restricted reminding procedure). A remote recall trial, trial 7, was conducted after the subjects engaged in 5 minutes of nonmemory tasks. This test provided two scores: (1) the total number of items correctly identified through free recall on all seven trials, and (2) the total number of items correctly recalled through both free and cued recall over all trials. The data for this test are shown in table 6–11.

From the Luria-Nebraska Neuropsychological Test Battery (LNNB), five variables from two tests were chosen: the number of words recalled in the 5th trial of Word Learning; the total of words recalled on all trials (including the 5th trial); Design Reproduction; Design Recall—immediate; and Design Recall—delayed format. Though a relatively new battery of tests, the construction and validity of this test have been described (Golden, Hammeke, & Purische, 1978) as well as the clinical utility for describing residual functioning in elderly samples (Kane et al., 1981; Mittenberg, Kasprisin, & Farage, 1985). In addition, the LNNB has been successfully employed with samples of elderly patients (Gillen, Golden, & Eyde, 1982; Sulkava et al., 1983).

To examine the discriminant validity of these NPT measures for our

Table 6–12. Means ($\bar{X}$) and standard deviations (SD) for the normal elderly (NE) and malignant memory disorders (MMD) groups on selected subtests of the Luria Nebraska Neuropsychological Battery

	GROUPS		
Variable	NE	MMD	F value
Word Learning, 5th Trial			
$\bar{X}$	4.46	.77	99.83
SD	2.13	1.87	
N	71	52	
Total Word Learning			
$\bar{X}$	31.62	15.17	142.19
SD	2.85	11.37	
N	71	101	
Design Recall			
$\bar{X}$	4.14	2.12	107.86
SD	.85	1.58	
N	71	290	
Design Reproduction			
$\bar{X}$	4.96	4.28	15.02
SD	.21	1.47	
N	71	291	
Delayed Reproduction			
$\bar{X}$	4.65	2.32	104.63
SD	.69	1.84	
N	68	236	

samples, the performance of our NE subjects was compared to that of the MMD groups. The results of our one-way analysis of variance for the NPT variables are contained in tables 6–8 to 6–12. All comparisons were highly significant, with the NE subjects performing in an intact fashion on all measures of cognitive functioning. The consistently higher level of functioning associated with the NE subjects indicated that this group is a benign group. On the other hand, the fact that the MMD subjects scored, on average, at a significantly lower level than the NE groups across all areas of cognitive functioning indicates that this group had more problems than just memory disorders. This may reinforce the need for using a comprehensive battery of tests to assess many areas of functioning even though the client may be referred for psychological assessment with respect to solely memory problems.

METHOD

Once the reliability of the PFQ was established by correlational techniques, it was possible to examine the pattern of subscale scores to determine if certain problems associated with everyday tasks were related in some meaningful way to professional ratings of functioning and performance on objective tests on neuropsychological functioning. Many techniques exist to derive empirical groups. Rourke (1985) reviewed the problems associated with using "canned" statistical programs and, in turn, demonstrated how useful an intelligent application of these techniques may be. The current authors' experiences (Crockett, 1977; Crockett, Clark, & Spreen, 1981; Clark et al, 1983) have indicated that applications of hierarchical analysis programs (Veldman, 1967) to neuropsychological test data confirmed the clinically obvious fact that most patients can be differentiated in terms of severity of illness. Differentiating patients on the basis of severity of illness can provide meaningful information such as response to treatment (Clark, Crockett, & Klonoff, 1979). This is a very useful prediction when one is faced with allocating scarce hospital resources. It is essentially important when one considers that neuropsychological patients admitted to hospital for either cognitive assessment or rehabilitation can typically demand substantial input from many hospital departments.

The statistical method used in this study involved employing the data contained in table 6–3 describing the psychometric characteristics of the PFQ. These data were combined with those in table 6–4 (the level of functioning associated with the NE group on the individual subscales of the PFQ). Standard errors of measurement were calculated following Nunnally (1967). The standard error of measurement of these subscales was used to construct 95% confidence intervals. This figure was used because it implies that any group of individuals falling beyond that confidence interval would have a significant difference between its mean and the mean for the NE sample. As this is a conservative estimate, it is likely that some combinations of subtle symptoms might be overlooked. However, the use of this confidence interval is justified in that it provides a theoretical estimate of the number of times an individual might show this amount of impairment or more on the basis of pure chance even though that person still might, most appropriately, belong to the NE group.

Once the appropriate standard error of measurement and confidence intervals were computed for each of the scales of the PFQ, the data for the NE and MMD subjects were combined to determine whether a subject's score fell beyond the 95% confidence interval. The number of times a particular subject's score fell beyond this range for the five subscales was computed. This resulted in the subjects being classified as showing deficits on none of the areas (group 1), on one of the areas (group 2), on two of the areas (group 3), on three of the areas (group 4), on four of the areas (group 5), and on all five areas (group 6) of everyday functioning as measured by this questionnaire. These six groups were used to examine differences in functioning as rated on the FRS and measured by the battery of neuropsychology tests.

RESULTS

Present Functioning Questionnaire

Using the method already described, each of the five scales of the PFQ was converted into dichotomous scores reflecting the presence or absence of impairment on a particular scale. Subsequently, patients were classified into one of six groups on the basis of whether they showed impairments on no tests, one test, two tests, three tests, four tests, or all five tests. Since these groups were constructed in a nonparametric fashion (i.e., without reference to how extreme the deviation or deficit might have been), it was necessary to compare the mean profile for these groups on their actual scores for the five subscales. These data are contained in table 6–13. This table contains the mean for the total group and the Z-score transformation for each of the individual six groups. From the data in this table, it can be seen that the subjects who were classified as showing deficits on none of the tests were indeed a benign group. The most salient feature for this group is the relative absence of any

Table 6–13. Analysis of Present Functioning
Questionnaire subscales using Z-score transformations

Group defined by impairment on:	Personality total	Everyday tasks total	Language skill total	Memory total	Self-care total
No areas	−1.06	−1.25	− .99	−1.50	− .59
One area	−0.58	−1.18	− .77	− .62	− .58
Two areas	−0.40	−0.65	− .47	− .19	− .59
Three areas	−0.18	−0.02	.09	.10	− .39
Four areas	0.39	0.59	0.19	0.54	0.23
Five areas	1.00	1.15	1.01	.89	1.01
Total mean	4.67	4.36	2.32	6.85	1.69
Total SD	3.32	3.37	2.31	4.29	2.86
F value	80.29	165.06	71.70	162.36	49.83

Note: All Z score transformations are based on means and standard deviations derived from all subjects.

difficulties with memory reported by the significant other (Z score $= -1.50$). Subjects in groups showing no deficits, one deficit, and two deficits were similar in that none of the subjects in these groups were described as showing *any* problems with self-care. Subjects in the group reported as having one deficit had a significant feature in that this was the first group to show an emergent problem with memory functioning (i.e., they reported an average of 4.2 problems in this area as compared to only 0.4 problems reported by the subjects in the group with no impairment on any of the scales of the PFQ). They also tended to show a small but reliable increase in a number of problems reported in the areas of present functioning, suggesting that although this group had some problems with memory functioning, they were not significantly impaired in their general ability to cope with everyday life. The subjects in the group showing deficits in two areas showed even more problems with respect to memory (i.e., MEMTOT-6.04) but still were able to cope with problems of everyday life. Subjects in the group showing deficits on three areas of the PFQ revealed the emergence of problems in almost all areas of functioning. The only area of relative preservation of functioning was in terms of their ability to cope with problems of self-care. Subjects showing deficits on four areas of the PFQ had relatively severe problems with memory and everyday functioning (MEMTOT $= 9.2$ and ETOT-6.4, respectively) but with relatively preserved language skills (LSTOT $= 2.8$). Finally, those subjects falling in the group with deficits on all five areas measured by the PFQ reported a high frequency of problems in all areas. It is important to note the covariance of problems reported by collaborative informants in the areas of memory and everyday functioning. Severity of impairment regularly increased as more and more difficulties were reported in these two areas. It should also be noted that individuals in these groups could maintain their levels of functioning with respect to personality, language skills, and self-care despite the observed problems with everyday functioning and memory.

Since the patients' levels of described functioning on the PFQ were used in constructing these groups, the F tests associated with the subscales of the PFQ were inflated. Therefore, the ratings obtained from professionals who have assessed these patients were of extreme interest. The mean of the eight scales of the Functional Rating Scale are contained in table 6–14. Once again it can be seen that individuals who were described by significant others as having no significant problems on any of the five areas measured by the PFQ functioned at the highest level. Subjects in this group were very intact with respect to levels of perceived functioning in the area of memory, social, home and hobbies, and orientation. Z-score transformations of the means for the personal care (range $= -.78$–1.23) and language skills (range $= -.92 - .87$) groups are artificially low due to the relatively low overall rate of assessed problems in these two areas. Subjects who showed deficits on one of the subtests of the PFQ maintained their good level of orientation (Orientation $=$

Table 6–14. Analysis of Functional Rating Scale using groups based on the Present Functioning Questionnaire and Z-score transformatios

Groups defined by failure on:	Memory	Social	Home & Hobbies	Personal Care	Language Skills	Problem Solving	Affect	Orientation
No area	-1.32	-1.40	-1.30	- .78	- .92	-1.12	-1.11	-1.28
One area	- .79	- .88	- .92	- .78	- .73	- .79	- .61	-1.08
Two areas	- .17	- .34	- .47	- .71	- .45	- .43	- .15	- .84
Three areas	.16	.25	.27	- .28	.07	.19	- .11	- .19
Four areas	.40	.47	.47	.28	.28	.35	.43	.11
Five areas	.90	.95	.91	1.16	.87	.50	.84	.64
Total mean	2.92	2.95	2.85	2.04	2.29	2.66	2.94	2.49
Total SD	1.35	1.29	1.38	1.34	1.34	1.47	1.40	1.47
F value	104.40	162.90	148.63	93.20	50.35	74.98	60.04	71.53

Note: All Z-score transformations are based on means and standard deviation derived from all subjects.

1.3) but had more problems in the area of affect and control of mood (Affect = 2.1). Perhaps this is a response, on part of the subjects, to the insight into the nature of their problems. They were also described as showing emergent problems with their memory (Memory = 1.9). Subjects with failure in three areas of the PFQ showed definite problems with their memory (Z score = 3.1), social functioning (Z score = 3.3), and involvement with home and hobbies (Z score = 3.2). Subjects with failures on four tests had difficulties in these three areas (Z score = 3.5, 3.6, and 3.5, respectively) plus increased problems in terms of their affect (Z score = 3.5). Finally, subjects who fell in the group defined as having significant deficits on all five areas of the PFQ were judged by the professional staff as having problems on all areas of the FRS including personal care (Z score = 3.8). This finding is in contrast to the levels of problems reported by significant others and suggests that perhaps those individuals associated with the subjects in this group were helping the patient to cope in more ways than they realized.

Group differences on the PFQ and FRS run the risk of being the result of biases in either the report of the collaborative informant or the observation of the professionals who have come in contact with them. Such distorting factors may include the family's denial of problems or the risk of "halo effects." An examination of the patient's performance on neuropsychological tests, therefore, provides an opportunity to validate the perception of the significant others and professionals against objective test data. Table 6–15 includes the data for word learning—fifth trial, design recall—delayed format, word learning total, design reproduction, and design recall—immediate. These variables were derived from the Luria-Nebraska Neuropsychological Test Battery. The subjects who were categorized as showing no deficits on the PFQ maintained a high level of functioning on these measures of verbal and nonverbal learning. Subjects in the groups showing deficits on one scale of the PFQ had an intact level of overall functioning on most of the objective tests but began to show problems in engaging in verbal learning tests, as indicated by their relatively low score on the word learning test (WL—5th = 3.2). Problems in this regard continue to emerge in subjects classified as showing deficits on two areas of the PFQ (WL—5th = 2.5) along with deficits in their ability to engage in new verbal learning on all five trials (WL—Tot = 17.4). Subjects classified into the group showing deficits on three areas of the PFQ showed an interesting pattern. They maintained their ability to reproduce designs (Des-Repro = 4.6), suggesting an intact set of complex psychomotor skills, but had a significant salient difficulty on the last trial (WL—5th = .21) and over all trials (WL-Tot = 17.4) on the Word Learning Test. This deficit persisted and intensified, with subjects showing deficits on either four or five tests of the PFQ (WL—5th = .91 and .07, respectively). Subjects showing deficits on five tests had a collateral deficit in terms of their ability to engage in word learning over all the trials (WL—Tot = 6.1). The pattern of results on this test shows that word learning difficulty is often the first and

Table 6–15. Analysis of neuropsychological variables using groups based on the Present Functioning Questionnaire and Z-score transformations

Groups defined by failure on:	Word Learning 5th Trial	Word Learning Total	Design Recognition	Design Reproduction	Design Delayed	Buschke Total Free Recall	Buschke Total Recall
No areas	.65	.84	1.07	.41	1.00	1.03	.59
One area	.09	.73	.74	.44	.63	.53	.37
Two areas	– .15	.48	.33	.39	.19	– .21	– .07
Three areas	– .98	– .34	– .23	.21	– .32	– .40	– .04
Four areas	– .73	– .57	– .34	– .19	– .38	– .67	– .32
Five areas	–1.04	–1.26	– .86	– .71	– .82	– .94	–1.19
Total mean	2.90	21.47	2.47	4.38	2.82	44.5	74.1
Total SD	2.73	12.21	1.68	1.39	1.92	24.85	16.51
F value	24.31	66.22	49.21	16.72	44.64	57.75	14.10

Note: All Z-score transformations are based on means and standard deviations derived from all subjects.

most reliable deficit on neuropsychological tests to emerge with increasing difficulty in coping with everyday life.

Also included in table 6–15 are the results from the Buschke's Cued Recall procedure for assessing memory in the elderly. All groups showed significant differences in terms of the number of words they could recall (i.e., had acquired and learned to retrieve) and in terms of how many words they could recall with the provision of semantic cues. Subjects in the group showing no impairment could recall almost all of the words (i.e., 99.8%) presented to them with the provision of cues, whereas the subjects showing impairment in three areas (i.e., 87.4%), four areas (i.e., 82.0%), and five areas (i.e., 64.8%) were able to recall significantly fewer words. That subjects in the group showing impairment in the most areas could still retrieve a majority of the material presented to them suggests that these group differences were not exclusively due to general conditions such as aphasia or depression. Moreover, the low rates of recall during the FR condition indicated the problem these subjects were experiencing was with retrieval rather than acquisition. In fact, subjects with no impairment in everyday functioning as reported by significant others recalled most of the material (i.e., 84.2%) without the aid of semantic cues, and those with impairment in two areas recalled less than half (i.e., 46.7%) of the material.

The data in table 6–16 provide some indication regarding the intactness of psychomotor functioning in these subjects. Subjects in the group showing no impairment functioned in a relatively robust fashion with respect to their finger tapping speed and strength of grip. By the time the subjects were described as having two problems on the PFQ, difficulties with strength of grip began to emerge. It is of interest to note the salient feature of problems of production and regulation of fine motor movement using the left, nondominant hand amongst the subjects. These problems coexist with problems

Table 6–16. Analysis of psychomotor variables using groups based on the Present Functioning Questionnaire and Z-score transformations

Group defined by failure on:	Tapping, right hand	Tapping, left hand	Dynamometer, right hand	Dynamometer left hand
No areas	.57	.49	.41	.38
One area	.28	.20	.26	.28
Two areas	.30	.32	.09	.03
Three areas	− .06	.00	.00	.09
Four areas	− .28	− .15	− .12	− .14
Five areas	− .46	− .53	− .36	− .38
Total mean	37.91	35.20	27.23	24.94
Total SD	15.64	13.81	12.22	11.21
F value	11.35	10.02	5.12	5.31

Note: All Z-score transformations are based on means and standard deviations derived from all subjects.

Table 6–17. Analysis of expressive and receptive measures using groups
based on the Present Functioning Questionnaire and Z-score transformations

Group defined by failure on:	Word fluency	Tactile naming, right	Tactile naming, left	Visual naming
No areas	.94	.52	.52	.44
One area	.87	.47	.63	.40
Two areas	.14	.31	.38	.20
Three areas	− .16	− .27	− .41	− .10
Four areas	− .36	− .02	− .28	− .06
Five areas	− .78	−1.02	−1.05	− .94
Total mean	22.97	13.67	12.72	14.27
Total SD	15.97	3.95	4.43	3.89
F value	43.90	19.08	22.53	12.89

Note: All Z-score transformations are based on means and standard deviations derived from all subjects.

regulating the movements of the right index finger. This may suggest a generalized pattern of dysfunctioning.

The data presented in table 6–17 describe the subjects' performance on a variety of verbal fluency and naming tasks. These tests use materials drawn from the Neurosensory Center Comprehensive Examination for Aphasia (NCCEA). The most discriminating feature among these patients was their ability to generate units of expression as measured by the Word Fluency Test (WFT). That is, subjects classified as showing either no deficits or deficits on only one area as assessed by the PFQ generally maintained their level of functioning on the WFT (mean = 37.9 and 36.8, respectively). Subjects showing deficits in only two areas as measured by the PFQ showed a dramatic decline in their ability to generate units of expression on the WFT (mean = 25.2). Groups showing impairment in all five areas of the PFQ were also characterized as having difficulty with tactile naming using their dominant (TN-R = 9.6) and nondominant hands (TN-L = 8.1). However, their lowered scores on the WFT (mean = 10.7) suggest that at least part of their problem on these tests may to be due to acquired expressive difficulties.

The subjects' performance on the selected subtests of the WAIS-R was examined using the same groupings defined by number of areas of impairment (see table 6–18). The subjects falling in the group showing no impairment on the PFQ performed at a very good level (i.e., above scale score = 11.0) as did the subjects in the groups defined as having problems in one area. However, by the time the patients were described as having problems in two areas measured by the PFQ, their performance showed a relative impairment. This impairment was most notable on the subtest measuring their ability to engage in a coding task (i.e., Digit Symbol = 8.42), followed by their ability to define words on a vocabulary test (i.e., Vocabulary = 10.85) and on a task measuring their ability to integrate parts into a meaningful whole (i.e., Object Assembly

Table 6–18. Analysis of WAIS-R age-scaled scores using groups based on the Present Functioning Questionnaire and Z-scores transformations

Groups defined by failure on:	Information	Digit span	Similarities	Vocabulary	Block-design	Object assembly	Digit-symbol
No areas	.97	.77	.95	.52	.81	.55	.65
One area	.63	.64	.75	.31	.66	.27	.75
Two areas	.19	.34	.18	− .47	.12	− .32	− .51
Three areas	− .01	− .04	− .14	− .26	− .44	− .65	− .57
Four areas	− .35	− .23	− .35	− .98	− .47	− 1.19	− 1.37
Five areas	− .82	− .82	− .75	− 1.24	− 1.00	− .81	− 1.27
Total mean	8.46	9.35	9.01	12.67	9.25	10.47	11.18
Total SD	4.73	4.54	5.25	3.91	4.95	4.05	5.41
F value	43.38	32.43	39.75	16.38	34.82	16.83	50.48

Note: All Z-score transformations are based on means and standard deviations derived from all subjects.

= 9.17). These problems were joined by a new set of problems with respect to patients who were classified as having problems in at least three areas showing an additional problem on the subtest measuring their ability to reproduce geometric designs using colored blocks (i.e., Block Design = 7.08). Subjects in the group defined as having four problem areas on the PFQ showed dramatic deficits with respect to their ability to integrate parts into a meaningful whole (Object Assembly = 5.67) and their ability to engage in a coding task (Digit Symbol = 3.75). Subjects having difficulties in at least five areas as measured by the PFQ showed generalized decline across the subtests in the intellectual test battery. The sensitivity of the Object Assembly and Digit Symbol tests to increasing levels of problems in everyday functioning appears to support the use of these subtests as part of Fuld's formula for detecting the presence of DAT.

Finally, the subjects' performance on the MAS was examined with respect to the number of reported problem areas. Cutoff points were established for all of the subscales of the MAS with the exception of MAS4 (Tuokko et al., 1987). These cutoff points were based on a discriminant validity study using three elderly samples at varying levels of functioning ranging from independent living, community dwelling patients referred to a memory disorder clinic, and, finally, a sample of residents of an extended care facility. The results, as shown in table 6–19, indicated that abnormal functioning, defined by levels of functioning that fell at or below each cutoff on three or more of the subscales, was strongly related to problems maintaining oneself in the community. All six groups were above these established cutoff points on the subscale measuring social behavior (MAS1) and mood (MAS5). As such, the scales appear to be relatively insensitive to increases in and levels of reported problems. In contrast, only the group with no reported problems had an average level of functioning that fell above the cutoff point on expressive language (MAS6). This suggests that even subjects with failure in just one area of functioning as measured by the PFQ were experiencing a decline in their general adaptive functioning. Average levels of functioning on the subtest measuring mental status (MAS3) fell below the cutoff point for a group showing two or more problem areas. Subjects with problems in three or more areas had impaired functioning on the subtests measuring receptive language functioning—auditory stimuli (MAS2) and receptive language functioning—visual stimuli (MASVIS). Finally, subjects had to be impaired in all five areas measured by the PFQ in order to have average levels of functioning that fell below the cutoff point for the scale measuring accessibility (MAS8).

The relationship of the two measures of everyday functioning, the FRS and the PFQ, to the neuropsychological variables was examined using canonical correlation analysis (CCA). The presence of a significant correlation between the FRS and PFQ ($R = .64$; $df = 1$; $p < .001$) suggested significant overlap between these two measures of everyday functioning. However, the results of the Roy-Bargman Stepdown F-Test indicated the presence of two significant

Table 6–19. Analysis of the Multifocus Assessment Scale using groups based on the Present Functioning Questionnaire and Z-score transformations

Groups defined by failure on:	Social behavior	Receptive	MASVIS	Mental Status	Orientation	Mood	Expressive	Accessibility
No areas	.29	.40	.59	.94	.47	.32	.59 ★	.52
One area	.29	.60	.56	.77 ★	.60	.29	.44	4.3
Two areas	.19	.41 ★	.49 ★	.60	.48	.05	.42	.45
Three areas	.09	.09	.01	− .10	.03	.04	− .09	.22
Four areas	.01	− .04	− .09	− .31	− .56	− .10	− .07	.04 ★
Five areas	− .47 ★	− .72	− .83	− .94	−1.05	− .33 ★	− .71	− .87
Total mean	10.68	6.75	7.33	6.63	7.49	20.49	2.54	9.11
Total SD	1.12	1.96	2.72	3.54	3.05	6.07	.78	1.43
F value	6.04	17.63	26.82	65.07	56.21	3.68	19.23	27.32

Note: No cut off points were available for Orientation subtest. All Z-score transformations are based on means and standard deviation for all subjects.
★ = cutoff points.

components to these measures ($F = 27.1$; df $= 19/238$; $F = 12.29$; df $= 19.237$; $p < .001$), suggesting that the pattern of correlation among the measures of everyday functioning and the neuropsychological test variables should be analyzed separately.

The next step was to examine the relationship between the subscales of the PFQ and the subjects' performance on the NPT variables. The Roy-Bargman Stepdown F tests indicated that PTOT ($F = 8.88$; df $= 19/239$), ETOT ($F = 13.51$; df $= 19/238$), LSTOT ($F = 4.70$; df $= 19/237$), MEMTOT ($F = 3.80$; df $= 19/236$), and SCTOT ($F = 8.92$; df $= 19/235$) were significantly related to performance on the NPT variables ($p < .001$). A majority of the variance between these two data sets (54.0%) was accounted for by a linear relationship between them. An analysis of the individual components of the PFQ and the NPT-variables revealed the presence of significant univariate relationships.

Problems with personality were significantly associated with Receptive Language-Oral Stimuli (t value $= 2.16$; $p < .03$); Receptive Language Skills—Visual Stimuli (t value $= 2.06$; $p < .04$); Orientation (t value $= 4.84$, $p < .001$); Mood (t value $= 5.59$; $p < .001$); and Accessibility (t value $= 2.72$, $p < .007$). Problems of personality functioning may be related to fundamental problems in communication with respect to the patient's ability to understand spoken/written communications within the environment, since they may impinge on the ability to gain information regarding the social milieu.

Problems with everyday functioning were mostly closely related to the WFT (t value $= 2.63$; $p < .009$); Mental Status (t value $= 2.14$; $p < .03$); and Orientation (t value $= 5.04$; $p < .001$). This suggests that problems with completion of everyday tasks may be related to the person's ability to communicate concise pieces of information regarding their environment.

Language skills as measured by the PFQ were associated with psychomotor speed as reflected by scores on the dominant and nondominant Finger Tapping Test (t value $= 2.17$; $p < .03$; t value $= 1.92$, $p < .05$, respectively); WFT (t value $= 2.24$; $p < .03$); Receptive Language Skills—Visual Stimulus (t value $= 2.53$; $p < .01$); and Mood (t value $= 2.28$; $p < .02$). Since at least three of these tests are timed tasks, the results may reflect an underlying dimension of "robustness." Moreover, these tests are well known to be related to language functioning.

Problems of memory were related to Delayed Designs Recall (t value $= 2.68$; $p < .008$); tapping scores for the right and left index finger (t value $= 2.70$; $p < .007$; and t value $= 2.57$; $p < .01$, respectively); WFT (t value $= 2.67$; $p < .008$); Orientation (t value $= 3.35$; $p < .001$); Mood (t value $= 1.91$; $p < .05$); and Accessibility (t value $= 1.90$; $p < .05$). Clearly, problems with memory were associated with actual difficulties on both verbal and nonverbal memory tasks as well as problems with distractibility of the patient in everyday life.

Problems of self-care were associated with Design Reproduction (t value $= 6.73$; $p < .001$); the dominant and nondominant strength of grip (t value $= 2.35$; $p < .02$; t value $= 2.42$; $p < .02$, respectively); WFT (t value $= 2.24$;

$p < .03$); Social Behavior (t value $= 4.74$; $p < .001$); and Orientation (t value $= 2.82$; $p < .005$). This suggested that individuals with problems with self-care should be carefully evaluated with respect to their psychomotor robustness as well as their hand–eye coordination as reflected in copying tasks, as these measures will be highly related to their ability to engage in appropriate social intercourse and maintain their orientation.

CCA of the FRS and the NPT variables suggested that there were significant multivariate relationships between each of the scales and the neuropsychological test variables ($F = 43.27$, df $= 19/240$, $F = 4.03$, df $= 19/239$, $F = 3.44$, df $= 19/238$, $F = 4.43$, df $= 19/237$, $F = 2.46$, df $= 19/236$, $F = 4.11$, df $= 19/235$, $F = 4.07$, df $= 19/234$, and $F = 13.45$, df $= 19/233$, $p < .001$, respectively). An analysis of the amount of variance held in common between these two data sets (67.5%) suggested that the FRS was more closely related to the NPT variables than the PFQ. Analysis of the individual components of the FRS and NPT variables revealed significant univariate relationships.

Memory functioning was related to Design Reproduction—Delayed Format (t value $= 3.91$; $p < .001$); WAIS-Information (t value $= 3.22$; $p < .001$); Mental Status (t value $= 2.93$; $p < .004$); Orientation (t value $= 2.63$; $p < .009$); and Accessibility (t value $= 2.28$; $p < .02$). The relationship between the subject's ability to recall information from long-term memory and his or her mental status to problems of memory appears to support the general usage of these variables to assess patients suspected of having malignant memory disorders.

Ratings of the patient's social, occupational, and community function were related to Design Recall—Delayed Format (t value $= 2.25$; $p < .02$); Dominant Finger Tapping Speed (t value $= 2.62$; $p < .009$); WFT (t value $= 2.94$; $p < .004$); WAIS-Information (t value $= 2.04$; $p < .04$); WAIS-Similarities (t value $= 2.20$; $p < .03$); Mental Status (t value $= 2.02$; $p < .04$); Orientation (t value $= 2.26$; $p < .02$); Mood (t value $= 4.12$; $p < .001$); and Accessibility (t value $= 2.62$; $p < .009$). These results suggest that in order to maintain one's functioning in the general social environment, the patient not only needed simple memory skills but also to maintain and act on information from long-term memory and to engage in a certain level of self-directed activity.

Patients' ability to engage in activities around the home or in hobbies was related to their ability to recall designs they have been previously exposed to (t value $= 4.52$; $p < .001$); to tap the right index finger (t value $= 2.18$; $p < .03$); to produce units of expression on the WFT (t value $= 3.01$; $p < .003$); to recall personally relevant information (t value $= 2.57$; $p < .01$); to control mood levels (t value $= 4.91$; $p < .001$); and maintain their accessibility (t value $= 2.34$; $p < .02$). The profound effect of a subject's mood on ability to cope with problems in the home, as well as the intact ability to retrieve stored information, was revealed by this analysis.

The patients' ability to engage in personal care was related to Design Recall-Immediate as reflected by their ability to reproduce geometric design from visual memory (*t* value = 2.35; *p* < .02); to exhibit nondominant motor strength (*t* value = 1.90; *p* < .05); to provide units of expression on the WFT (*t* value = 2.04; *p* < .04); to maintain their social behavior (*t* value = 2.71; *p* < .007); to be aware of their surroundings (*t* value = 2.63; *p* < .009); and to be accessible (*t* value = 2.41; *p* < .02). Perhaps the significance of the measure of the nondominant motor strength indicates the importance of dominant hemispheric functioning in determining level of personal care. That is, if patients have not only language problems but also problems with their nondominant skills, their level of personal care may be very impacted. Not surprisingly, the patient's rating of language function was related not only to verbal skills but also to measures of intactness of the dominant hemisphere.

The patient's language functioning was related to ability to recall designs (*t* value = 2.09; *p* < .04); to tap their dominant index finger (*t* value = 2.37; *p* < .02); to engage in verbal reasoning task as measured by WAIS-Similarities (*t* value = 2.29; *p* < .02); to their receptive skills for Visual Stimuli (*t* value = 2.09; *p* < .04) and to their Mood (*t* value = 2.19; *p* < .03). At least part of these patients' problems using language in everyday life, then, seems to stem from an underlying deficit in their ability to verbally encode information from their environment and to retain this encoding in their memory. The problems with mood and lowered dominant motor speed are felt to be of secondary consequence to the disruption of their sensory-motor strip.

Problem-solving ability was significantly related to the patient's ability to reproduce designs after a significant delay (*t* value = 3.54; *p* < .001); produce units of expression on a WFT (*t* value = 2.03; *p* < .04); and engage in a verbal reasoning task (*t* value = 3.74; *p* < .001). This relationship may be based on deficits in the patient's ability to maintain, organize, and manipulate verbally encoded information from the environment.

Staff rating of the affective status of these patients was most strongly related to the patient's self-reported mood and orientation (*t* value = 5.94; *t* value = 3.54; *p* < .001, respectively), followed by the subject's ability to engage in a verbal reasoning test and their ability to derive meaning from visual/verbal stimuli as measured by the receptive language skills tasks (*t* value = 3.47; *p* < .001; *t* value = 3.37; *p* < .001, respectively). The patients' affective status was also related to physical robustness, as indicated by their ability to tap either their dominant or nondominant index finger, as well as their access-ibility (*t* value = 2.69; *p* < .008; *t* value = 2.80; *p* < .006; *t* value = 2.91; *p* < .004, respectively).

Finally, the patients' orientation was most strongly related to their mental status and their orientation as measured by the MAS (*t* value = 10.14; *p* < .001; *t* value = 4.23; *p* < .001, respectively). Their orientation was also related to their level of residual social behavior (*t* value = 3.22; *p* < .001) and their ability to engage in a simple visual memory task, Design Recall—Delayed Format (*t* value = 3.59; *p* < .001). These relationships reflect not only the common content of the orientation scales but also the accepted relationship between fundamental social skills and accessibility to procedures designed to access orientation.

DISCUSSION

Implicit within the diagnosis and description of dementia is the assumption that everyday functioning will be affected. The three leading diagnostic systems—ICD9, DSM3, and NINCDS-ADRDA—all require a reduction in the patient's everyday status in order to establish the diagnoses of dementia. To date, our measures of everyday functioning have been either too limited or too broadly defined. Clinical scales have been developed that focus on limited aspects of a patient's functioning and have been applied to various samples of patients with the degenerative disease in order to establish the correlation between level of functioning and ability to cope with everyday life. In other circumstances, longer questionnaires have been developed and applied within samples designated to reflect various research interests. Unfortunately, these scales have often been too cumbersome to apply in a clinical situation and have not been related to a specific diagnostic criterion. Moreover, both types of batteries frequently have not been applied to impaired elderly subjects whose level of impairment falls within an intermediate range. These subjects, who are too intact to require institutionalized care yet are in need of assistance in their everyday functioning, are not adequately assessed by either type of battery. In this chapter, we described the development and application of several scales that we felt met the assessment needs of these elderly subjects who fall within this intermediate range of impairment.

In developing these scales, it was recognized that there were at least three major sources of data: the patients' self-reported level of problems, collaborative informants who were familiar with the patients' everyday functioning, and the professional observations of a multidisciplinary assessment team. Because of the unreliability inherent in the self-report of the impaired elderly due to denial, lack of awareness of important issues, and their confusion about their own status, we chose to use the patients' observed level of functioning on a battery of neuropsychological tests as the criterion variable (Baddeley, Sunderland, & Harris, 1982). The Present Functioning Questionnaire was developed as a quick, convenient, and reliable means of obtaining comprehensive information regarding the collaborator's perception of the elderly patient's ability to function within everyday situations. Psychometric analyses of this questionnaire revealed high levels of reliability, and inter-area correlations that were high enough to provide consistent estimates of the patients' performance and low enough to indicate the areas making up the heterogeneous concept of everyday functioning were sampled. The Functional Rating Scale was developed to provide objective definitions of the major areas of impairment required for establishing the diagnosis of dementia. This scale facilitated the integration of information from multidisciplinary sources as well as provided descriptions of anchor points that enhance the discrimination of patients of varying degrees of impairment. This scale also demonstrated more than adequate reliability and discriminant validity for use within the context of assessing the elderly patients at an intermediate level of dysfunctioning. Finally, a battery of neuropsychological tests used in other research settings was applied to this group in order to provide objective evidence with respect to their level of functioning and how it might affect the elderly patients' ability to perform everyday tasks. As a consequence, we believe that these measures met and exceeded the goals of providing assessment techniques related to signs and symptoms associated with dementing disorders, yet were behaviorally defined with objective definitions of various levels of functioning.

Our analyses indicated that these measures were related not only to gross differences among clinically defined groups such as the normal elderly in contrast to elderly samples with malignant memory disorders but, moreover, were strongly related to information from collaborative informants, professional assessors, and the neuropsychological tests employed. With respect to the perceptions of the collaborative informant, six groups of elderly patients could be defined on the basis of the number of areas measured by this questionnaire in which the patient was described as having significantly more problems than were typically encountered in our sample of normal elderly subjects. These groups were defined in terms of whether the patient showed problems in none of the areas measured by the PFQ, one, two, three, four, or all five areas. Everyday functioning, as described by the collaborative informant, appears to be relatively resilient to emerging problems in the areas of personality, language skills, memory, and self-care. However, once an elderly patient was described as having difficulties in more than three areas, his or her level of functioning showed a marked decline across all areas of everyday functioning. Language skills and memory appeared to emerge as specific problems, which then led to problems either with personality or everyday functioning. Problems in self-care were usually the last set of problems to emerge in elderly patients who were having difficulty maintaining their level of functioning in an independent context. That is, collaborative informants began to report problems emerging with self-care only after they had identified the elderly patient as having problems in all the other areas of the PFQ. Moreover, individual elderly subjects who had problems in none, one, two, and three areas of everyday functioning as measured by the PFQ reported similar levels of difficulties with self-care, typically reporting less than one problem with self-care for all of these groups. In contrast, patients with problems in four areas measured by the PFQ were described as having two problems with self-care, whereas elderly subjects with reported problems in all five areas had roughly double that number of reported problems.

The finding of a nonlinear relationship between levels of impairment and rates of problem areas identified by collaborative informants raises serious questions with respect to models of acquired impairment in elderly samples. We believe that the prospects for developing a salient model for impairment of everyday life are extremely poor. Other than demonstrating a progressive rate of increasing problems that leads to gradual emergence of problems coping with everyday life, it appears that there are a finite number of threshold points that, if exceeded, lead to the identification of increased numbers of problems with everyday functioning by significant others. Salient features that may be related to identified organic conditions may be lost in such dramatic changes. This finding, if replicated across other research groups, will have profound implications for other theoretical models of brain–behavior relations.

The most important finding associated with the Functional Rating Scale is the observation that multidisciplinary professionals often identify problems at a higher rate than do collaborative informants. This difference may be partially related to the insidious nature of the disease as well as the ability of elderly patients' families to compensate for these changes. By way of example, we noted that patients with problems in three or fewer areas measured by the PFQ report having less than one problem, on average, with their self-care, whereas on the Functional Rating Scale these patients have at least a questionable level of impairment with respect to their personal care. Once again, elderly patients show a dramatic increase in their rated levels of impairment when their number of problem areas exceeds three or more. The areas most likely to be affected were in terms of memory, social/occupational/community functions; home and hobbies; and affect. With increasing levels of rated impairment, problems with personal-care, language skills, problem-solving, and orientation became more obvious. Once again, these ratings are highly correlated, thus suggesting the limitations of a salient feature model for accounting for large portions of variance.

Perhaps the neuropsychological variables are the most problematic to interpret. Although they have the advantage of being equally novel to all subjects and demonstrate objective evidence of reliability and discriminant validity, they have major problems with respect to being sensitive to fluctuating levels of motivation and to the presence of sensory impairment, and may seem to the patients taking the test as only marginally related to their problems. Despite these difficulties, the measures of memory functioning were relatively sensitive to the emergence of problems as reported by the collaborative informant. Measures of expressive and receptive language functioning, though still permitting significant differentiation between high- and low-functioning elderly patients, seem to be less sensitive. This may be related to the homogeneity of problems of concern to patients attending a malignant memory disorders clinic, in that a majority of these patients are identified as having memory complaints, whereas only some of them reported problems with their language. Measures of intellectual functioning also provided relatively good discrimination among our patients, indicating that at least part of their problems with everyday functioning could be attributed to declining cognitive abilities. This interpretation was reinforced by results of our analyses of the subscales of the Multifocus Assessment Scale for the frail elderly. The scales most sensitive to emergence of problems in everyday functioning were Expressive Language, Mental Status, Receptive Language—Visual Stimulus, and Receptive Language—Auditory Stimuli. However, measures of psychomotor functioning provided less satisfactory discrimination among our groups, indicating that lateralized or focal deficits affecting psychomotor strength and fine motor speed have less to do with everyday functioning than do measures of memory or language.

In reviewing these results, it should be noted that there may be other means of grouping subjects than the statistically based progressive model we employed. Alternative means of examining the relationship of level of impairment could involve comparing groups from different diagnostic categories. These diagnostic categories could involve comparing groups having dementia with different etiological bases (e.g., multi-infarct versus Alzheimer type) or contrasting groups with diverse disorders (e.g., depressed versus demented patients). On the other hand, comparisons could be made of the relationships between everyday functioning and groups based on salient features reflecting a priori model of how symptoms might emerge. Such models might be based on a regression hypothesis speculating that problems with everyday functioning may reflect the reverse order of developmental stages of skill acquisitions. Alternatively, groups may be based on data acquired through other investigative procedures such as Positron Emission Transaxial Tomography, Regional Cerebral Blood Flow, or Magnetic Resonance Imaging.

We do not wish to discourage these alternative approaches prematurely, but we believe several features of our results are worth noting. First, all rating scales showed substantial correlation among the subtests of the data, indicating the presence of a general factor associated with the perception of the collaborative informant or the assessment team. The presence of a general factor does not necessarily rule out the value of other possible models, but it does have important implications for the magnitude of variance these alternative models, based on specific impairment, might be associated with and thus their generalizability to clinical settings. In addition, multivariate analysis of the maximal relationship between these data sets indicated that the improvement in our ability to predict everyday functioning would be quite small.

However, we firmly believe that whatever model is employed, researchers in this area should avoid canned statistical packages to generate groups based on empirical features. We also believe that it is necessary to develop local data bases that fit the needs and resources in a given region. That is, if a local site has special housing units available, there is a need to develop standards of everyday functioning that reflect special resources available within patients' environment in order to predict who will, and who will not, be capable of adapting to them. Finally, we believe that tasks involving new learning, either verbally or nonverbally mediated, will aid in differentiating patients who may or may not do well in those special situations.

Additional research in the area of everyday functioning of the elderly is necessary to identify those problem areas that may not affect everyday functioning. For example, it may be that some areas of cognitive or social functioning have less to do with determining overall adaptation than others. Memory, though playing a major role in the diagnosis of some types of dementia, may not have a crucial role in determining everyday functioning. This may be especially true in situations where subjects can rely on automatic, overlearned skills or where they may have prosthetic alternatives such as interested and involved relatives. In turn, it may be necessary to develop laboratory studies to provide measures of diverse functions such as decision making, the ability to meet competing demands in a flexible manner, and the ability to compensate for identified problems. Last, we believe that methods that might assess the patient's ability to learn and apply procedures involving one, two, and three stages might provide sensitive indices of how the patient may adjust to everyday life.

In general, this chapter showed that rating scales can be developed that provide stable estimates of levels of everyday functioning. These rating scales may be used to summarize data coming from many different sources. We presented rating scale data derived from significant others and from a variety of professionals who come in contact with the dementing patient. Other rating scales could be developed to capture information coming from a wide variety of sources such as treatment personnel, housing managers, or employers. The ratings of the demented patients showed substantial and significant agreement despite the heterogeneity in the observational basis for these judgments. However, the degree of fit between these data sources was less than perfect, indicating that data from other sources may enhance our assessment procedures of these patients and, correspondingly, improve our understanding of these patients. We have not yet had the opportunity to examine the changes in level of functioning over time. This type of observation, either as part of a longitudinal or cross-sectional study, will surely enhance our understanding of the disease course associated with the dementing process.

Both sets of rating scales of everyday functioning were significantly related to objective test performance. Functional ratings were more strongly tied to objective performance than were reports of problems by collaborative informants. The advantage of staff ratings over significant others' reports might be due to a psychosocial determinant of the perception of impairment by the collaborative informant. That is to say, this source of data may be limited by such factors as defensiveness, denial, or outright lack of information on behalf of the informant. On the other hand, neither data set provided absolute prediction of objective test performance. We believe that this observation is related to inherent difficulties associated with the testing procedure.

In objective testing, the examiner selects the behavior to be observed, regulates the pace of the examination, monitors the patient's problem-solving processes, and redirects the patient should he or she become distracted by irrelevant features within the examination procedures. In each case, the examiner fulfills an important role for the patient. The functions provided by the examiner are often the ones most important for determining the patient's level of functioning in everyday situations and the behaviors most likely to be impaired in the dementing process. This may mean that objective tests may never be able to assess the very factors that are most important to determining levels of everyday functioning. Objective testing may be critized at yet another level. These test procedures surely have a place in research, but within a clinical situation they may not be cost effective. At a simplistic level, if one wishes to know how well a patient maintains his room, it may be more efficient to develop a means of obtaining, from housekeeping staff, how much intervention is required than to attempt to develop a realistic method of assessing "room-keeping ability." Indeed, we believe that well-developed scales capable of obtaining information from a wide variety of sources have a much greater role to play in developing our understanding of everyday functioning in dementing patients than they currently enjoy.

NOTE

The authors thank the volunteers and staff of the University Hospital—UBC Site who made this study possible.

REFERENCES

Albert, M. S. (1982). Geriatric neuropsychology. *Journal of Consulting and Clinical Psychology* 49, 835–850.

Alzheimer, A. (1977). A unique illness involving the cerebral cortex. In D. A. Rottenberg & Hochberg (Eds.), *Neurologic classics in modern translation* (pp. 40–43). New York: Hafner Press. (Original work published 1907).

American Psychiatric Association. (1980). *Diagnostic and statistical manual of mental disorders (Third edition)*. Washington, D.C.: Author.

Baddeley, A., Sunderland, A., & Harris, J. (1982). How well do laboratory-based psychological tests predict patient's performance outside the laboratory? In S. Corkin et al. (Eds.), *Alzheimer's disease: A report of progress (Aging*, Vol. 19). New york: Raven Press.

Berger, E. Y. (1980). A system for rating the severity of senility. *Journal of the American Geriatrics Society* 28, 234–236.

Bigler, E., Steinman, D., & Newton, J. (1981). Clinical assessment of cognitive deficits in neurologic disorder. I: Effects of age and degenerative disease. *Clinical Neurology* 36, 5–13.

Blessed, G., Tomlinson, B. E., Roth, M. (1968). The association between quantitative measures of dementia and of senile change in the grey matter of elderly subjects. *British Journal of Psychiatry* 114, 797–811.

Brinkman, S., & Braun, P. (1984). Classification of dementia patients by a WAIS profile related to central cholinergic deficiencies. *Journal of Clinical Neuropsychology* 6 (4), 393–400.

Buschke, H. (1984). Cued recall in amnesia. *Journal of Clinical Neuropsychology* 6 (4), 433–440.

Clark, C., Crockett, D., & Klonoff, H. (1979). Empirically derived groups in the assessment of recovery from aphasia. *Brain and Language* 7, 240–251.

Clark, C., Crockett, D., Klonoff, H., & MacDonald, J. (1983). Analysis of the WAIS in brain damaged patients. *Journal of Clinical Neuropsychology* 5(2), 149–158.

Coblentz, J. M., Mattis, S., Zingesser, L. H., Kasoff, S. S., Wisniewski, H. M., & Katzman, R. (1973). Presenile dementia: Clinical evaluation of cerebrospinal fluid dynamics. *Archives of Neurology* 29, 299–308.

Coval, M., Crockett, D., Holliday, S., & Koch, W. (1985). A Multifocus Assessment Scale for use with frail elderly populations. *Canadian Journal on Aging* 4 (2), 101–109.

Crockett, D. (1977). A comparison of empirically derived groups of aphasic patients on the N.C.C.E.A. *Journal of Clinical Psychology* 33, 194–198.

Crockett, D., Clark, C., Spreen, O., & Klonoff, H. (1981). Severity of impairment on specific types of aphasia: An empirical investigation. *Cortex* 17, 83–96.

Cronbach, L. (1951). Coefficient alpha and the internal structure of tests. *Psychometrika* 16, 197–334.

Cummings, J. L., & Benson, D. F. (1986). Dementia of the Alzheimer type: An inventory of diagnostic clinical features. *Journal of the American Geriatrics Society* 34, 12–19.

Duke University Center for the Study on Aging. (1978). *Multidimensional functional assessment: the OARS methodology* (2nd ed.). Durham, NC: Duke University Press.

Folstein, M. F., Folstein, E., & McHugh, P. R. (1975). Mini-mental state: A practical method for grading the cognitive state of patients for the clinician. *Journal of Psychiatric Research* 12, 189–198.

Fuld, P. (1984). Test profiles of cholinergic dysfunction and Alzheimer's type dementia. *Journal of Clinical Neuropsychology* 6 (4), 380–392.

Gillen, R., Golden, C., & Eyde, D. (1982). Use of the Luria-Nebraska Neuropsychological Battery with elderly populations. *Clinical Gerontologist* 1 (2), 3–21.

Golden, C. J., Hammeke, T., & Purisch, A. (1978). Diagnostic validity of a standardized neuropsychological battery derived from Luria's neuropsychological tests. *Journal of Consulting and Clinical Psychology* 46 (6), 1258–1265.

Golden, R. R., Teresi, J. A., & Gurland, B. J. (1984). Development of indicator scales for the comprehensive assessment and referral evaluation interview schedule. *Journal of Geronotology* 39, 138–146.

Gurland, B., Golden, R. R., Teresi, J. A., & Challop, J. (1984). The SHORT-CARE: An efficient instrument for the assessment of depression, dementia and disability. *Journal of Gerontology* 39, 166–169.

Gurland, B., Kuriansky, J., Sharpe, L., Simon, R., Stiller, P., & Birkett, P. (1977–1978). The comprehensive assessment and referral evaluation (CARE)—rationale, development, and reliability. *International Journal of Aging and Human Development* 8, 9–41.

Hughes, C. P., Berg, L., Danziger, W. L., Coben, L. A., & Martin, R. L. (1982). A new clinical scale for the staging of dementia. *British Journal of Psychiatry* 140, 566–572.

Kane, R., Sweet, J., Golden, C., Parsons, O., & Moses, J. (1981). Comparative diagnostic accuracy of the Halstead-Reitan and standardized Luria-Nebraska neuropsychological batteries in a mixed psychiatric and brain-damaged population. *Journal of Consulting and Clinical Psychology* 49 (3) 484–485.

Kozma, A., & Stones, M. J. (1980). The measurement of happiness: Development of the Memorial University of Newfoundland Scale of Happiness (MUNSH). *Journal of Gerontology* 35 (6), 906–912.

Lawton, M. P. (1971). The functional assessment of elderly people. *Journal of the American Geriatric Society* 19, 465–481.

Lawton, M. P., & Brody, E. M. (1969). Assessment of older people: Self-maintaining and instrumental activities of daily living. *Gerontologist* 9, 179–186.

Lawton, M. P., Moss, M., Fulcomer, M., & Kleban, M. H. (1982). A research and service-oriented multi-level assessment instrument. *Journal of Gerontology* 37, 91–99.

Linn, M. W. (1967). A rapid disability rating scale. *Journal of American Geriatrics Society* 15, 211–214.

Linn, M. W., & Linn, B. S. (1981). Problems in assessing response to treatment in the elderly by physical and social function. *Psychopharmacology Bulletin* 17 (4), 74–81.

Linn, M. W., & Linn, B. S. (1982). The Rapid Disability Rating Scale-2. *Journal of the American Geriatrics Society* 30, 378–382.

Lawton, M. P. (1983). Assessment of behaviors required to maintain residence in the community. In T. Crook, S. Ferris, & R. Bartus (Eds.), *Assessment in geriatric psychopharmacology*. New Canaan, CT: Mark Powley.

Linn, M. W., & Linn, B. S. (1983). Assessing activities of daily living in institutional settings. In T. Cook, S. Ferris, & R. Bartus (Eds.), *Assessment in geriatric psychopharmacology* (pp. 97–110). New Canaan, CT: Mark Powley.

Linn, M. W., & Linn, B. S. (1984). Self-evaluation of life (SELF) scale: A short comprehensive self-report of health for the elderly. *Journal of Gerontology* 39, 603–612.

Martin, A., Brouwers, P., Lalonde, F., Cox, C., Teleska, P., & Fedio, P. (1986). Towards a behavioral typology of Alzheimer's patients. *Journal of Clinical and Experimental Neuropsychology*

8 (5), 594–610.

Mattis, S. (1976). Mental status examination for organic mental syndrome in the elderly patient. In L. Bellack & B. Karasu (Eds.), *Geriatric psychiatry* (pp. 77–121). New York: Grune & Stratton.

McKhann, G., Drachman, D., Folstein, M., Katzman, R., Price, D., & Stadlan, E. M. (1984). Clinical diagnosis of Alzheimer's disease: Report of the NINCDS-ADRDA work group under the auspices of the Department of Health and Human Services task force on Alzheimer's disease. *Neurology* 34, 939–944.

Miller, E. (1971). On the nature of the memory disorder in presenile dementia. *Neuropsychologia* 9, 75–81.

Mittenberg, W., Kasprisin, A., & Farage, C. (1985). Localization and diagnosis in aphasia with the Luria-Nebraska Neuropsychological Battery. *Journal of Consulting and Clinical Psychology* 53 (3), 386–392.

Nunnally, J. (1967). *Psychometric theory*. New York: McGraw-Hill.

Plum, F. Dementia. (1979). *Nature* 279, 372–375.

Reisberg, B., Ferris, S. H., DeLeon, M., & Crook, T. (1982). The Global Deterioration Scale for assessment of primary degenerative dementia. *American Journal of Psychiatry* 139 (9), 1136–1139.

Reitan, R., & Davison, L. (1974). *Clinical neuropsychology: Current status and applications* (p. 382). New York: John Wiley.

Rourke, B. (Ed.). (1985). *Neuropsychology of learning disorders: Essentials of subtype analysis*. New York: Guilford Press.

Schneck, M. K., Reisberg, B., & Ferris, S. H. (1982). An overview of current concepts of Alzheimer's disease. *American Journal of Psychiatry* 139, 165–173.

Spreen, O., & Benton, A. (1969). *Neurosensory centre comprehensive examination for aphasia*. Unpublished manuscript. University of Victoria, Neuropsychology Laboratory, Department of Psychology, Victoria.

SPSS—X. (1983). *Statistical packages for the social sciences—User's guide*. New York: Author.

Sulkava, R., Haltia, M., Paetau, A., Wikstrom, J., & Palo, J. (1983). Accuracy of clinical diagnosis in primary degenerative dementia: Correlation with neuropathological findings. *Journal of Neurology, Neurosurgery, and Psychiatry* 46, 9–13.

Tuokko, H., Crockett, D., Beattie, B. L., Horton, A., & Wong, W. (1986). *The use of rating scales to assess psycho-social functioning in demented patients*. Paper presented at the International Neuropsychological Society Annual Meeting, Denver, CO.

Tuokko, H., & Crockett, D. (1987). *Performance of normal and demented elderly on the Buschke cued recall test of memory*. Paper presented at the International Neuropsychological Society Annual Meeting, Washington, D.C.

Tuokko, H., Crockett, D., Holliday, S., & Coval, M. (1987). The relationship between performance on the multi-focus assessment scale and functional status. *Canadian Journal on Aging* 6 (1), 33–45.

Vitaliano, P. P., Breen, A. R., Albert, M. S., Russo, J., & Prinz, P. N. (1984). Memory, attention, and functional status in community-residing Alzheimer-type dementia patients and optimally healthy aged individuals. *Journal of Geronotology* 39 (1), 58–64.

Veldman, D. (1967). *Fortran programming for the behavioral sciences* (pp. 303–337). New York: Holt, Rinehart and Winston.

Wechsler, D. (1981). *Wechsler Adult Intelligence Scale—Revised*. New York: Harcourt, Brace, Jovanovich.

Weintraub, S., Baratz, R., & Mesulam, M. M. (1982). Daily living activities in the assessment of dementia. In S. Corkin (Ed.), *Alzheimer's disease: A report of progress* (pp. 189–192). (Aging. Vol. 19). New York: Raven Press.

Wells, C. E. (1982). Chronic brain disease: An update on alcoholism, Parkinson's disease, and dementia. *Hospital and Community Psychiatry* 33, 111–126.

Winograd, C. (1984). Mental status and activities of daily living. *The Geronotologist* 24, 257.

World Health Organization. (1978). *Mental disorders: Glossary and guide to their classification in accordance with the Ninth Revision of the International Classification of Diseases*. Geneva: Author.

7. LIFE SPAN PERSPECTIVE ON PRACTICAL INTELLIGENCE

SHERRY L. WILLIS AND MICHAEL MARSISKE

INTRODUCTION

The relatively brief history of the study of human intelligence reflects a continuing tension between identifying the most basic processes or units of cognition, on the one hand, and describing and predicting complex human behavior, on the other. Some eight decades ago, Binet (Binet & Simon, 1905) sought to predict performance on complex academic tasks via the assessment of a small group of basic mental abilities. Since Binet's time, research and debate has continued unabated on the relationship between basic cognitive processes and complex forms of intelligence. During the past two decades, the study of basic skills and cognitive processes has been reflected in the information-processing approach to cognition (Newell & Simon, 1972; Rybash, Hoyer, & Roodin, 1986; Salthouse, 1985), in the study of artificial intelligence (Hillman, 1985), and in the development of componential models of intelligence (Sternberg, 1982). The study of complex forms of human performance has been reflected in recent research on topics, such as expertise (Hoyer, 1985), practical or everyday intelligence (Sternberg & Wagner, 1986), and ecological and construct validity concerns within clinical psychology and neuropsychology (Crook, 1979; Kasniak & Davis, 1986; West, 1986).

In this chapter, we will consider the relationship between basic and complex forms of cognition from a life span perspective. We will begin by presenting a conceptual framework for defining the relationship between basic and complex forms of intelligence. Second, we will selectively review research on changes in performance on basic cognitive abilities that have been studied within a life span perspective. Findings on basic mental ability performance are of particular importance in this chapter, since we will propose that the individual's levels of functioning on basic units of cognition are important precursors of performance on many complex cognitive tasks. Third, we will review the limited literature on adults's performance on tasks of daily living. Everyday task performance is the aspect of practical intelligence of particular concern in this chapter. Finally, we will consider the implications of a life span approach for the study of practical intelligence in adulthood.

MULTIPLE INTELLIGENCE THEORIES

Several theorists propose that intelligent behavior involves multiple forms of intelligence, including a practical intelligence domain and a mechanistic domain. Baltes, Dittman-Kohli, and Dixon (1984) distinguished between the "mechanics" of intelligence involving basic mental abilities and cognitive processes, and the "pragmatics" of intelligence concerned with everyday cognition. In Sternberg's (1982) triarchic theory, the contextual part of intelligence is concerned with adaptation to one's environment and the componential part with cognitive mechanisms and processes. Several of those proposing multiple intelligence models consider practical intelligence to be the most salient form of intelligence in adulthood.

Practical intelligence is said to involve intellectual competence in naturalistic settings or in worldly affairs (Neisser, 1976; Wagner, 1986). Charlesworth (1976) defined practical intelligence as "behavior under the control of cognitive processes and employed toward the solution of problems which challenge the well-being, needs, plans, and survival of the individual" (p. 150). Definitions of practical intelligence have often focused on its distinction from one form of mechanistic or componential intelligence, namely academic intelligence. Academic intelligence has been measured in terms of tasks found on IQ tests and in school settings, and thus has been closely associated with the psychometric intelligence approach. Psychometric intelligence tasks have been characterized as (1) being disembedded from an individual's ordinary experience; (2) having little intrinsic interest; (3) being well defined in that all needed information is available; (4) being formulated by other people; and (5) having only one correct answer and one method of correct solution (Neisser, 1976; Wagner & Sternberg, 1986).

The primary distinction between practical and psychometric intelligence is that psychometric intelligence is reflected by tasks associated with the academic or clinical setting whereas practical intelligence involves tasks encountered in the "real" world. However, we find some of the other characteristics attributed to psychometric intelligence to be less apt in differentiating psychometric and practical intelligence. For example, many tasks of daily living are formulated by society rather than by the individual (e.g., driving regulations, banking procedures). Moreover, many practical problems involve one correct or commonly agreed on solution or procedure (e.g., determining the correct departure time from an airline schedule, giving the correct currency when purchasing an item).

A major issue for multiple intelligence theories is the definition of the interrelationship among the various forms. Berg and Sternberg (1985) stated, "A mechanistic theory is needed to specify the cognitive processes by which contextually appropriate behavior is carried out" (p. 348). The question then arises whether the mechanistic constructs and measures (e.g., primary abilities, cognitive processes) traditionally studied by psychologists are relevant to the study of practical intelligence. Moreover, does the salience of different mechanistic constructs vary with age? Some contend that psychometric and practical intelligence are distinct, unrelated forms of intelligence (Ceci & Liker, 1986; Friedricksen, 1986), but others suggest a hierarchical relationship between psychometric intelligence and some forms of practical intelligence (Berry & Irvine, 1986; Willis & Schaie, 1986). Our view is similar to that of Berry and Irvine (1986) in that basic cognitive processes and abilities are believed to be universal across cultures. When nurtured and directed by a particular culture, cognitive processes and abilities develop into cognitive competencies that are manifested in daily life as cognitive performance.

Findings from our research suggest a hierarchical model of the relationship between psychometric and practical intelligence, as shown in figure 7–1. Our research based on this model has been guided by several hypotheses. First, basic abilities and cognitive processes are important precursors of certain forms of practical intelligence. That is, the skills and processes represented in basic abilities are involved in performance of many practical intelligence tasks. Second, practical intelligence tasks are complex, and practical intelligence dimensions will be related to more than one basic ability or process. Third, practical intelligence can be represented in terms of multiple general practical intelligence dimensions. Performance on various practical intelligence dimensions should be interrelated. The interrelationship among practical intelligence dimensions may be related to shared factual knowledge or task features, or to basic abilities and processes that are common to multiple practical intelligence dimensions. Finally, age-related change in performance on a practical intelligence dimension should also be reflected in a related pattern of change in underlying abilities and processes.

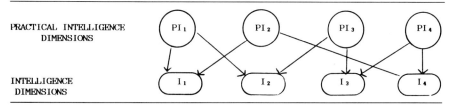

Figure 7–1. Hierarchical model of the relationship between basic abilities and processes (I) and dimensions of practical intelligence (PI).

DEVELOPMENTAL CHANGES IN BASIC MENTAL ABILITIES

Since in our conceptual framework, basic mental abilities and processes are hypothesized to underlie certain dimensions of practical intelligence performance, we will turn now to consideration of developmental changes in mental ability performance in adulthood. Within our model, changes in performance on basic cognitive abilities are of importance in understanding practical intelligence functioning in adulthood.

Much of the life span research on changes in basic cognitive processes has been conducted within a psychometric approach to the study of mental abilities (Botwinick, 1977; Schaie, 1983). Within the psychometric approach, intelligence is conceptualized in terms of a set of primary mental abilities. The question for the adult developmentalist is how performance on ability measures changes across adulthood.

Our understanding of developmental change in mental abilities is derived from findings of longitudinal studies, in which the same individuals are studied across time (Schaie, 1983). For the past decade we have have been involved in the Adult Development and Enrichment Project (ADEPT), a short-term longitudinal study of change in older adults' ability performance (Baltes et al., 1980; Willis, 1987). The ADEPT project has examined changes in mental ability functioning within the fluid–crystallized model of psychometric intelligence (Cattell, 1971).

According to this model, fluid intelligence is hypothesized to be the more elementary of the two intelligence dimensions and to be most closely associated with the neural substrate. Decline in fluid intelligence in old age is hypothesized, according to the model, to be associated with neural assaults or damage. Fluid intelligence involves the ability to reason with regard to novel and abstract problems. Fluid intelligence is a second-order dimension represented by primary abilities, such as Figural Relations and Inductive Reasoning. Measures of these abilities require the individual to determine a pattern of relationships in figural material or in a series of numbers or letters. Because the measures are administered under timed conditions, the individual is required to engage in abstract reasoning in a time-limited context.

In contrast to fluid intelligence, crystallized intelligence is hypothesized to reflect abilities and skills acquired within cultural institutions, such as schooling. In old age, crystallized intelligence is hypothesized to decline at a later age and at a slower rate than fluid intelligence. Crystallized intelligence is represented by primary abilities, such as verbal meaning and social intelligence. In addition, we have examined change in a third intelligence dimension, speed. The speed dimension assesses the individual's ability to make simple perceptual discriminations accurately under speeded conditions. The speed dimension is represented by the perceptual speed primary ability.

In the ADEPT project, we examined change in ability performance in older adults, 60 to 84 years of age. They were assessed at two occasions over a 7-year interval. Figure 7–2 presents short-term longitudinal data regarding change

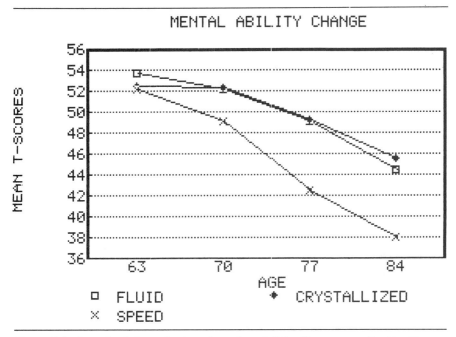

Figure 7–2. Age-related change for three dimensions: fluid intelligence, crystallized intelligence, and speed.

in performance on the fluid, crystallized, and speed dimensions for ADEPT participants.

Note that the pattern and rate of decline vary across the three intelligence dimensions. The steepest pattern of decline occurred for the speed dimension, as would be expected. There is considerable evidence within the gerontological aging literature regarding age-related decline in speed of responding (Salthouse, 1985). Across the age period studied, the magnitude of normative age-related decline on the speed dimension is approximately 2.50 standard deviation units. Note also that the magnitude of decline is less from 63 to 70 years than from 70 to 77 years.

On average, fluid intelligence also exhibits a relatively linear pattern of decline; however, the magnitude of decline from age 63 to 84 is approximately one standard deviation unit, much less than the magnitude of decline for the speed dimension. In contrast, note that decline does occur later, on average, for crystallized intelligence, as hypothesized by the G_f–G_c model; there is no reliable decline from 63 to 70 years. The magnitude of decline for crystallized intelligence from age 63 to 84 is approximately one-half of a standard deviation unit.

Research from ADEPT and other longitudinal studies suggests several findings with regard to age-related change in basic abilities. First, the average

age of onset of decline varies across intelligence dimensions. For example, decline on crystallized abilities, such as vocabulary, has been shown to begin later, on average, than for abilities involving abstract reasoning and speeded responding. In contrast, the earliest onset of decline occurs, on average, for highly speeded tasks, as represented by the speed dimension.

Second, the magnitude of performance decline varies across abilities. The greatest magnitude of decline was found for the speed dimension. In contrast, the magnitude of decline for the crystallized intelligence dimension was approximately one-fifth the magnitude of decline for the speed dimension.

These two findings suggest that a *multidimensional* approach to the study of developmental change in mental abilities is required (Willis & Baltes, 1980). Since onset and rate of age-related decline vary for different abilities, it is useful to conceptualize cognitive functioning as a multidimensional construct rather than as a global, unitary phenomenon. Global assessments of intellectual ability, such as the total score on the Wechsler Adult Intelligence Scale (WAIS; Matarazzo, 1972), mask the pattern of differential developmental change occurring for various abilities. Neuropsychologists are sensitive to the importance of a multidimensional approach, since different cognitive processes are affected by different neural structures and areas of the brain.

In addition, longitudinal findings indicate that there are wide individual differences, not only in the level of ability performance, but in the onset and rate of ability change. Figure 7–3 presents the proportion of adults who declined, remained stable, or improved on the three intelligence dimensions (fluid, crystallized, speed) over a 7-year period. The top graph presents the proportion of individuals who declined, remained stable, or improved on each intelligence dimension from 63 to 70 years of age; the middle graphs from 70 to 77; the bottom graph from 77 to 84 years of age. Note that although the proportion of individuals exhibiting age-related decline increases across the age intervals, in most instances half or more of the individuals did not show reliable decline over the 7-year period. Only for the fluid dimension did the majority of the individuals exhibit decline from 77 to 84 years. Thus the widest range of individual differences in the pattern of ability change is shown for the oldest age group (77–84 years). There is considerable evidence that range of individual differences in ability performance increases with age (Willis, 1985).

DEVELOPMENTAL CHANGE IN TASKS OF DAILY LIVING

We turn now from consideration of basic cognitive skills and processes to a discussion of developmental change in forms of practical intelligence. Despite agreement that practical intelligence involves activities performed in real-world contexts, the specific tasks and measures employed to study practical intelligence have varied widely. Research on practical intelligence has included the study of expertise in various professions, including business managers and academic psychologists (Wagner & Sternberg, 1986), typists (Salthouse,

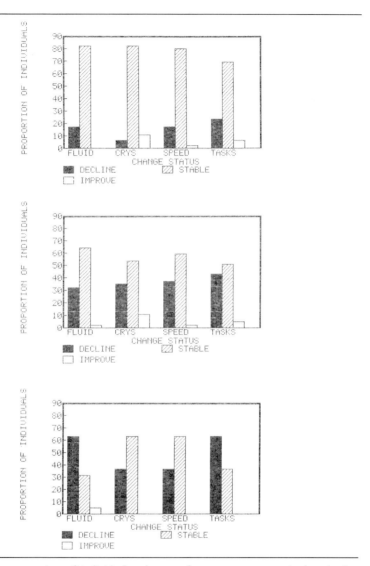

Figure 7–3. The proportion of individuals whose performance was categorized as having declined, remained stable, or improved on four intelligence dimensions: fluid intelligence, crystallized intelligence, speed, and everyday tasks. The top graph shows change status for age 63 to 70, the middle graph for 70 to 77, and the bottom graph for age 77 to 84.

1984), and lab technicians (Hoyer, 1985); expertise in leisure activities, such as chess and bridge (Charness, 1986); and the study of wisdom (Baltes, Dittman-Kohli, & Dixon, 1984).

Clinicians, however, are often concerned with the competence of patients to perform activities demanded in daily living within our society. Thus, in this chapter, we will consider practical intelligence in terms of activities of daily living. These activities are defined by the following characteristics: (1) the tasks involve cognitive problem solving; (2) they represent *common* activities experienced by "average" community-dwelling adults in their daily lives; (3) competency in many of these tasks is considered basic or essential to function effectively in our society; (4) the tasks may be defined by others (e.g., societal norms, legal regulations) rather than by the individual; and (5) many of these tasks involve one correct or commonly agreed on response.

In our research, we have studied adults' ability to perform everyday activities involving printed material. The tasks studied include (1) interpreting bottle labels, such as labels on prescription drugs or household cleaning products; (2) reading charts, schedules, and tables, such as bus schedules, employee benefit tables, or weight charts; (3) reading a road map; (4) interpreting advertisements, such as a "yellow page" ad; and (5) interpreting text material, such as the letter to the editor in a newspaper.

Previous research has shown that adults, particularly the elderly, have difficulty reading and interpreting printed material. Misinterpretation of printed material interferes with many adults' ability to carry out activities of daily living. Studies indicate that errors in self-administered medications are made by 40 to 60% of the elderly (Ouslander, 1981). Ability to comprehend prescription labels is a significant predictor of patient compliance; 24% of the elderly failed to understand the primary prescription label, and 39% misinterpreted the auxiliary label (Murray et al., 1986). In a national study 33% of adults could not comprehend a medicare form and 10% could not interpret a personal loan form (Robeck & Wilson, 1977). Studies indicate that adults also have difficulty with consumer-related tasks; only 33% of shoppers could determine the most economical size of product from information on the package (Capon & Kuhn, 1982).

Cross-sectional studies indicate that even young and middle-aged adults have difficulty with printed-material tasks, but there is the additional problem in later adulthood that performance may decline as a function of age-related change. In the following section, we will present data from our own research regarding age-related change in performance on everyday tasks involving printed materials.

Longitudinal Change in Everyday Task Performance

We examined 7-year change in performance of everyday tasks involving printed material in the same older adult population for which mental ability data were presented earlier in the chapter. Figure 7–4 presents average longitudinal change data for three groups: 63-year-olds retested at age 70; 70-year-olds retested at age 77; and 77-year-olds retested at age 84. Note that the pattern of age-related change is fairly linear but that the magnitude of change varies across the age groups. The 63-year-olds' decline was less than .2 of a

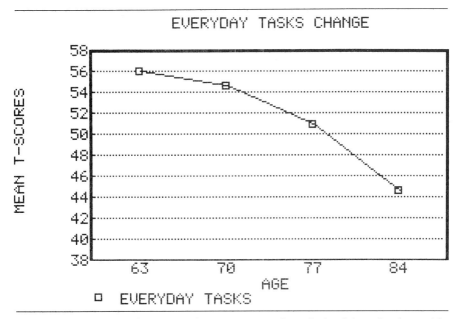

Figure 7–4. Age-related change in performance on everyday tasks involving printed material.

standard deviation over the 7-year interval. In contrast, the magnitude of decline was .40 and .60 standard deviation units for the 70- and 77-year-olds, respectively.

In our model of practical intelligence, we hypothesized that basic mental abilities and cognitive processes were some of the primary precursors of competence in everyday tasks performance. Therefore, it is of interest to compare patterns of age-related change for basic mental abilities (figure 7–2) with longitudinal change for everyday activities (figure 7–4). Comparison of the two figures suggests that change in everyday tasks involving printed materials most closely resembles the pattern of change exhibited by fluid intelligence. For both fluid intelligence and everyday tasks, age-related change is evident beginning at age 63, and the magnitude of decline increases over each 7-year age interval. The pattern of decline on everyday tasks differs from that for the other two mental ability dimensions, in that decline on everyday tasks begins somewhat earlier than decline shown for crystallized intelligence; however, decline on everyday tasks is less steep than that shown for speed.

Although figure 7–4 indicates a decline, *on average*, for older adults on everyday tasks involving printed material, further analyses of the data indicate wide individual differences in the rate and patterns of change. Each individual's scores were examined in terms of magnitude of change, and an individual's performance was categorized as having reliably declined, having remained stable, or having improved over the 7-year interval. On the right-hand side of figure 7–3, a bar graph shows the proportion of individuals in each of the three age groups exhibiting decline, stability, or improvement trajectories for everyday tasks. Note that approximately 70% of the subjects showed no reliable decline over the period from 63 to 70 years of age and that 38% showed reliable decline over this age period. Though 43% of the individuals showed reliable decline from 70 to 77 years, still half of those studied showed no decline. In the oldest age group, most individuals did show age-related decline from 77 to 84 years; however, the performance of 36% did not decline. These data demonstrate that comparison of group means, such as in figure 7–4, masks the wide individual differences in patterns and rate of change. Although the mean scores suggested decline, on average, across all age groups, scores of individuals indicate that at least half of the subjects showed no reliable decline from 63 to 70, or from 70 to 77 years of age.

Ability Correlates and Predictors of Everyday Task Performance

In our model, basic mental abilities and cognitive processes were hypothesized to be antecedents of performance on complex cognitive tasks. To test this hypothesis, we examined whether performance on basic mental abilities at the first assessment occasion was a significant predictor of everyday task performance 7 years later. The three mental abilities (fluid, crystallized, speed) at the first occasion of measurement were entered as independent variables in multiple regression analyses, conducted separately for each of the three age groups. Fluid and crystallized abilities were found to be significant predictors of everyday task performance for each of the three age groups. Substantial individual differences in everyday task performance were accounted for by the mental abilities for each of the three age groups: $R^2 = .80$; $R^2 = .61$; $R^2 = .69$.

To examine further the reciprocal relationship between abilities and everyday task performance, a series of structural equation analyses were conducted. That is, the directionality of the relationship between abilities and everyday tasks was examined by contrasting models of abilities as predictors of everyday task performance *versus* models of everyday task performance as predictors of abilities. Findings from the structural equation analyses indicated that fluid ability at the first assessment occasion predicted everyday task performance at the second assessment occasion 7 years later. However, subsequent analyses indicated that everyday task performance at the first assessment occasion predicted abilities at the second assessment occasion less well. Therefore, these findings provide strong support for our hypothesis that functioning on basic mental abilities is a significant antecedent of everyday task performance.

A significant relationship between basic abilities or cognitive processes and measures of daily activities has also been reported by several other investigators. Cavanaugh (1983) found verbal ability to be related to recall of TV program material. In a study examining differences in young and older adults' recall, he found no difference in recall for high verbal young and older adults; however, low verbal older adults recalled significantly less material. Furthermore, verbal ability was found to be particularly important for the initial comprehension of the TV program, thus influencing encoding rather than retrieval.

In a series of studies Kausler & Hakami (1983) examined age differences in recall of activities performed by subjects. Several laboratory measures of verbal learning (i.e., serial learning, paired-associates, verbal discrimination learning) were found to be significant predictors of older adults' ability to recall activities performed; however, no relationship between the verbal learning tasks and activity recall was found for younger adults. Camp and colleagues (1989) found inductive reasoning ability to be a significant correlate of older adults' performance on everyday problem-solving tasks (e.g., what to do when the refrigerator breaks down). Fluid and crystallized abilities were also related to solution of interpersonal conflict problems (Cornelius & Caspi, 1987; Cornelius, Kenny, & Caspi, 1989).

If everyday problem solving is broadly construed to include cognitively oriented leisure activities, the literature also indicates an association between frequency of game playing and performance on laboratory/clinical tasks. Rice, Meyer, and Miller (1988) examined the relationship between prose recall and the elderly's leisure activities. Over half of the variance in prose recall was explained by amount of time spent in playing word games; a positive association was found between recall and doing crossword puzzles; a negative relationship between recall and playing of bingo was found. Clark, Lanphear, and Riddick (1987) found that videogame playing resulted in significant improvement in the elderly's reaction time. Finally, our research also indicated self-reports of frequency of game playing to be predictive of mental ability performance (Tosti-Vasey et al., 1987).

On the other hand, several studies report little relationship between laboratory/clinical tasks and applied problems. Wagner and Sternberg (1986) found generally nonsignificant correlations between verbal ability and tacit knowledge regarding professional issues in academic psychology and business management for professionals in these disciplines. Ceci and Liker (1986) reported little relationship between a general IQ measure and race-track handicapping for expert racecourse bettors. Mercer, Gomez-Palacio, and Padilla (1986) reported nonsignificant relationships between social adaptive behavior and a general IQ measure.

The preceding discrepancies in research findings can be attributed to a number of factors. First, many of the studies reporting no relationship between laboratory tasks and everyday problem solving have focused on highly domain-specific tasks that involve a very specialized knowledge base (e.g., race-course handicapping). A second related problem is that a number of studies have in actuality been studies of expertise, in which performances of experts and novices in the same field have been compared. The expertise approach has focused on highly specialized domains of knowledge involving select occupational groups (e.g., senior management, psychology faculty) or activities (e.g., race-course handicapping) for which criteria regarding expertise can be documented. As Wagner (1986) acknowledged, it would be difficult to define expertise or to select experts for many aspects of everyday problem solving. Third, subjects have often represented very select samples (e.g., psychology faculty, MBA graduate students), such that there is likely to be a restriction in range for the laboratory or ability measures and/or for the criterion-practical intelligence tasks, resulting in lower correlations. Novices in the expertise studies are often graduate students in the same professional field. Fourth, many studies have measured academic intelligence in terms of a single laboratory measure (e.g., vocabulary test) or a global intelligence test (e.g., WISC). However, everyday problem-solving tasks are complex and would be expected to involve multiple abilities; thus the relationship between a wide array of abilities and a given task of daily living needs to be examined.

It is worth noting that a number of the studies reporting a significant relationship between laboratory ability tasks and everyday problem solving involve older adult samples and less select populations. In two studies (Cavanaugh, 1983; Kausler & Hakami, 1983) a significant relationship was found for the older adult group but not for the younger adult group. A larger correlation between ability measures and everyday problem solving in old age may be partially due to the fact that individual differences in cognitive functioning tend to increase in later adulthood, as some older adults begin to experience cognitive decline and others remain stable in performance (figure 7–3).

SUMMARY AND IMPLICATIONS

A life span approach to the study of practical intelligence involves a focus on three issues. First, the researcher and clinician must be attentive to developmental *change* occurring within the individual. Individuals continue to develop and change across the life course. The researcher and clinician must be knowledgeable regarding normative patterns of age-related change for various cognitive abilities and processes. Longitudinal research indicates that the rate and pattern of change differ across various abilities. As illustrated in our research, abilities and skills involving novel, abstract reasoning (e.g., fluid intelligence) and speeded responses show an earlier and steeper pattern of decline than abilities and skills (e.g., crystallized intelligence) that are more meaningful and routinely exercised. Our data indicated that decline in crystallized problems occurred later than for novel, fluid reasoning tasks. Many older adults function adequately in familiar, routinized contexts, but they function less effectively and are vulnerable to mishaps when required to reason and respond to unfamiliar, abstract problems that require quick (speeded) responses.

Second, a life span approach emphasizes the importance of *individual differences* in the study of development. Variability in cognitive performance often increases with increasing age, as illustrated in figure 7–3. For all of the abilities and skills examined, 70 to 80% of individuals remained stable from 63 to 70 years of age. However, over the age period of 70 to 77 years, an increasing proportion of individuals experience reliable decline, thus increasing the variability in performance within this age group. This pattern of increasing variability continued in the oldest age group (77–84 years). The implication of greater variability with age is that the study and treatment of the older adult needs to become increasingly individualized. Greater attention needs to be given to the prior developmental history of the individual in diagnoses and treatment, since in old-old age there is no one universal developmental pattern. For example, a low level of performance may indicate that the older adult has suffered significant decline, *or* it may be that the individual's performance is stable and that he or she has performed at a low level for many years; information on the individual's prior developmental history is needed to differentiate between the two diagnoses.

Third, a *multidimensional* approach to the study of both basic and complex forms of cognition is indicated within a life span perspective. That is, the basic units of cognition involve multiple abilities and skills that have different patterns and rates of change across the adult life course. Global or unitary measures of cognition mask the multidimensionality and multidirectionality of cognitive change. A multidimensional approach to the study of practical intelligence is indicated. Our model and research findings indicate that practical intelligence problems are complex and that multiple basic abilities serve as predictors or precursors of performance on complex cognitive tasks. For example, in the data presented in this chapter, both fluid and crystallized abilities were found to be predictors of everyday tasks involving printed material; both verbal ability and reasoning skills were required to perform tasks, such as interpreting medicine bottle labels or reading a bus schedule. The specific abilities and skills that underlie various complex tasks will vary with the nature of the tasks. However, we believe that most tasks of daily living will involve multiple basic abilities and skills.

Finally, we have presented data to suggest that significant relationships do exist between laboratory or clinical assessment measures and at least some tasks of daily living. In terms of multiple intelligence theories, our findings suggest a relationship between the "mechanics" and the "pragmatics" of intelligence. The challenge for the researcher and clinician lies in further examination of the interface between basic cognitive processes and practical intelligence activities required to function effectively in our society.

NOTE

Preparation of this chapter was supported by research grants AGO3544 and AGO5304 from the National Institute on Aging.

REFERENCES

Baltes, P., Cornelius, S., Spiro, A., Nesselroade, J., & Willis, S. (1980). Integration vs differentiation of fluid-crystallized intelligence in old age. *Developmental Psychology* 16, 625–635.

Baltes, P., Dittman-Kohli, R., & Dixon, R. (1984). New perspective on the development of intelligence in adulthood: Toward a dual-process conception and a model of selective optimization with compensation. In P. Baltes & O. Brim, Jr. (Eds.), *Life-span development and behavior* (Vol. 6, pp. 33–76). New York: Academic Press.

Berg, C., & Sternberg, R. (1985). A triadic theory of intellectual development during adulthood. *Developmental Review* 5, 334–370.

Berry, J., & Irvine, S. (1986). Bricolage: Savages do it daily. In R. Sternberg & R. Wagner (Eds.), *Practical intelligence* (pp. 271–306). New York: Cambridge University Press.

Binet, A., & Simon, T. (1905). Methodes nouvelles pour le diagnostic du niveau intellectual des anormaux. *L'Anee Psychologique* 11, 191–244.

Botwinick, J. (1977). Intellectual abilities. In J. E. Birren & K. W. Schaie (Eds.), *Handbook of the psychology of aging*. New York: Van Nostrand Reinhold.

Camp, C., Doherty, K., Moody-Thomas, & Denney, N. (1989). Practical problem solving in adults: A comparison of problem types and scoring methods. In J. Sinnott (Ed.), *Everyday problem solving: Theory and applications*. New York: Praeger.

Capon, N., & Kuhn, D. (1982). Can consumers calculate best buys? *Journal of Consumer Research* 8, 449–453.

Cattell, R. (1971). *Abilities: Their structure, growth, and action*. Boston, MA: Houghton-Mifflin.

Cavanaugh, J. C. (1983). Comprehension and retention of television programs by 20- and 60-year olds. *Journal of Gerontology* 38, 190–196.

Ceci, S., & Liker, J. (1986). Academic and nonacademic intelligence: An experimental separation. In R. Sternberg & R. Wagner (Eds.), *Practical intelligence* (pp. 119–142). New York: Cambridge University Press.

Charlesworth, W. (1976). Intelligence as adaptation: An ethological approach. In L. Resnick (Ed.), *The nature of intelligence* (pp. 147–168). Hillsdale, NJ: Ablex.

Charness, N. (1986). Expertise in chess, music, and physics: A cognitive perspective. In L. K. Obler & D. A. Fein (Eds.), *The neuropsychology of talent and special abilities*. New York: Guilford.

Clark, J., Lanphear, A., & Riddick, C. (1987). The effects of videogame playing on the response selection processing of elderly adults. *Journal of Gerontology* 42, 82–85.

Cornelius, S., & Caspi, A. (1987). Everyday problem solving in adulthood and old age. *Psychology and Aging* 2, 144–153.

Cornelius, S., Kenny, S., & Caspi, A. (1989). Academic and everyday intelligence in adulthood: Conception of self and ability tests. In J. Sinnott (Ed.), *Everyday problem solving: Theory and applications*. New York: Praeger.

Crook, T. (1979). Psychometric assessment in the aged. In A. Raskin & L. F. Jarvik (Eds.), *Psychiatric symptoms and cognitive loss in the elderly*. Washington, D.C.: Hemisphere.

Frederiksen, J. (1986). A componential theory of reading skills. In R. Sternberg (Ed.), *Advances in the psychology of human intelligence* (Vol. 1). Hillsdale, NJ: Erlbaum.

Hillman, D. (1985). Artificial intelligence. *Human Factors* 27, 21–31.

Hoyer, W. (1985). Aging and the development of expert cognition. In T. M. Shlecter & M. Toglia (Eds.), *New directions in cognitive science* (pp. 69–87). Norwood, NJ: Ablex.

Hultsch, D., & Dixon, R. (1984). Memory for test materials in adulthood. In P. B. Baltes & O. G. Brim (Eds.), *Life-span development and behavior* (Vol. 6). New York: Academic Press.

Kasniak, A., & Davis, K. (1986). Instrument and data review: The quest for external validators. In L. Poon (Ed.), *Handbook for clinical memory assessment*. Washington, D.C.: American Psychological Association.

Kausler, D., & Hakami, M. (1983). Memory for activities: Adult age differences and intentionality. *Developmental Psychology* 19, 889–894.

Matarazzo, J. (1972). *Wechsler's measurement and appraisal of adult intelligence* (5th ed.). Baltimore: Williams & Wilkins.

Mercer, J., Gomez-Palacio, M., & Padilla, E. (1986). The development of practical intelligence in cross-cultural perspective. In R. Sternberg & R. Wagner (Eds.), *Practical intelligence* (pp. 307–337). New York: Cambridge University Press.

Murray, M., Darnell, Weinberger, M., & Martz, B. (1986). Factors contributing to medication noncompliance in elderly public housing tenants. *Drug Intelligence and Clinical Pharmacy* 20, 146–151.

Neisser, U. (1976). General, academic, and artificial intelligence. In L. Resnick (Ed.), *Human intelligence: Perspectives on its theory and measurement* (pp. 179–189). Norwood, NJ: Ablex.

Newell, A., & Simon, H. (1972). *Human problem solving*. Englewood Cliffs. NJ: Prentice-Hall.

Ouslander, J. (1981). Drug therapy in the elderly. *Annals of Internal Medicine* 95, 711–722.

Rice, G., Meyer, B., & Miller, D. (1988). Relation of everyday activities of adults to their prose recall performance. *Educational Geronotology* 14, 147–158.

Robeck, M., & Wilson, J. (1977). *Psychology of reading: Foundations of instruction*. New York: Wiley.

Rybash, J., Hoyer, W., & Roodin, P. (Eds.). (1986). *Adult cognition and aging*. New York: Pergamon.

Salthouse, T. (1984). Effects of age and skill in typing. *Journal of Experimental Psychology: General* 113, 345–371.

Salthouse, T. (1985). *A theory of cognitive aging*. Amsterdam: North Holland.

Schaie, K. W. (1983). *Longitudinal studies of adult psychological development*. New York: Guilford.

Sternberg, R. (1982). A componential approach to intellectual development. In R. Sternberg (Ed.), *Advances in the psychology of human intelligence* (Vol. 1). Hillsdale, NJ: Erlbaum.

Sternberg, R., & Wagner, R. (Eds.). (1986). *Practical intelligence*. New York: Cambridge University Press.

Tosti-Vasey, J., Willis, S., Christina, R., & Jay, G. (1987). *Cognitive abilities and frequency of game playing in the elderly*. Paper presented at the annual meeting of the American Psychological Association, New York.

Wagner, R. (1986). The search for intraterrestrial intelligence. In R. Sternberg & R. Wagner (Eds.), *Practical intelligence*. New York: Cambridge University Press.

Wagner, R., & Sternberg, R. (1986). Tacit knowledge and intelligence in the everyday world. In R. Sternberg & R. Wagner (Eds.), *Practical intelligence*. New York: Cambridge University Press.

West, R. (1986). Everyday memory and aging. *Developmental Neuropsychology* 2, 323–344.

Willis, S. L. (1985). Towards an educational psychology of the adult learner. In J. Birren & K. W. Schaie (Eds.), *Handbook of the psychology of aging* (2nd ed). New York: Van Nostrand Reinhold.

Willis, S. (1987). Cognitive interventions in the elderly (1987). In K. Schaie (Ed.), *Annual review of gerontology and geriatrics* (Vol. VII, pp. 159–188). New York: Springer.

Willis, S. L., & Baltes, P. B. (1980). In L. W. Poon (Ed.), *Aging in the 1980s: Psychological Issues* (pp. 260–272). Washington, DC: American Psychological Association.

Willis, S., & Schaie, K. (1986). Practical intelligence in later adulthood. In R. Sternberg & R. Wagner (Eds.), *Practical intelligence*. New York: Cambridge University Press.

II. ISSUES IN REHABILITATION

8. A RATIONALE FOR FAMILY INVOLVEMENT IN LONG-TERM TRAUMATIC HEAD INJURY REHABILITATION

HARVEY E. JACOBS

INTRODUCTION

Advances in medical treatment and rehabilitation have improved outcomes for many survivors of traumatic head injury. Once medical sequelae are controlled however, many survivors face complex problems that preclude the opportunity for self-sufficient living. Newly developing therapies can address some of these issues, but this treatment is not available to all due to cost, geographic location, and the inability to address the broad multitude of problems faced by this population. In the absence of professional treatment, family members frequently find themselves serving as therapists, despite lack of training and problems that they may be experiencing with their own personal adjustment to the catastrophic injury. However, research with other populations of disabled persons has demonstrated that family members can be trained to be effective therapeutic agents to meet a broad range of issues and learn how to advocate for needed services beyond their capabilities. It is likely that this technology can also be used to help meet some of the long-term needs of persons with traumatic head injuries.

Traumatic head injuries are one of the leading causes of death and disability in the United States. Each year more than 100,000 people die from head trauma, 50,000 to 90,000 experience significant intellectual and physical impairments that precludes their return to independent living, and more than 200,000 experience continuing sequelae that interfere with normal life (Anderson et al., 1980; Caveness, 1979; Jennett & MacMillan, 1981; Kalsbeek et al., 1980; Kraus,

1978; Olson & Henig, 1983). Head injury ranks third as a leading neurologic cause of disability, behind cerebrovascular disease and epilepsy, and ahead of other more commonly recognized disorders such as Parkinson's disease, primary brain tumor, spinal cord injury, multiple sclerosis, cerebral palsy, and congenital muscular distrophy (National Head Injury Foundation, 1982). It is the primary cause of neurologic disability for individuals under 34 years of age (Kraus et al., 1984).

Although major advances in the acute medical management of head injury patients have developed over the past decade, advances in long-term rehabilitation have not followed as rapidly. Immediately following a traumatic head injury, the patient can expect comprehensive and competent medical care from interdisciplinary treatment teams. Medical developments over the past decade have helped to improve the prognosis for once considered terminal cases (Bakay & Glasauer, 1980; Jennett & Teasdale, 1981). Psychosocial treatment is also generally available during the initial months of adjustment to help patients accept their disability and adapt to a new life-style, help them locate sources of financial support, and encourage them to continue treatment (Bond, 1979; Govthier, 1980; Panting & Merry, 1972).

Early intervention is also directed toward helping the family unit adjust to major changes in roles, expectancies, and interaction as a result of the trauma. Similar to other chronic and traumatic medical disorders, family members need special help in adjusting to the catastrophe as well as to the beginnings of a new and significantly altered life (Kubler-Ross, 1969; Muir & Haffey, 1984; Rosenthal, 1984).

POSTDISCHARGE SERVICES

Once acute treatment ends, however, many patients and families find themselves in compromised situations due to the number and complexity of posttraumatic sequelae. For example, in a study of 50 severely head-injured patients 12 to 70 months posttrauma, Thomsen (1974) noted than 70% still experienced physical disabilities ranging from minor motor dysfunctions to severe gait disturbances, and 38% remained aphasic. Only 8% were able to return to their previous job, and 72% were unable to even enter a sheltered workshop setting. Eighty-four percent of the patients had significant psychological and behavior problems, including irritability, uncontrolled tempers, unresponsiveness, lethargy, pathological laughing/weeping, and psychiatric or emotional disturbances. Only 14 were able to live independently, with the remaining patients dependent on their families for perpetual support. Most other studies of severe traumatic head injury patients have noted similar outcomes (Brooks & Aughton, 1979; Jennett et al., 1981; Lezak et al., 1980; Mauss-Clum & Ryan, 1981; Najenson et al., 1980, 1974; Oddy et al., 1978a; Weddell et al., 1980).

Although some patients may receive continuing physical, occupational, or speech therapy after leaving the hospital, the level and variety of outpatient services are drastically reduced for a variety of reasons. Many patients have sustained extended hospital stays that have exhausted their insurance benefits. Others find that their policies do not cover continuing rehabilitation programs or services deemed educational or psychosocial rather than medical in nature (National Head Injury Foundation, 1982). Frequently, the types of services required posthospitalization are different and more involved than those required during the initial phases of recovery. Because an insufficient number of long-term neurological rehabilitation programs are available, many clients simply do not have access to proper treatment (Gagnon, 1984). This is especially unfortunate since recovery following severe head injury is a long-term process that does not end with hospital discharge or even after a one- or two-year period of "spontaneous recovery." In fact, continued recovery among traumatic head injury patients has been documented for periods of up to 30 years (Thomsen, 1981; Thorp, 1956, 1983).

Advances in the field of cognitive rehabilitation and skill integration (Ben-Yishay & Diller, 1983; Gianutsos, 1980; Trexler, 1982) have also demonstrated significant improvement in patient functioning years after neurological regeneration has theoretically plateaued (Institute of Rehabilitation Medicine, 1978, 1979, 1980, 1981; Najenson et al., 1984). Major changes in the philosophy and direction of long-term treatment are evolving as a result of these findings, with greater emphasis placed on long-term and more complex skills acquisition (Rosenthal et al., 1983).

Even in the absence of continuing neurological recovery, rehabilitation programming can help the individual and family members circumvent fixed deficits and address problems that will not go away through environmental and social engineering procedures (Bond & Brooks, 1976). Lindsley (1964) called this process behavioral prosthetics, in reference to physical prosthetics. Much as a physical prosthesis can help a person overcome the disability incurred through loss of a limb, behavioral prostheses can help the individual overcome the loss of intellectual, cognitive, and behavioral abilities by structuring the environment and people around the person to compensate for the deficit. For example, family members can help the patient with memory deficits, or special mapping systems can be set up in the environment to help the individual with perceptual deficits. Aggressive behavior episodes may be similarly managed by controlling the amount and diversity of stimulation that the impaired person receives. Unlike the physical prosthesis that can often be independently managed by the patient, however, behavioral prostheses often require the continuing work of others in the environment and therefore suggest the need for lifetime care.

FAMILY INVOLVEMENT

In the absence of available long-term rehabilitation services, the responsibility for continuing care often falls on family members (Jacobs, 1984; Muir & Haffey, 1984; National Head Injury Foundation, 1981; Rosenthal, 1984).

Although many families are willing to accept this responsibility, they are often ill-equipped to meet the associated challenges. Caring for a family member with a head injury involves maintaining one's ongoing commitments, assuming the responsibilities of the disabled family member, recognizing the special needs the patient now presents, and acquiring expertise in medical and psychosocial treatment protocols that are relevant to patient care. The changes in daily life that the nonimpaired family members often experience can also have profound influences on the development, growth, and stability of each person in the household (Jacobs, 1985; Lezak, 1978; Rosenbaum & Najenson, 1976). Roles, responsibilities, opportunities, socialization, and almost every other area of each family member's daily life are affected.

Family members must also deal with the impact of a head-injured member in the family unit. The stress imposed by the added demands of the family frequently exacerbate existing problems or promulgate new ones. For example, the loss of a breadwinner's ability to provide for the family may incur financial uncertainty and feelings of incompetency or jealousy. The survivor's psychological, behavioral, and emotional problems may impact on the family more than the physical impairments regardless of how understanding they may be (Bond, 1979; Brooks & Aughton, 1979; Oddy et al., 1978a, b). Patients who exhibit no physical symptoms but do exhibit less easily assessed cognitive and behavioral sequelae are often misunderstood as being lazy, stubborn, or apathetic, which in turn breeds family resentment and anger. These problems, combined with frustration over insufficient resources, poor knowledge, and unavailable programs to meet immediate needs, further increase the toll on the family. Although some families are able to "pull together" and help their impaired member, many families have been noted to suffer a variety of serious consequences, including break-up, separation, divorce, alienation of specific family members, and increased psychosomatic, emotional, and physical illness (Lezak, 1978; Liberman et al., 1980; Mauss-Clum & Ryan, 1981; Oddy et al., 1978a, Thomsen, 1974).

Finally, there are the dynamics of adjustment to the catastrophe that family members also experience. Although the paradigms used to describe this course of adjustment have met with varying levels of acceptance, there is general acknowledgment of an adaptation process and its effects on the family's ability to function as a unit, care for each other, and help the patient (Fink, 1967; Kubler-Ross, 1969; Pearson, 1973; Weisman, 1972). During early phases of adjustment when family members have not yet acknowledged (or deny) the extent of the injury, they often have difficulty accepting the advice of others and caring for the patient. Intervention beyond general support at this stage is generally unsuccessful (Romano, 1974; Rosenthal & Muir, 1983). As families move toward acceptance, they may gradually begin to take greater responsibility for the head-injured member and accept the advice of others. The likelihood of successful family intervention increases with such acceptance.

The development of this acceptance, however, is not an absolute or linear process. The amount of time required to move through these phases can vary significantly—sometimes taking years; not all family members progress through the phases at the same rate, and it is not clear that all families pass through all of the acknowledged phases. In addition, the rate of progress toward acceptance is often influenced by factors such as family typology, shock of the catastrophic event, available family resources, the premorbid family situation, past history of coping, and the age and familial role of the patient (Fisher, 1977; Power & Dell Orto, 1980). The development of acceptance may also be more of a dynamic than a direct process, especially when dealing with the nondefinitive nature of traumatic head injury. With the lack of an "ultimate" resolution, the family members may fluctuate between levels of acceptance according to the progress and setbacks that their injured family member continues to face over their lifetime (Muir & Haffey, 1984).

Family Contributions to Rehabilitation

Despite these concerns there are a number of reasons to consider the family as a logical and potent force in long-term traumatic head injury rehabilitation programming.

First, supportive family members can often provide more integrated contact hours to the patient than outpatient treatment programs (Mace & Rabins, 1982). Even moderately functioning families can be available almost constantly, compared to the limited hours of costly professionals.

Second, family members may be more motivated to continue long-term and intensive treatment in search of small but important gains when others have given up. The significant effect that a concerned and a caring family member can have on the quality of a patient's outcome has been repeatedly acknowledged in the rehabilitation literature (Muir & Haffey, 1984; Power & Dell Orto, 1980; Wright, 1980) as well as in Hollywood.

Third, experience in other clinical areas such as child management (Becker, 1971; Falloon & Liberman, 1983; Patterson, 1975) has demonstrated that many daily training and rehabilitation programs can be conducted by the family, with proper guidance, at a lower cost than professional service delivery.

Fourth, clinical evidence indicates that family members may personally benefit through a sense of understanding and accomplishment when they are actively involved in the rehabilitation process (Sbordone, 1983). Families are often able to work out problems of guilt, helplessness, and anger by becoming a productive force in the patient's recovery (Grief & Matarazzo, 1982; Seligman, 1975).

Fifth, the level of positive support provided by the family has been noted to favorably influence outcome, whereas negative family roles can retard progress if not treated (Galloway & Goldstein, 1971; Lindenberg, 1977; Meff, 1959; Olshansky & Beach, 1975).

Sixth, there is the financial reality of the cost of rehabilitation to society. With the exception of major breakthroughs in either treatment or financial aid, there are few alternatives to family members for extended treatment beyond the level of custodial care (Gagnon, 1984).

Finally, informed and concerned family members are typically stronger advocates for the disabled person than anyone else. In the absence of needed services, groups of affected families of other disabled populations have historically organized to provide or lobby for appropriate treatment. The history of the Association for Retarded Citizens and correspondent changes in treatment for persons with developmental disabilities is perhaps the best working model of this approach today. The concerted efforts of this group of families in conjunction with involved professionals over the past 25 years has helped to bring about dramatic changes in services, helping many previously institutionalized individuals take their rightful place in the community (Matson & McCartney, 1981; Ruegamer et al., 1982).

PREVIOUS RESEARCH BY OTHERS

Research and clinical reports have also noted the importance of family involvement and the positive impact that family members can have. During acute inpatient rehabilitation, family therapy is usually an integral component of treatment, and family members may become involved in at least some aspect of patient care (Bond, 1979; Grothier, 1980; Lezak, 1978; Rosenthal, 1984). Unfortunately, family therapy does not generally continue after discharge, when the problems differentiate and become more severe. The importance of teaching families goal setting and long-term planning has also been recognized (Kreger & Whealon, 1981; Sbordone, 1983) but not consistently implemented in long-term head injury rehabilitation. As specifically noted by Rosenthal and Muir (1983):

To date, some research performed has documented the need for family intervention, but none has demonstrated that successful family intervention differentially affects outcome. Despite this lack of scientific evidence, clinicians are reporting that the inclusion of family intervention into the broad spectrum of rehabilitative treatment for head injured persons is essential. The tasks that are yet to be accomplished involve more controlled research into the effects of head injury on the family system and determining the most effective and reliable methods of intervention to maximize patient and family acceptance.

More advanced family therapy research among other populations such as dementia (Mace & Rabins, 1982; Zarit & Zarit, 1982), marital therapy (Liberman et al., 1980), childhood disorders (Becker, 1971; Masten, 1979), alcoholism (Steinglass, 1976), drug dependency (Stanton, 1979), and psychiatric disabilities (Falloon et al., 1982) has noted the impressive contributions that families can make. For example, the 3-year tightly controlled study by

Falloon et al. (1982) demonstrated that families of persons with schizophrenia could significantly reduce the likelihood of symptom relapse when they were taught how to communicate with one another, were provided with basic factual information about schizophrenia, and learned how to use problem solving and behavior management techniques to control daily affairs. Once families developed these abilities they continued to use them with minimal professional intervention, preventing relapse in all patients within the treatment families as compared to less than half the patients in the control group families. These results were especially significant because they reversed a long-held view that families of persons with schizophrenia were more likely to exacerbate than reduce symptoms (Jacobs et al., 1985). In addition, this study represented one of the most rigorously controlled evaluations of family intervention processes across all areas of psychosocial and physical rehabilitation.

Although it is obvious that the etiology, course, and early management of schizophrenia (Strauss & Carpenter, 1981) are much different from those of traumatic head injury, there are also many differences between head injury and frequently associated major medical disorders. Head injury is neither a medical nor a psychosocial disorder, but a unique and complex disability that affects both of these domains.

Similar to other medical disorders, traumatic head injury has a readily identifiable biophysiological base and relies on existing medical facilities during the initial phases of treatment. Even medical insurance reimbursement immediately postinjury is similar to that for other illnesses.

Following hospital discharge, however, significant differences begin to appear. Because of the greater amount of prognostic information available for many other chronic medical disorders, it is usually easier to identify a probable course for other medically involved patients. Due to the diversity of the brain, its executive functions, and our incomplete knowledge about its operation, there is typically no generally recognized course of recovery for the traumatically head-injured patient. Part of this problem is due to the broad range of poorly defined factors that can influence recovery (Gilchrist & Wilkinson, 1979; Smits, 1974). In addition, there are still no good and articulate predictors of long-term recovery following head injury. Instruments such as the Glasgow Coma and Outcome Scales (Jennett & Bond, 1975; Teasdale & Jennett, 1974) provide only general medical indicies of recovery and little information regarding social, vocational, educational, or behavioral outcome. Other available neuropsychological and functional assessment protocols do not yet provide the necessary validity and reliability to articulate the nuances of long-term recovery (Bond, 1983). In the absence of articulate prognostic indicators, both family members and the rehabilitation professional must deal with a greater quantity of unknowns than may be typical of other high-incidence medical disorders. This high degree of uncertainty and lack of "landmarks" to measure client progress make long-term rehabilitation management much more difficult and uncertain.

Psychosocial treatment within major medical rehabilitation is also generally directed toward counseling and supportive adjustment to the disability. For the head-injured patient, psychosocial treatment must also assume a primary role of direct intervention by virtue of the behavioral, emotional, and cognitive sequelae that are noted in head injury. Although helping the patient and family members understand the nature of the disability remains important, they also require direct intervention to treat these issues.

Finally, the amount of time required to resolve the disability is uncertain in head injury. Not only is the course of rehabilitation highly variable, it is often not clear how far the person will progress or how long such progress will take. In many situations treatment is an active, lifetime process that requires the family's continued and complete efforts. This is especially significant due to the high incidence of head injury among young adults. With a potential postinjury life span similar to that of the nondisabled population, continuing care and rehabilitation of a traumatic head injury survivor can be a 35- to 60-year process.

Not surprisingly, some of these problems are similar to the issues that practitioners, patients, and families face in managing mental illness. Although the etiology and onset of these two classes of disorders are remarkably different, some of the issues faced in long-term management may be similar. These issues include a variety of the behavioral, emotional, and cognitive problems noted, the emotional toll of the disability on family members, the lack of prognostic indicators, uncertainty about the course or duration of the disability, and the lack of needed resources (National Head Injury Foundation, 1981; 1982). Similar comparisons can be drawn between specific issues in head injury and other disability groups as well.

These comparisons are not designed to argue for the adoption of any established system to address the unmet needs of this population. Instead, these comparisons help to acknowledge the fact that head injury patients face a wide range of issues that are individually similar to a broad base of disability groups. This in turn makes long-term head injury rehabilitation programming unique and subject to special consideration. Special programs are required to match the unique combination of unmet needs for this population. Even though many of these programs do not presently exist for the head injured, their development does not have to be costly. Because of the similarity of individual issues to other disability groups, it should be possible to adapt previously developed intervention strategies to meet some of the needs of persons with head injuries in a cost–effective and systematic manner that avoids the cost of "re-inventing the wheel."

ROLE OF THE FAMILY

It is evident that families can play a crucial role in this process. Many families already spend considerable "treatment" time with the survivor and, in the absence of other available services, frequently serve as the primary service delivery agent, regardless of their training. This role frequently results in "spinning one's wheels" in an attempt to fulfill a basic need of being useful and supportive to the survivor in the absence of help from others. By helping families identify the long-term needs of severe traumatic head injury survivors and teaching them how to address those needs they are capable of administering, it should be possible to redirect some of this energy to meet some of the crucial issues facing both patients and families.

To some extent, this assistive process is already being developed through support groups of head-injured survivors, families, and professionals; many as regional chapters of the National Head Injury Foundation and related organizations. Similar to families of other disabled populations, many of these groups developed out of a grass-roots need for peer support and in an attempt to provide or find rehabilitation services to meet the needs of their impaired family members. Professionals and laypersons have also become involved as recognition of the need has developed (in part through the efforts of families and survivors). To be effective, however, more specific direction and education are needed.

At the individual level, this effort involves more intensive training and hands-on experience for families and survivors in the management of long-term sequelae. When appropriate, family members can and should get involved in treatment while the survivor is still in the rehabilitation program. Training must be directed toward more than instruction in how to perform daily tasks; it must teach how to assess changes and progress, modify treatment, problem solve, and seek help and resources as needed. In this manner, family members can begin to become helpful and contributing team members rather than passive persons on the periphery of care. Such training can also help the family begin to assume the central role that most will find themselves in the post-discharge environment.

At the group level, families continue to need advanced education and training in areas such as long-term sequelae of head injury, how to operationalize the needs of their impaired family members into objective goals, how to identify resources to meet family and patient goals, how to develop objective and realistic measurement criteria for assessing progress, and how to provide competent care and treatment in areas within their capability. They also need help developing programs and locating resources for services they can't provide. In this manner individual families can begin to work together and address the broader issues they all face.

Finally, at the social and community level, more help is required to teach and encourage advocacy and consumerism among all who are involved with head injury rehabilitation in order to facilitate long-term development. This includes professionals as well as families and survivors. Using the model of the Association of Retarded Citizens, this combined group of concerned individuals can make significant inroads into the social and political arena to address the needs of this growing population.

SUMMARY

In summary, a significant number of advances have facilitated opportunities for medical recovery among traumatic head injury victims who would have previously died of their injuries. Similar progress in long-term rehabilitation efforts has been just as promising, but not as productive, due in part to the diversity of problems associated with such recovery. While initial traumatic head injury recovery focuses on medical restoration, long-term issues span all life areas including social, familial, educational, vocational, community, financial, and interpersonal arenas. The absence of broad-spectrum programs to address these issues can be ameloriated, in part, through the use of technology and systems developed for other populations of disabled persons. Based on this past experience, family members can become a significant member of long-term treatment team programming and assume a more effective role in service delivery and advocacy for the development of needed programs, if they are given the proper support and direction.

REFERENCES

Anderson, D. W., Kalsbeek, W. D., & Hartwell, T. D. (1980). The national head and spinal cord injury survey: Design and methodology. *Journal of Neurosurgery* 53, S11–18.

Bakay, L., & Glasauer, F. E. (1980). *Head injury*. Boston: Little, Brown.

Becker, W. C. (1971). *Parents are teachers*. Champaign, IL: Research Press.

Ben-Yishay, Y., & Diller, L. (1983). Cognitive remediation. In M. Rosenthal, E. R. Griffith, M. R. Bond, & J. D. Miller (Eds.), *Rehabilitation of the head injured adult*. Philadelphia: F. A. Davis.

Bond, M. R. (1979). The stages of recovery from severe head injury with special reference to late outcome. *International Rehabilitation Medicine* 1, 155–159.

Bond, M. R. (1983). Standarized methods of assessing and predicting outcome. In M. Rosenthal, E. R. Griffith, M. R. Bond, J. D. Miller (Eds.), *Rehabilitation of the head injured adult*. Philadelphia: F. A. Davis.

Bond, M. R., & Brooks, D. N. (1976). Understanding the process of recovery as a basis for the investigation of rehabilitation for the brain injured. *Scandinavian Journal of Rehabilitation Medicine* 8, 127–133.

Brooks, N. & Aughton, M. E. (1979). Psychological consequences of blunt head injury. *International Rehabilitation Medicine* 1, 160–165.

Caveness, W. F. (1979). Incidence of craniocerebral trauma in the United States with trends from 1970 to 1975. In R. Thompson and J. Greene (Eds.), *Advances in neurology* (Volume 22). New York: Raven Press.

Falloon, I. R. H., Boyd, J. L., McGill, C. W., Razani, J., Moss, H. B., & Gilderman, A. M. (1982). Family management in the prevention of exacerbations of schizophrenia: A controlled study. *New England Journal of Medicine* 306, 1437–1440.

Falloon, I. R. H., Liberman, R. P. (1983). Behavioral therapy for families with child management problems. In M. R. Textor (Ed.), *Helping families with special problems*. New York: Jason Aronson.

Fink, S. (1967). Crisis and motivation: A theoretical model. *Archives of Physical Medicine and Rehabilitation*, 592–597.

Fisher, L. (1977). On the classification of families. *Archives of General Psychiatry* 34, 422–433.

Gagnon, R. (1984). *The AARC: A model for effective long term care for the traumatically head injured*. Unpublished manuscript. Los Angeles: American Head Trauma Alliance.

Galloway, J. P., & Goldstein, H. K. (1971). *A follow-up study of the influences of group therapy with relatives on the rehabilitation potential of rehabilitation clients*. New Orleans: Delgado Community College.

Gianutsos, R. (1980). What is cognitive rehabilitation? *Journal of Rehabilitation*, 27–40.

Gilchrist, E., & Wilkinson, D. M. (1979). Some factors determining prognosis in young people with severe head injuries. *Archives of Neurology* 36, 355–359.

Gouthier, J. L. (1980). Rehabilitation problems of disabled persons. *Canada's Mental Health* 29, 19–21, 40–41.

Grief, E., & Matarazzo, R. G. (1982). *Behavioral approaches to rehabilitation: Coping with change.* New York: Springer.

Institute of Rehabilitation Medicine. (1978). *Working approaches to remediation of cognitive deficits in brain damaged. Monograph #59.* New York: NYU Medical Center.

Institute of Rehabilitation Medicine. (1979). *Working approaches to remediation of cognitive deficits in brain damaged. Monograph #60.* New York: NYU Medical Center.

Institute of Rehabilitation Medicine. (1980). *Working approaches to remediation of cognitive deficits in brain damaged. Monograph #61.* New York: NYU Medical Center.

Institute of Rehabilitation Medicine. (1981). *Working approaches to remediation of cognitive deficits in brain damaged. Monograph #62.* New York: NYU Medical Center.

Jacobs, H. E. (1984). *The family as a therapeutic agent.* Palm Springs, CA: Models of Care and Rehabilitation in Head Injury, 2nd Annual Southwestern Symposium.

Jacobs, H. E. (1985). Los Angeles head injury survey: After effects of head injury are assessed. *Independent Living Forum* 2, 12–14.

Jacobs, H. E., Donahoe, C. P., & Falloon, I. R. H. (1985). Rehabilitation of the chronic schizophrenic: Areas of intervention. In E. Pan, T. Backer,C. Vash, & S. Newman (Eds.), *Annual Review of Rehabilitation Volume IV.* New York: Springer.

Jennett, B., & Bond, M. R. (1975). Assessment of outcome after severe brain damage. Lancet 1, 480–484.

Jennett, B., & MacMillan, R. (1981). Epidemology at head injury. *British Medical Journal* 282, 101.

Jennett, B., Snock, J., Bond, M. R., & Brooks, N. (1981). Disability after severe head injury: Observations on the use of the Glasgow Outcome Scale. *Journal of Neurology, Neurosurgery, and Psychiatry* 44, 285–293.

Jennett, B., & Teasdale, G. (1981). *Management of head injuries. Contemporary neurology series* (Vol. 20). Philadelphia: F. A. Davis.

Kalsbeek, W. D., McLauren, R., Harris, B. S. H., et al. (1980). The national head and spinal cord injury survey: Major findings. *Journal of Neurosurgery* 53, S19–31.

Kraus, J. F. (1978). Epidemiologic features of head and spinal cord injury. In B. S. Schoenberg (Eds.), *Advances in neurology.* New York: Raven Press.

Kraus, J., Black, M. A., Hessol, N., et al. (1984). *The incidence of acute brain injury and serious impairment in a defined population.* Manuscript under review. Los Angeles: UCLA School of Public Health.

Kreger, S. M., & Whealon, R. C. (1981). A procedure for goal setting: A method for formulating goals and treatment plans. *Rehabilitation Nursing* 23–25, 30.

Kubler-Ross, E. (1969). *On death and dying.* New York: MacMillian.

Lezak, M. D. (1978). Living with the characterologically altered brain injured patient. *Journal of Clinical Psychiatry* 39, 592–598.

Lezak, M. D. (1979). Subtle sequelae of brain damage. *American Journal of Physical Medicine* 57, 9–15.

Lezak, M. D., Cosgrove, J. N., O'Brien, K., & Wooster, N. (1980). *Relationships between personality disorders, social disturbances, and physical disability following traumatic brain injury.* San Francisco: International Neuropsychological Society.

Liberman, R. P., Wheeler, E. G., deVisser, L. A. J. M., Kuehnel, J., & Kuehnel, T. (1980). *Handbook of marital therapy: A positive approach to helping troubled relationships.* New York: Plenum Press.

Lindenberg, R. E. (1977). Work with families in rehabilitation. *Rehabilitation Counseling Bulletin* 20, 67–76.

Lindsley, O. R. (1964). Geriatric behavioral prosthetics. In R. Kastenbaum (Ed.), *New thoughts on old age.* New York: Springer.

Mace, N. L., & Rabins, P. V. (1982). *The 36 hour day: A family guide to caring for a person with disease, related dementing illness and memory loss in later life.* Baltimore: Johns Hopkins Press.

Masten, A. S. (1979). Family therapy as a treatment for children: A critical review of outcome research. *Family Process* 18, 323–336.

Matson, J. L., & McCartney, J. R. (Eds.). (1981). *Handbook of behavior modification with the mentally retarded.* New York: Plenum Press.

Mauss-Clum, N., & Ryan, M. R. (1981). Brain injury and the family. *Journal of Neurosurgical Nursing* 13, 165–169.

Muir, C. A., & Haffey, W. J. (1984). Psychological and neuropsychological interventions in the mobile mourning process. In B. A. Edelstein & E. T. Couture (Eds.), *Behavioral assessment and rehabilitation of the traumatically brain damaged*. New York: Plenum Press.

Najenson, T., Groswasser, Z., Mendelson, L., & Hackett, P. (1980). Rehabilitation outcome of brain damaged patients after severe head injury. *International Rehabilitation Medicine* 2, 17–22.

Najenson, T., Mendelson, L., Schechter, I., et al. (1974). Rehabilitation after severe head injury. *Scandinavian Journal of Rehabilitation Medicine* 6, 5–14.

Najenson, T., Rahmani, L., Elezar, B., & Averbuch, S. (1984). An elementary cognitive assessment and treatment of the crainocerebrally injured patient. In B. A. Edelstein & E. T. Couture (Eds.), *Behavioral assessment of the traumatically brain damaged patient*. New York: Plenum Press.

National Head Injury Foundation. (1981). *The silent epidemic*. Framingham MA: Author.

National Head Injury Foundation. (1982). *Help for the head injured and their families*. Framingham, MA: Author.

Neff, W. R. (1959). *Success of a rehabilitation program: A follow-up study of the vocational adjustment center*. Monograph 3. Chicago: Jewish Vocational Service.

Oddy, M., Humphrey, M., & Uttley, D. (1978a). Stresses upon the relatives of head-injured patients. *British Journal of Psychiatry* 133, 507–513.

Oddy, M., Humphrey, M., & Uttley, D. (1978b). Subjective impairment and social recovery after closed head injury. *Journal of Neurology, Neurosurgery and Psychiatry* 41, 611–616.

Olshansky, S., Beach, D. (1975). Special report. *Rehabilitation Literature* 36, 251–253.

Olson, P. A., & Henig, E. (1983). *A manual of behavior management strategies for traumatically brain injured adults*. Chicago: Rehabilitation Institute of Chicago.

Panting, A., & Merry, P. H. (1972). The long term rehabilitation of severe head injuries with particular reference to the need for social and medical support for the patient's family. *Rehabilitation* 38, 33–37.

Patterson, G. R. (1975). *Families: Applications of social learning to family life*. Champaign, IL.: Research Press.

Pearson, J. (1973). Behavioral aspects of Huntington's chorea. *Advances in Neurology* 1, 701–712.

Power, P. W. & Dell Orto, A. E. (Eds.), (1980). *Role of the family in the rehabilitation of the physically disabled*. Baltimore: University Park Press.

Romano, M. D. (1974). Family response to traumatic head injury. *Scandinavian Rehabilitation Medicine* 6, 1–4.

Rosenbaum, M. & Najenson, T. (1976). Changes in life patterns and symptoms of low mood as reported by wives of severely brain-injured soldiers. *Journal of Clinical and Consulting Psychology* 44, 881–888.

Rosenthal, M. (1984). Strategies for intervention with families of brain injured patients. In B. A. Edelstein & E. T. Couture (Eds.), *Behavioral assessment and rehabilitation of the traumatically brain damaged*. New York: Plenum Press.

Rosenthal, M., Griffith, E. R., Bond, M. R., & Miller, J. D. (Eds.). (1983). *Rehabilitation of the head injured adult*. Philadelphia: F. A. Davis.

Rosenthal, M., & Muir, C. A. (1983). Methods of family intervention. In M. Rosenthal, E. R. Griffith, M. R. Bond, & J. D. Miller (Eds.), *Rehabilitation of the head injured adult*. Philadelphia: F. A. Davis.

Ruegamer, L. C., Kroth, R., & Wagonseller, B. R. (1982). *Public Law 94–142: Putting good intentions to work*. Champaign IL.: Research Press.

Sbordone, R. (1983). *The emotional reaction of family members of head injured patients*. International Traumatic Head Injury Conference, London, England.

Seligman, M. E. P. (1975). *Helplessness: On depression, development and death*. San Francisco: W. H. Freeman.

Smits, B. J. (1974). Variables related to success in a medical rehabilitation setting. *Archives of Physical and Medical Rehabilitation* 55, 449–454.

Stanton, M. D. (1979). Family treatment approaches to drug abuse problems: A review. *Family Process* 18, 251–280.

Steinglass, P. (1976). Experimenting with family treatment approaches to alcoholism, 1950–1975: A review. *Family Process* 15, 97–124.

Strauss, J. S., & Carpenter, W. T. (1981). *Schizophrenia*. New York: Plenum.

Teasdale, G. & Jennett, B. (1974). Assessment of coma and impaired unconsciousness. *Lancet* 2, 81.

Thomsen, I. V. (1974). The patient with severe head injury and his family. *Scandinavian Journal of Rehabilitation and Medicine* 6, 180–183.

Thomsen, I. V. (1981). Neuropsychological treatment and longtime follow-up in an aphasic patient with very severe head trauma. *Journal of Clinical Neuropsychology* 3, 43–51.

Thorp, M. J. (1956). An exercise program for the brain injured. *Physical Therapy Review* 36, 664–675.

Thorp, M. J. (1983). Thirty year brain trauma follow-up. American Congress of Rehabilitation Medicine, Los Angeles.

Todd, J., & Satz, P. (1980). The effects of long-term verbal memory deficits: A case study of an adolescent and his family. *Journal of Marital and Family Therapy* 6, 431–438.

Trexler, L. E. (Ed.). (1982). *Cognitive rehabilitation: Conceptualization and intervention.* New York: Plenum Press.

Weddell, R., Oddy, M., & Jenkins, D. (1980). Social adjustment after rehabilitation: A two year follow-up of patients with severe head injury. *Psychological Medicine* 10, 257–263.

Weisman, A. (1972). *On death and dying.* New York: Behavioral Publications.

Wright, G. N. (1980). *Total rehabilitation.* Boston: Little, Brown.

Zarit, S. H., & Zarit, G. M. (1982). Families under stress: Interventions for caregivers of senile dementia patients. *Psychotherapy: Theory, Research and Practice* 19, 461–471.

9. PSYCHOSOCIAL CONSEQUENCES OF SIGNIFICANT BRAIN INJURY

MARY PEPPING AND JAMES R. ROUECHE

INTRODUCTION

This chapter is a clinically driven description, with literature citations and case examples intermingled, that attempts to pull together what is known about the psychosocial consequences of severe brain injury. Hopefully, with this combination of what has been discovered and integrated from past study (e.g., Goldstein, 1942, 1952; Lishman, 1968, 1973; Lezak, 1978; Weddell, Oddy, & Jenkins, 1980; Levin, 1978; Brooks, 1984; Fordyce, Roueche, & Prigatano, 1983; Prigatano, 1985, 1986), and what is continuing to unfold in current work, clinically useful and theoretically stimulating ideas will be found.

It might be helpful to begin by defining what we mean when we talk about psychosocial in the context of the brain-injured person. We are addressing here those organically and emotionally based changes in thinking, personality, communicative ability, and physical and functional skills that will alter per-manently the character of who this person is and will be. These changes affect the individual both as an intrapsychic entity (sense of self, connection with self) and as an interpersonal or social creature. In this latter instance, we include relating to others and to the environment as a physical entity.

In no way is this definition intended to rob persons who have suffered brain injury of their integrity, value, humanity, or hope. At the same time, based on what we have experienced in our work with these courageous individuals and their families, we feel bound to convey the seriousness and the pervasiveness of the changes they must face and integrate to regain or achieve wholeness. It is worth noting that people with somewhat more mild to moderate brain injuries

215

also face a significant number of adjustment issues. Our focus in this chapter will be primarily on the more severely (coma greater than 24 hours) injured individual.

In any review of the brain injury literature, including information about survivors of either traumatic or vascular types of damage, one finds frequent reference to the challenges of "living with the characterologically altered" (Lezak, 1978) individual. Regardless of etiological event, length of time postinjury, nature of preinjury relationships, and levels of adjustment, it seems the "final common pathway" (Akiskal & McKinney, 1974) in the case of brain injury is significant change in psychosocial adjustment. In reviewing 22 years (1965–1987) worth of published material on this topic, one finds a wide variety of specific contributory factors to changes in overall adjustment. Some of these changes are noted as perceived by the families of patients (e.g., McKinlay et al., 1981; Oddy, Humphrey, & Uttley, 1978; Thomsen, 1974), the patients themselves (Labaw, 1969), and the rehabilitation therapists (Prigatano, 1986c; Gans, 1983; Ben-Yishay et al., 1979, 1982) who work with these patients and their families. Many of these factors will be listed in more detail in the sections to follow, documenting cognitive and personality change following brain injury. In addition, a broad and valuable historical perspective on these issues can be found in two of Prigatano's recent publications (1986a, 1986b).

From a more global perspective at this point in the text, the following model might be useful to consider in conceptualizing three broad categories of factors that will determine ultimate level of psychosocial functioning. As can be seen in figure 9–1, the pie chart includes factor I, preinjury assets and liabilities, which breaks into three specific divisions relating to personality, work, and family. The second broad parameter is the brain injury itself, specifically its nature and severity and how these factors determine long-term residual effects in the areas of cognition, personality, communicative ability, and physical functioning. Finally, the last but not least category belongs to reaction to difficulties, and under this general rubric would be included issues related to awareness, emotional reactions, acceptance, realism, hope, and the use of compensatory techniques and strategies.

The challenge of rehabilitation following severe brain injury becomes abundantly more apparent with this rather concretized diagram. Patients, families, and therapists are attempting significant change in a situation in which one factor (I) is relatively fixed, another factor (II) can often be only moderately improved, and the third factor (III) is powerfully affected by I and II. In addition, the patient and family's ability to improve their coping ability vis-à-vis factor III is strongly influenced by the cohesiveness and quality of the rehabilitation intervention.

It is also worth adding that at this juncture in the development of rehabilitation approaches, we are struggling still with how to help brain-injured people bring about positive and lasting change. This latter issue is certainly not unique to the brain-injured population. Anyone working within a therapeutic enterprise confronts it, whether as patient or therapist. What makes the challenge of positive and lasting change in adjustment particularly difficult for the person who has suffered significant brain damage is that the very organ that allows them to analyze, perceive accurately, synthesize, integrate, and question has been significantly compromised.

It has been our experience that in a well-structured environment, with much redundancy built into the cues and concepts used, brain-injured patients can handle all of the issues that are pertinent to their understanding of what has happened to them. A therapeutic climate that fosters the honest, clear, and respectful exchange of ideas and opinions, even if in colorful or heated terms at times, is the climate in which people of all needs and persuasions may grow.

One can't write a chapter on psychosocial adjustment following brain injury without including at least a brief comment on the importance of staff examining their own motivations for doing this particular type of work. All people, whether therapists or patients, are likely to be a blend of healthy and unhealthy parameters. Therapists must be able to keep the needs of the patient as their paramount concern at work, with the continuing review of staff needs and issues an important part of ultimate honesty, fairness, and effectiveness. Staff members who attempt to teach brain-injured patients about honesty, clarity, awareness, acceptance, and respect for others must make these precepts an integral part of their own way of being. A "do what I say, not what I do" approach to rehabilitation is not likely to be effective.

THE THREE-FACTOR MODEL FOR PSYCHOSOCIAL CONSEQUENCES OF BRAIN INJURY

Factor I: Preinjury Assets and Liabilities

Any attempt at brain injury rehabilitation that does not carefully account for the factors predating the injury is probably doomed, if not to flamboyant failure, then to quiet ineffectiveness. This doesn't mean that years of psychoanalytically oriented psychotherapy must be undertaken, nor that a vast sociological analysis of the family or current Zeitgeist be attempted or fully comprehended. It does mean that some appreciation for the following issues should be included in both the assessment and ongoing treatment of brain-injured patients:

1. *Personality and coping style*
   a. Preinjury personality style, including nature of relationships with others
   b. Coping style with respect to stressful events
   c. The patient's role in his or her accident
2. *Work experience and cognitive assets.* Level of preinjury work or school adjustment, which would include information on preinjury IQ, degrees, and work functioning.

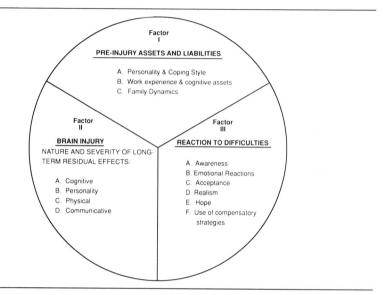

Figure 9–1. A three-factor model for psychosocial consequences following brain injury.

3. *Family dynamics.* The nature of the family system, on a spectrum from healthy to significantly dysfunctional.

Although facets of both personality and coping style that are characterologically based are not expected to change dramatically in the process of therapy, identifying these factors as they affect each individual's attempt to get better is important. In some instances, the more maladaptive ways of coping can be altered. In other situations, the kind of limitation that a particular way of dealing with reality is going to impinge on someone's ability to cope simply needs to be honestly and consistently addressed. This can be as critical a component to effective rehabilitation as improvements in speech, gross and/or fine motor functions, or memory and thinking strategies.

Preinjury personality style

It is not the purvue of this chapter to compare and contrast the various theories of personality that exist; there are many fine and useful models. We will define personality in the context of this chapter as "the pattern of emotions and behaviors that develop over time" (Prigatano, 1986c), some tendencies of which are biologically based, some of which are rather powerfully determined by environmental factors. These latter factors can be both conscious and unconscious in origin, and all aspects noted can be modified in the light of later experience.

Some of the personality characteristics that one might consider can be derived from clinical history and from interview. Other aspects of personality functioning can be obtained via extended observation. Further aspects may be delineated through a variety of personality instruments, including the Minnesota Multiphasic Personality Inventory, the California Personality Inventory, the Myers-Briggs, and a variety of adjective checklists. The Katz Relative's Rating Scale can also be a useful adjunctive measure, allowing family members to provide some consistent observational data. These measures cover a spectrum of parameters, including such tendencies and behaviors as outgoingness versus somewhat more introverted styles; anxious, tense, or worried behaviors versus those with tendencies to be somewhat more blithe, cheery, or unconcerned; tendencies to be rather blunt and direct versus more circumspect or indirect, and so on.

Taken all together, results of the patient and family report, clinical observations of interpersonal behaviors, and these personality tests will help form a useful picture of the individual and his or her personality style. It has been our observation, both clinically and from a research outcome standpoint, that personality factors very powerfully affect an individual's ability to struggle effectively with the changes in self and with the rehabilitation process.

It is important to note that preinjury personality will also combine with organically mediated personality syndromes or changes (e.g., frontal lobish behavior, limbic dyscontrol, perceptually based paranoia, and suspiciousness). These factors will be described in more detail in later sections. In general, it is fair to say that brain injury tends to exacerbate or intensify preexisting personality difficulties. On occasion, it produces changes (e.g., being more affectionate or talkative) that the patient's family may find to be positive.

Preinjury personality style also overlaps to some extent with coping ability. Much of what we will say here is common sense to those in the helping professions, but it is still worth repeating. Individuals who have a history of difficulty coping as measured by previous psychiatric hospitalization or disturbance, incarceration, arrest records, significant involvement with alcohol or other drugs, and/or significant histories of multiple traumas incurred as a result of recklessness on their part are likely to have highly intensified difficulty coping with the kinds of changes that accompany brain injury. The degee to which head trauma patients may represent a high risk taking segment of the population is a question that continues to be raised in family studies (e.g., Kreutzer, 1988). If one's sense of self was not well and healthily established prior to this kind of devastating change, one's chances for coping effectively with severe problems at a time when cognitive, physical, and social assets may be seriously compromised are fairly poor.

This doesn't mean that treatment cannot be provided, nor does it guarantee treatment failure. It does mean that the nature of intervention—its course, the rapidity with which change for the better is possible, and the ultimate cost to all concerned in terms of time, resources, and amount of improvement possible—needs to be acknowledged. These factors must be included as a continuing part of the therapeutic dialogue. They are not excuses for continued difficulty, nor reasons for hopelessness. They do need to be recognized as powerful forces that strongly modify and affect ultimate levels of psychosocial functioning.

Personally, we have found it helpful to look at the degree to which an individual was prone to denial or minimization of difficulties prior to any kind of brain injury. In addition, the individual whose outlook tends to be somewhat rigid and defensive is probably at risk for adjustment problems following significant brain injury. Persons who have had difficulty coping productively with stress in general will likely have difficulty coming to terms with the catastrophic effects of severe brain injury. Finally, individuals with significant preinjury characterologic disturbances (e.g., antisocial personality, hysterical personality disorder) are likely to find it difficult to acknowledge problems and/or to benefit from awareness/acceptance-oriented rehabilitation.

In addition to preinjury personality and coping style, another important parameter to consider is the individual's role in his or her accident. We refer to this in part as the "level of masochism" (Wienecke, 1986, personal communication) in the etiology of the events surrounding the injury. The purpose of obtaining this information is certainly not to blame someone or exonerate someone else for the tragic circumstances that have brought them to this point in their lives. We simply want to try to understand as clearly as possible what some of the forces may have been that were bearing on this person, from a psychological standpoint, and that may still be potent forces in that person's rehabilitation process and life. Some examples of events we believe to be significant are fairly straightforward, while many seem more esoteric. For example, the 17- or 18-year-old youth who is the youngest of a series of children, and having much difficulty separating from "the nest," may be at somewhat greater risk for a serious accident than would be an older sibling. This latter individual may feel somewhat different pressures (for example, to achieve, to make his or her mark in the world). In our group of patients over the last eight and a half years, there appears to be a disproportionately greater number of younger or only sons and daughters, versus oldest sons and daughters. The son-mother bond or daughter-father bond is sometimes characterized by the mutual unconscious placement of this child into the role of surrogate spouse. Prior to the accident, the child who has subsequently become a brain-injured patient may have been accorded more respect and intimacy than was the same sex parent. Questions about the degree to which this child feels that he or she must remain in the home, to take care of mother or father, remain to be answered.

One has to question the role of early experience, programming, pain, and fairness, as well as current pressures, in situations such as these. The man in his late 20s who was beaten and traumatized through much of his young life and who manages to establish a fairly healthy relationship with a spouse and children of his own is another case in point. When on a clear day, with dry road conditions and no other vehicles, this gentleman's vehicle simply leaves the road, following an argument with his wife earlier that morning, questions abound. In this situation, chaos resulted, with a moderate degree of brain injury, severe depression, increased jealousy and suspiciousness, greatly heightened anger and outbursts at home, leading to separation, divorce, and continuing inability to choose appropriate levels of work.

In other instances, a man or woman may be driving to work and be struck head-on by a drunk driver in an unavoidable set of circumstances. The individuals who sustain significant brain injury while belted into their seats raise a different kind of question. And patients who are wheeled into the trauma units of local hospitals wearing T-shirts that read "Born to Raise Hell" certainly deserve the best of treatment. The role they have played in their own near-demise must be considered in the long-term struggle to recover. It will affect, and to some extent dictate, the nature and success of interventions as we currently know them.

Work experience and cognitive assets

The next major preinjury factor to consider is level of work and/or school achievement and adjustment. This factor includes people working primarily as homemakers as well. This factor also provides some perspective on preinjury levels of cognitive assets.

People who were functioning well above average in a number of thinking areas prior to their injuries are at some advantage as compared to peers who may not have had such a generous helping of these attributes. This advantage does not necessarily mean that the person with a high IQ preinjury is guaranteed an optimal long-term outcome. Our data suggest that the IQ factor is not the best predictor in and of itself of postinjury success. The IQ factor can, however, often allow a given individual more "degrees of freedom" regarding postinjury adjustment. An individual who was good at a wide variety of tasks prior to an accident has a better chance of retaining/preserving some of these abilities in functional form. This factor can enhance employability, self-esteem, and opportunities for interaction with other people.

Level of education can also be an advantage in this paradigm, not so much because a degree per se predicts ultimate level of return to productivity or happiness. It is more related, in our opinion, to factors such as the capacity for commitment to a goal and reflects a broad base of thinking skills and interests.

With respect to work performance preinjury, we are most interested in the quality of work functioning, for example, reliability as an employee, conscientiousness with respect to quality of work, ability to get along well with co-workers, ability to make and maintain a commitment to a given position. People who are high-level executives prior to brain injury do not necessarily make for the best work outcomes. People who were laborers do not necessarily make for the worst work outcomes.

This information is and must be sought retrospectively, through interview with the patient, the family, and, where possible, previous employers. In addition to the basic facts of one's work history, it is also critical to assess work's importance in someone's life. The patient's attitudes about work and productivity as they relate to personal definitions regarding the "meaning of life" can figure rather prominently in ultimate return to work.

Certainly, the postinjury degree of deficit overall will play an extremely powerful role in determining who can and cannot work competitively. Among those individuals deemed to be capable of some level of work, the preceding factors noted are very important. Perhaps it goes without saying, but it has been our experience that individuals whose lives preinjury have been characterized by a very lengthy series of briefly held unskilled jobs, or those individuals who have never been a part of the labor force, are the two populations that may have the most difficulty achieving or resuming some realistic level of employment.

Family dynamics

The third broad preinjury factor that can figure prominently in ultimate level of psychosocial adjustment is the nature of family functioning. In this regard, we are interested generally in the degree of health versus dysfunction present in this family's ability to support and interact with its member. The patient's family can include both spouse and children as well as the patient's own parents and siblings. Generally, the family with whom one was living at the time of the accident is likely to be the family of focus in treatment.

If the nuclear family is unwilling or unable to participate actively in the rehabilitation process, the patient's ability to achieve and maintain optimal levels of psychosocial adjustment is very seriously at risk. Probably the only exception to this general rule would be the family that was so pervasively dysfunctional prior to the accident that the patient might do somewhat better without their influence. Clinically, we have identified three major types of family involvement. These include the following situations:

1. *Families* who are *present*, fairly *healthy* with respect to their psychological functioning, and committed to the patient's best interest and their own. These individuals are generally willing to speak up with their observations, questions, concerns, and comments. They are not always necessarily in agreement with staff or the patient, but they are marked by a willingness to discuss and negotiate. It is also important to note that this healthy type of family is not necesssarily devoid of posttrauma divorce or separation. In our experience, we have seen a number of fine and helpful spouses who, after years of effort and much soul-searching, have made the very difficult decision to proceed on their own. In these instances, the brain-injured spouse has been universally offered an opportunity to continue to play the role of parent and to interact with any children who were present.

2. *Present* but fairly *unhealthy* families who may not be particularly committed to the patient's return to productivity, and in fact may have somewhat

different or hidden agendas. These families may participate consistently, but they tend to use the time in family groups and family meetings as forums for anger, blaming, and hopelessness that goes beyond what one might expect in the process of grieving and venting one's feelings. Many of these families may actively or passively undermine both staff and patient efforts for consistency of treatment, whether out of fear, anger, personal frustration, exhaustion, or depression. Attempts to work with these family members on an individual basis are characteristically either rejected or wholeheartedly embraced, to the exclusion of much productive focus on the needs and issues of the patient.

3. The *absent* family who generally refuses to participate in any aspect of treatment. This type of family is not as rare as one might expect, at least as we find in a postacute, relatively chronic population. The frustrations of the very acute family may relate to lack of information, apprehension about the future, and factors related to immediate crisis. The postacute family that comes in for treatment some two years postinjury knows what the future is likely to hold. These families share all of the feelings of many of the families in the first two categories, the primary difference being that they do not appear to be able to participate in any discussion of their feelings or the issues at hand. These families may be pleasant when one contacts them on the phone, they may agree to involvement, and then consistently cancel appointments, forget meetings, have trouble returning phone calls, or not respond to letters. In some instances, they will appear for the initial neuropsychological assessment, and participate in discussions up to and including the day of their brain-injured relative's program admission, and then become unavailable.

From a rehabilitation perspective, almost any form of contact with families is preferred to no contact at all. None of us enjoys being yelled at or blamed during the course of a 6-month, full-time program. Yet even under those circumstances we do have the opportunity to see, listen, support, confront, and ally to the best of our ability with whatever family is present. Sometimes, even under adverse conditions, the seeds for a more trusting and helpful relationship are laid during this period.

Perhaps it goes without saying, but generally family type 1 is the best harbinger of long-term positive psychosocial outcome. The nature of their participation in the program is often consistent with the nature of the healthy kinds of relationships they have established in the past. Family norms appear to promote people doing the best that they can with what they have, in a climate of support. Interestingly, some patients from type 3 families do eventually achieve a fair number of their rehabilitation goals, in spite of lack of nuclear family support. In these instances, the patients may have formed a strong therapeutic alliance with the rehabilitation team as surrogate family and, on the basis of this support, are able to establish a foundation, from which other interpersonal relationships and work relationships can be established.

Finally, although patients from type 2 families may not be characterized by out and out failure, from a productivity standpoint, as a group they tend to be the "underachievers." That is, they would generally be described by staff as individuals with more potential than they are currently using in their day-to-day life. Their ability to get along with others is noted as improved, but their levels of productivity are often less than reasonable.

It is also extremely important to note that given individuals, by combination of their own preinjury factors, nature of brain damage, and their own emotional reaction, may find themselves in a failure or less than optimal category, in spite of consistently strong family participation and support.

Combined with information on factor I, preinjury assets and liabilities (personal, work, family), factor II, the nature of brain injury suffered, is critical to note. Type, location, and severity will all have important residual effects on cognition, communication, personality, and physical functioning. We have gone into some detail in this chapter on the pathophysiology of brain injury. If this seems a little unusual in a description of psychosocial adjustment following brain injury, it is because we feel it is critical to have this degree of emphasis on the organic substrait of dysfunction. In the day-to-day application of rehabilitation efforts, this emphasis is often a fine line clinically distinguishing organic from more functionally (i.e., psychiatrically) based factors in overall adjustment. Although we may never know the exact percentage of each broad contributor (i.e., amount of factor II/organic versus some combination of factors I/preinjury and III/emotional reaction versus factor II's organic impact as it can be modified by preinjury and emotional reaction issues), we can attempt to do justice to the patient in this regard.

It is our feeling that unless rehabilitation specialists have some degree of education and sophistication regarding the role and nature of organicity as it determines behavior, it is easy to slip into an attitude of blame, unrealistic expectations, and/or frustration vis-à-vis a particular patient's progress. Knowledge of brain function and dysfunction has a direct effect, or should, on the kind of rehabilitation strategies one chooses. A frontal lobe based memory disturbance is a far different commodity than a limbic system memory disturbance, in our opinion. Awareness problems that are psychiatrically based with respect to denial and difficulty coping need to be approached in a different way than right hemisphere based anosognosia. In its most severe form, these problems may be easy to distinguish. In the more chronic brain-injured population, in more subtle forms, the underpinnings of these problems can be very difficult to distinguish, yet they remain critical to treatment planning.

Factor II: Brain Injury, The Organic Substrate

In describing the general impact of organic conditions, one is generally safe in stating that the extent of structural damage to the brain is closely tied to the significance of overall behavioral and psychosocial disruption (Levin et al., 1979; Rimel et al., 1981, 1982). However, this statement is far too broad to have much clinical utility and lends little specificity as to the influences of nature, extent, and location of injury.

Nature of injury quite simply refers to the mechanism or mechanisms whereby brain tissue is damaged, destroyed, or otherwise disturbed. Extent of injury refers to the total amount of brain tissue that is affected, and location of injury relates to the various regions, lobes, or structures that may be compromised.

Numerous means of disturbing the normal functions of brain tissue are known under the general label of neuropathologies. Certainly, this discussion is not intended as a detailed review of neuropathology, but rather a description of disorders common to the rehabilitation setting (for a more thorough review of this topic, the reader is referred to *Organic Psychiatry*, Lishman, 1978). Broad categories of neuropathology would include head trauma, vascular disturbance, degenerative disorders, toxic conditions, infectious processes, neoplastic disturbance, anoxic conditions, metabolic and endocrine disorders, and nutritional deficiency (Lezak, 1983).

Certain issues relative to the various neuropathologies are important to consider in assessing the neurobehavioral ramifications of brain injury. These would include (1) local versus diffuse effects, (2) processes that permanently destroy tissue versus rendering it temporarily nonfunctional or semifunctional, (3) primary versus secondary effects of a given process, (4) the longitudinal clinical course of a given neuropathology, (5) at what point in the ontogenetic development of the organism damage occurs, and (6) the cumulative effect of preexisting disorders. We will not attempt in this chapter to describe in detail how each of these issues relates to specific neuropathological conditions; rather we will attempt to confine our discussion to those entities most commonly encountered in the rehabilitation setting.

Numerous assumptions are held with respect to the impact of these issues, particularly in clinical practice. A somewhat more scientifically based set of notions, and certainly similar ones, has come from animal research. Some of these are: (1) There is generally a consistent and regular recovery curve (or at least predictable course). (2) Given comparable lesions, younger subjects tend to exhibit less persistent behavioral disturbance. (3) Heavily overlearned skills are less likely to be disturbed by brain injury and are more likely to recover postinjury. (4) Older skills tend to be less affected and recover more quickly than recently acquired skills. (5) More severe lesions tend to have greater effects on neurobehavioral performance and tend to be associated with less overall recovery. (6) Slowly progressive lesions result in less severe deficits with better long-term recovery. (7) Experience following brain injury influences recovery and ultimate outcome. (8) Interventions that influence the extent and rate of recovery tend to be more effective when applied closer to the time of injury.

Thus far, fairly generally statements have been made relative to the organic underpinnings of brain injury. At this point, it may be worthwhile to go into more detail regarding the pathophysiology of organic brain injury. Again, due to the overall breadth of this topic, we will attempt to confine our remarks to the two major areas of neuropathology that present for neuropsychological rehabilitation. These are the areas of head injury/head trauma and vascular disorders.

Head trauma

Head trauma consists of two major classes: closed head injury and open head injury. The pathophysiologies of these injury types are quite different as they relate to the primary and secondary effects, and there are considerably different expectations in terms of neurobehavioral outcome.

Head trauma is perhaps the most common disturbance necessitating rehabilitation in younger individuals. Estimates suggest that 74% of the total incidence of head trauma can be accounted for in individuals between the ages of 10 and 39 (Rosenthal et al., 1983). Additionally, these injuries are approximately two to three times more common in males (Rimel & Jane, 1983).

Open head injuries are those in which the integrity of the bony enclosure of the brain is compromised. This type would include such injuries as gunshot wounds (missile wounds), depressive skull fractures, or other penetrating injuries. Open head injury tends to lead to fairly local or circumscribed damage to brain tissue in the immediate area of penetration, that is, just beneath a depressive skull fracture or along the track of a bullet wound (Newcombe, 1969). More diffuse or widespread brain damage is possible in these injuries, however, primarily as a result of shock waves, pressure effects, intracerebral hematoma, or infection (Grubb & Cox, 1978). These diffuse effects of trauma are more common to closed head injuries and will be further discussed in that section. Of primary significance in open head injury is the attenuation or dissipation of mechanical energy as the bony skull is disrupted. This force would otherwise be applied in a more diffuse fashion to the more vulnerable structures of the brain itself. Open head injuries are likely to be associated with more specific and predictable patterns of neuropsychological deficit (e.g., Luria, 1965; Newcombe, 1969, 1979; Semmes et al., 1960, 1963; Teuber, 1962; 1964), and the recovery course is relatively rapid in the first 1 to 2 years postinjury (Walker & Jablon, 1961). This is not to say that certain specific deficits may not in fact persist on a more permanent basis.

Closed head injury is a condition in which numerous potential mechanisms for brain damage exist. These are logically divided into primary and secondary effects. Primary impact to the brain results in intense acceleration, deceleration, and rotational forces to the contents of the skull. The architecture of the inner skull is irregular in contour and rigid in structure, quite the reverse of the brain itself. Miller (1983) referred to any of three possible types of primary injury. First, local brain damage refers to focal or localized contusion or laceration concentrated at the site of impact. This may be accompanied by greater or lesser degrees of surrounding tissue edema and/or hemorrhage. Second, lesions remote from the primary site of impact (coup) are referred to as contrecoup injuries. These lesions may present at a site that appears to be opposite the primary site of impact. The force of the initial blow is hypothesized to bounce the brain off the opposite side of the skull, resulting in contusion or laceration. Some believe that the incidence of contrecoup lesions is quite high (Smith, 1974), and others, that the mechanism of contrecoup injury is much less prevalent and more a result of skull architecture (Ommaya et al., 1971; Adams et al., 1980). Third, polar brain damage is the result of comparatively soft vulnerable brain impacting the rigid and irregular contours of the inner skull. Apparently due to the architechtonics of the skull, contusion and/or laceration are commonly seen in the polar regions of the brain, including the frontal poles, orbital frontal region, temporal poles, and mesial temporal lobe. It is not uncommon to find these lesions bilaterally, though severity of insult may be greater on one side (Teasdale & Mendelow, 1984). The occipital regions are less commonly the site of polar brain damage. Polar lesions can also be associated with variable degrees of hemorrhage and swelling, which in turn adds to overall brain volume.

A third, and perhaps most important form, of primary damage (Teasdale & Mendelow, 1984) is diffuse brain injury. This injury occurs with widespread shearing forces on white matter and resulting axonal tearing. This form of injury is diffusely present in white matter, but may be comparatively greater in the corpus callosum, upper brain stem, and frontal and temporal areas (Grubb & Cox, 1978; Teasdale & Mendelow, 1984).

Secondary damage to the brain can largely be attributed to two factors. The first factor is the effect of increases in the total volume of the brain. Because the cranial vault is in essence a "closed box," it has little tolerance for an increase in volume or in the elevated intracranial pressure that is a direct result of increased volume. Intracranial hemorrhage, edema, or brain swelling (Zimmerman et al., 1978) all may contribute to elevations in intracranial pressure. As pressure increases, space normally occupied by cerebral spinal fluid is filled. Progression leads to herniation of the brain from one intracranial compartment to another. Medial portions of the temporal lobes are particularly vulnerable to this effect, as they are pressed downward through the tentorial notch. This further compression of brain stem structures results in abnormal posturing, ocular motor disturbances, loss of consciousness, and disturbance to basic vital functions (Broe, 1982). Certain extracranial factors may also play a role in determining cerebral volume, including systemic respiratory failure, other causes of arterial hypoxia (Miller, 1983), or arterial hypotension either secondary to blood volume loss or disturbance to auto-regulation systems (Overgaard & Tweed, 1974; Fieschi et al., 1974).

The second major factor in secondary damage to the brain relates to the interruption of the steady supply of nutrients, as in cerebral ischemia/hypoxia. This pathology tends to be widespread through the brain, though regions commonly involved include the hippocampus, basal ganglia, the primary arterial distribution regions and watershed regions of the cortex, and the cerebellum (Miller, 1983). Systemic injuries that produce arterial hypoxemia and/or hypotension are common in head trauma. Other sources of ischemia/ hypoxia include elevation of intracranial pressure, cerebral vasospasm, and disturbance to normal autoregulation of cerebral blood flow and cerebral profusion pressure. A progressive rise in intracranial pressure has been shown experimentally to produce a fall in cerebral blood flow (Johnston & Rowan, 1974). In the absence of compensatory autoregulation of vasodilation, the brain is significantly at risk for the diffuse effects of ischemic damage.

Less common secondary effects of head trauma include intracranial infection and hydrocephalus. The dural covering of the brain, when intact, is an effective barrier to infectious processes of the brain. Compromise of this covering, as might occur in association with skull fracture or postsurgical intervention, is the primary source of intracranial infection. Hydrocephalus secondary to blockage of normal flow of cerebral spinal fluid is apparently uncommon following severe head injury (Miller, 1983). When present, it may contribute to effects of elevated intracranial pressure, as the fluid filled ventricles should normally function in a compensatory fashion to offset increased intracranial pressure. More common is the presence of hydrocephalus secondary to the diffuse loss of white matter, as in hydrocephalus ex vacuo, or focal tissue loss with localized dilation of a portion of the ventricular system, as in porencephaly.

Vascular disorders

Vascular disorders are typically characterized by local or specific brain lesions. Common vascular abnormalities include occlusion of vessels through thrombotic or embolic events or rupture of vessels as occurs with aneurysms, arteriovenous malformations, and spontaneous hemorrhage secondary to hypertension. Sudden onset of vascular insufficiency (as is common with cerebral emboli) is not well tolerated by the brain, and infarction of the corresponding region of distribution is resultant. Extent of infarct is proportionate to the size of the occluded vessel and to a lesser degree is influenced by the vulnerability of tissues to the anoxic effect. Larger infarcts may be accompanied by cerebral edema and mass effect with possible secondary vascular disturbance due to pressure (Greenfield, 1958).

Reductions in blood flow that occur more gradually, as in progressive occlusive arterial sclerotic disease, may be somewhat better tolerated as anastomotic vessels dilate and compensate for blood flow reduction. Both thrombotic and embolic strokes, when large, and particularly when precipitous in onset, produce significant brain injury. In the acute stage of stroke, indications of diffuse damage may be present as a result of reactive edema and other physiologic response to necrosis of cerebral tissue (Lezak, 1983). Swelling and other secondary effects of stroke, when severe, may cause greater damage with more distant effect than might be expected from the stroke alone. For the most part, however, a more focal or lateralized disturbance characterizes the long-term consequences of ischemic infarct as more diffuse swelling and physiologic response resolves.

Hemorrhage in the brain may have variable effects on brain tissue. Blackwood (1958) describes an anatomic difference between hemorrhage that dissects surrounding tissue with tissue separation rather than destruction, versus hemorrhagic infarction in which tissue supplied by a hemorrhaging vessel is infarcted. Large hemorrhages may produce elevations in intracranial pressure with associated secondary effects. In addition, nerve tissue surrounding a hemorrhagic clot undergoes physiologic response that may include edema, necrosis, and small "petechial" hemorrhages. Thus the effects of hemorrhage may be more widespread than that seen in ischemic infarction and may be accompanied by somewhat less predictable neurobehavioral sequelae (Lezak, 1983).

Nature and severity of long-term residual effects

In traumatic head injury, one often sees a combination of frontal-temporal effects (Adams & Victor, 1977) leading to the changes in cognition, personality, language functioning, and physical functioning, as will be discussed. Vascular injuries tend to produce more focal effects, depending on location, size of lesion, and the other factors noted in the previous section.

COGNITIVE CHANGES. Considering preinjury levels of functioning as one major factor and the nature of brain pathology as the second major factor affecting psychosocial outcome, let us take a closer look at the changes in cognition that proceed from organically based brain disturbance. The most commonly cited cognitive deficits we have found from a review of studies published during a 22-year period (Barth et al., 1983; Bond, 1975; Brennon, 1981; Bruckner & Randle, 1972; Crosson, 1987; Dennerll et al., 1966; Dikmen & Morgan, 1980; Gilchrist & Wilkinson, 1979; Levin et al., 1979; Lezak, 1978; Prigatano & Fordyce, 1986; Rimel et al., 1981, 1982) include the following:

1. Reduced attention and concentration
2. Heightened distractibility
3. Memory problems
4. Reduced learning capacity
5. Slowness in thinking and performance
6. Problems with flexibility of thinking
7. Trouble with planning
8. Difficulty with organization
9. Problems in initiation and follow-through
10. Reduced abstract reasoning capacity
11. Impaired complex information processing skills
12. Problems in judgment
13. Difficulties with perception, including but not limited to visual-spatial deficits per se

14. Communication disturbances, including aphasic problems as well as nonaphasic tendencies toward verbal expansiveness and tangentiality
15. Basic intellectual deficits as measured by IQ scores
16. Confusion and perplexity
17. Impulsivity
18. Disinhibition
19. Major problems with awareness of deficit

All of these difficulties are believed to be organically mediated and to stem directly from brain injury. There are also a variety of changes in personality, some organically mediated, which will be considered in the next section.

At times, people who have not suffered brain injury will tell us, "Well, I forget things too sometimes; you don't have to have a brain injury to have a problem with forgetting." Or, family members might say, "You should see the patient's brother; now there is a real problem in judgment!" There is no question that there are broad similarities among all humans with respect to their cognitive processes and weaknesses within those processes. The overriding concern with the person who has suffered significant brain injury is that she or he experiences far more profound and extensive difficulties that are not simply transient in nature (e.g., due to fatigue) or primarily a function of preexisting assets and difficulties (e.g., "I've never been good at math").

Instead, the severely brain-injured individual is faced with a panoply of disturbances, some possibly reflecting preexisting difficulty, but more reflecting new problems or further intensification of difficulties. One can imagine the psychosocial adjustment issues in both work and interpersonal life faced by an individual with attentional deficits, memory disturbance, inappropriateness, difficulty planning and organizing, and/or problems with impulsivity. Add to this the basic stress of dealing with a major catastrophe at a point when one's skills have been significantly reduced, and the challenge of brain injury is again made understandable.

The degree of confusion that brain-injured patients face, even among those who seem relatively high level, is significant, in our opinion, and frequently underestimated. In the structure of a rehabilitation program or a very familiar routine work setting, these patients may perform adequately. In more novel or complex situations, however, behavior can rapidly deteriorate. Ultimately, it will be the unique blend of residual cognitive, personality, and physical strengths and difficulties that will play such a major role in ultimate level of work placement and interpersonal functioning.

An example of the kind of confusion and behavioral deterioration we mention, as seen on a work trial, may help exemplify this point. A gentleman in his early 40s, with a year of college, who had worked successfully as a corporate pilot as well as a business manager for a number of years suffered severe bifrontal injury in an automobile accident when he was struck head-on by another car. This individual, whom we will call Glenn, suffered somewhat greater right frontal injury and maintained excellent verbal skills. His verbal

IQ scores postinjury were in the high average range, and his performances on memory tests, particularly recall for paragraphs and word pairs, was actually above average as compared to the normal population. Glenn was and is a very pleasant person, is able to maintain good conversations, and generally behaves appropriately in a one-on-one interaction.

Glenn was placed on a work trial in a library, where it was his task to move a series of bound journals, in alphabetical order, to a new location some 20 feet away. This job had to be done a section at a time, loading the cart, keeping the journals in order, placing them on the shelf in their proper sequence, using both alphabetic and numerical (volume number) cues to keep things straight. He was also asked to leave space for 5 additional years of each journal.

In spite of extensive training and supervision, Glenn was unable to consistently perform this task. He knew his alphabet very well, and his numbers. He could explain to you in excellent detail what he was supposed to be doing, but he could not do it accurately over the long haul. Glenn would sometimes get distracted and would only inconsistently use his compensations. If asked him to recite the list of steps on the compensation sheet, he could recite the list. He had a left visual field defect that sometimes contributed to "not seeing" a certain volume or group of volumes. Glenn was aware of his visual difficulties but not particularly aware of the degree of cognitive disturbance. From an organically based standpoint, this gentleman seemed unable to appreciate the importance or salience of some of these problems as they affected his everyday life.

Since these difficulties did not seem very important to Glenn, based on his perception of reality, he was somewhat reluctant to use the strategies that were coached and provided. He honestly felt he could remember what to do, and he was right about the memory part of it. He did remember what he was supposed to do. The fact that he couldn't carry it out seemed like a somewhat mild problem to him. One can imagine how perplexing his work difficulties were to him, to some extent; these problems were perplexing for the staff at the library who were assisting us in supervising Glenn. He is a classic example of how major disturbances in cognition that nonetheless may not be very apparent immediately in a nice person with good verbal skills still can have a very profound and deleterious effect on the individual's ability to work.

This chapter cannot cover all the types of cognitive difficulty, with examples from each as they relate to work and interpersonal functioning, and still cover all that needs to be mentioned from a psychosocial impact standpoint. Hopefully, the examples that are given will clarify some of the points with respect to brain injury, its effects, and implications on people's overall level of long-term functioning.

Finally, although we often view problems in cognition as those likely to affect the more private processes of thinking or problem solving, they extend far beyond the pale of test performance, ability to read and remember, and/or ability to follow instructions on a job site. Major changes in cognitive function will affect both the ability to work and the ability to love. It may well be in this latter realm of interpersonal relationships that these changes in cognitive status have their most devastating impact.

The example of Glenn can be extended here to give a fuller flavor to what this man and his family were up against in their struggle to find a balance in overall adjustment. As indicated, Glenn had problems with planning and organization and difficulty with judgment, but he was reluctant to use lists of compensations to check his follow-through on items that he could otherwise remember. On one occasion, he wrote 40 checks in the space of a month, each in the amount of 40 cents to about one dollar, all for entering a series of contests throughout the nation. It was at a time when his family was under significant financial duress, and the discovery of 40 missing checks, not all of which were entered in the check register, had a rather upsetting effect on family dynamics. When Glenn's wife, Sandy, attempted to discuss this with him, it was difficult for Glenn to see why she was so upset. In somewhat concrete terms, he felt that the overall amount was not very significant and shouldn't be a worry. He was right about this specific fact, for $35.00 was not a large amount. The more global issue—the effect 40 missing checks would have on his wife—was hard for Glenn to appreciate. The fact that the family questioned his judgment in general was also difficult for him to understand.

In addition to this kind of problem, Glenn had also suffered changes in hormonal functioning, secondary to some pituitary disturbance, that made it extremely critical for him to take a series of medications on a very routine and daily basis. Again, he could tell you all he was supposed to be taking but he didn't always follow through to take the medicine, which in his case could be life-threatening. After much discussion over a series of months, Gleen was finally persuaded to use a checklist. He used it inconsistently, feeling it was not really needed, and one day his wife discovered that Glenn didn't check off the medication at the time he took it. He simply waited until the end of the day, and went back and filled in 15 checkmarks for all the various dosages. Needless to say, this put further strain on the relationship. His wife felt that she was turning into a combination warden, policeman, and mother, and not at all in the role of wife, companion, and lover that she had previously enjoyed.

At the present time, both Glenn and Sandy are saddened by the loss of intimacy that has developed over time in their relationship, in spite of significant effort on both sides to understand and come to grips with what has happened. Although Glenn trusts that what his wife and therapists say is true with respect to his deficits, it is difficult for him to feel as strongly about them as they do. In part, this state of affairs stems directly from some organically based factors secondary to frontal lobe damage, an inability to differentiate "important" from "not important" facts. In part, it probably also relates to Glenn's preinjury tendencies to "look on the bright side."

PERSONALITY CHANGES. In this latter respect, our discussion leads to another important area to consider in the psychosocial consequences of brain injury:

organically based changes in personality. As these combine with the preinjury personality, they form a powerful constellation of influence on ultimate outcome.

In reviewing the common personality problems cited in the brain injury literature over a 22-year period (Bond, 1975; Fordyce, Roueche, & Prigatano, 1983; Gjone, Kristiansen, & Sponheim, 1972; Heaton & Pendleton, 1981; Lezak, 1978; McKinlay et al., 1981; Oddy et al., 1978; Oddy & Humphrey, 1980; Prigatano & Fordyce, 1986; Weddel et al. 1980; Crosson, 1987), a list emerges that many will recognize from their clinical work and/or from their personal relationships with people who have suffered significant brain injury. Among the factors that would be considered organically based—that is, a direct result of physical damage to a region of the brain—the following are noted:

1. Loss of ability to show empathy; a tendency to become self-centered (frontal)
2. Poor social judgment; inappropriate remarks and behavior (frontal)
3. Increased irritability and aggressiveness (temporal)
4. Loss of the self-critical attitude (frontal)
5. Childlike or childish behaviors, silliness, euphoria (frontal)
6. Emotional lability, mood swings (frontal, temporal, frontotemporal)
7. Moved easily to laughter or tears, or laughing and crying inappropriately (frontal)
8. Apathy, lack of concern, lack of interest (frontal)
9. Suspiciousness, paranoia, tendency to misperceive the intentions or behaviors of others (parietal, temporal, temporal-parietal)
10. Disinhibition (frontal)
11. Catastrophic reactions (may be subserved by a variety of locations of brain injury)

Many of these organically based changes in personality have been described in terms of syndromes, such as "frontal lobish" behavior. We have early reports describing the behavior of the unfortunate Phineas Gage, who became rude and loutish after taking a tamping rod through his frontal lobes. More recent portrayals would include one such as Jack Nicholson as a lobotomized patient in *One Flew over the Cuckoo's Nest*. There is a wide and fascinating variety of evidence, including scientific, cinematic, and clinical lore for frontal lobe based personality changes. Those factors that relate to inappropriateness, disinhibition, loss of the self-critical attitude, childlike behavior, and apathy can all be traced to this region. In addition to these, tendencies to be emotionally labile, problems with judgment, and difficulty with empathy or a tendency to be increasingly self-referenced would be added to the list.

As noted previously in the text, on some occasions family members find frontal lobe based personality change to be positive factors. For example, if the person in question had a relatively constricted range of emotional expression, or was unlikely to display feelings of affection for other members of the family, frontal lobe injuries may disinhibit the individual just enough to allow more overt exchanges of warmth among family. Conversely, some patients who preinjury were "wild and woolly" may be mildly subdued after frontal lobe damage, again to a degree that the family finds more livable.

Generally speaking, however, disturbances in frontal lobe functioning are quite distressing to family members and the patient's co-workers and friends. Young people who are socially insensitive, slow to pick up subtle cues, or who draw more than the average amount of attention to themselves by acting inappropriately or in a childlike way are likely to find their preinjury friends withdrawing. When the brain-injured individual attempts to establish new friendships, he or she may find it a rather difficult task, for all of the reasons noted. In this situation, unless significant rehabilitation efforts are mounted, and are successful, the brain-injured patient is likely to become withdrawn and depressed (Fordyce, Roueche, & Prigatano, 1983; Pepping & Epler, 1988).

When the temporal/parietal regions are involved, a different kind of personality disturbance is typically seen. This may frequently involve the underlying limbic system, including such regions of the brain as the amygdala, thalamus, and hypothalamus. In addition to some heightened irritability, these patients may suffer from true disturbances of perception. Their ability to interpret the nature of their surroundings, including other people's facial expressions, intentions, and behaviors, is often markedly affected.

In time, this can lead to the development of paranoid thinking and extreme levels of suspiciousness, mistrust, and overreactivity. The patients' reality, based upon their perceptions, or rather misperceptions, is truly different from that of their peers. If they trust their own perceptions, they are at odds with all around them. If they abandon their own perceptions and trust others, they are cast into a sea of doubt and confusion. Paranoid patients cling tenaciously to their view of reality and are among the most difficult patients to treat post-injury. Long-term therapeutic relationships, carefully developed over a period of years, with very frank discussions of the differences in opinion and respect for the patient's needs and outlook, can be of some benefit. At the same time, prognosis from a work adjustment standpoint and with respect to development of meaningful personal relationships outside of the patient's parents and therapists, is likely to be somewhat limited.

Distinct from the misperception and paranoia that may be seen with temporal-parietal disturbance, or limbic lesions, patients with temporal lobe/limbic system disturbance may also be susceptible to rage reactions. These intense episodes of anger can flash very quickly, with apparently little overt provocation, and may subside fairly quickly as well. They are quite frightening to family, friends, staff, and other patients when they occur, and they can be humiliating in their aftermath for the patient who explodes in this way. For patients who have children, this kind of disturbance can be particularly serious, as their ability to maintain composure and fairness during times of stress may be seriously breached. The volatile nature of this response can also make these patients unpredictable, and children and spouses over time will grow understandably wary.

In contrast to the rage reaction, which is believed to be more limbic in origin, most brain-injured patients, regardless of site of lesion, may be susceptible to the development of a catastrophic reaction (Goldstein, 1942) given the "right" set of circumstances. In this situation, when faced with tasks or demands that prove too difficult for them and render their deficiencies more apparent, they may initially become uncomfortable or flushed. Restlessness may appear heightened. Heart rate and breathing increase, and with time, if the offending stimulus is not removed (e.g., the difficult task stopped, the person confronting them backing down), the brain-injured person may momentarily break down. This catastrophic reaction can take the form of anger, weeping, "shutting down" (not talking), or running from the scene. As described by Kurt Goldstein (1942) in his early work with brain-injured soldiers, the organism's limits have been exceeded, and in a sense they are in an overload situation.

Under the right circumstances, any individual, with or without injury, could probably be brought to this kind of breaking point. The difference among brain-injured persons is that their point of catastrophic reaction occurs with levels of stress or confrontation that nonbrain-injured persons would probably not find intensely disturbing.

In review then, all the difficulties we have discussed have a very strong organic component vis-à-vis personality change and/or emotional distress in the brain-injured individual. Another set or constellation of feeling reactions following brain injury would be considered typical psychological effects of coming to grips with catastrophe, rather than stemming from organically based disturbances in brain structure and function. These are the feeling reactions that people have to their changed condition, and can include the full range or gamut of human emotion. Under these circumstances, anger may be a very normal reaction, not the organically based type of limbic/rage reaction we were discussing earlier. Sadness, grief, depression, hopelessness, helplessness, anxiety, fright, and humiliation, all of these feelings and more can be expected.

Patients themselves have mentioned lowered self-esteem, feeling envious of others, feeling defeated or dumb, becoming very discouraged, at times feeling very much rejected, and wanting to reject or hurt others in return. Embarrassment at some of these difficulties is also a common reaction. The depth and degree of shame (Baker, 1982, personal communication) brain-injured persons experience also merits continuing appreciation by all concerned.

Other factors mentioned in the studies cited earlier include a tendency to become more dependent on others, some reductions in the amount of personal responsibility taken, tendencies to become more socially withdrawn, major problems with social competence or the ability to get along with others, tendency at times to blame others for problems, along with some increased impatience, or at times, agitation. Clinically, we have found this latter problem somewhat more characteristic of patients who may seem fairly unaware of their changed circumstance or the degree and importance of these changes. The agitation may be the one behavioral clue initially revealed that the person on some level does recognize that something is definitely wrong and is most likely having an important if unconscious (in the psychiatric sense) reaction to it. We have also found that increases in physical symptomatology, along with heightened sleep disturbances, may be another clue that a given individual is in some turmoil if all other aspects of waking behavior may not appear that much different from usual.

Of critical importance is the finding that these emotional reactions tend to get worse with time rather than better (Fordyce, Roueche, & Prigatano, 1983) if left untreated. Although the notion that "time heals" applies to some aspects of recovery, "time festers" would be more apropos for those emotional issues not addressed postinjury.

In summary then, when attempting to predict an individual's behavior/ personality change following brain injury, one must take into account three things: (1) the nature of preinjury personality, (2) the organically based contributions to personality disturbance, and (3) the nature of the individual's emotional reactions to all that has befallen him or her. As noted, whether these reactions have been therapeutically addressed postinjury can also exacerbate the situation.

PHYSICAL CHANGES.[1] To this point then, we have discussed the organically based cognitive and personality changes that can occur, as well as a wide variety of emotional reactions that develop in response to these difficulties. Another area that is frequently not mentioned in discussions of psychosocial adjustment relates to the physical arena or spectrum of motor disturbances.

Although it is not the purpose of this chapter to provide a very detailed review of physical disturbances, it has been our experience that changes in physical functioning do have very significant impact on psychosocial adjust-ment. In and of themselves, these changes may not be the single most powerful predictive factor of who succeeds and who does not. There is no question, however, that individuals with very significant ataxic disturbances, and/or dense hemiparesis, have some aspects of their work and personal life more significantly affected than do patients with the same kinds of cognitive strengths and weaknesses but little in the way of motor difficulty.

While the more profound motor disturbances remain a challenging problem for all concerned, other more subtle disturbances in tone and gait, as well as loss of "the kinetic melody," can continue to play an important role in less obviously physically impaired patients. These individuals over time gradually give up or stop playing the sports and other leisure physical pursuits that gave them pleasure and brought them into social contact with others. In our work, we have found that young adults in particular who have no glaringly apparent motor deficits have subtle and not so subtle deficiencies in the areas of complex motor movements. These deficiencies are critical to their involvement in activities such as dancing, tennis, aerobics, raquetball, softball, and volleyball.

Finally, because we can be so focused on the functional outcomes for these people, we may fail to appreciate the degree to which changes in sensory functioning, including smell, taste, vision, hearing, and tactile sensitivity, profoundly affect the day-to-day quality of their lives. When many foods taste the same, when favorite foods or drinks have become aversive, the sense of who one is and has been continues to undergo alteration. The simple pleasures taken from the smell of freshly baked bread, of apples, or flowers may all be dulled or reduced. Other fragrances long enjoyed, such as a favorite perfume or roasting coffee, may become noxious. Even going out to dinner may become an exercise in futility from a sensory standpoint.

Struggling with a visual field defect, which may not be very obvious to others, but frustratingly present for the brain-injured person, can be another aggravation. Diminishment of hearing, loss of acuity secondary to rupture of the tympanic membrane, or changes in hearing secondary to skull fractures, and so forth also alter the nature of sensory experience. The degree to which these changes in peripheral sensation are contributing to some reductions in speed of information processing, in the ability to attend to relevant cues, and in many other aspects of cognitive and emotional functioning probably continues to be underappreciated by the nonbrain-injured population.

COMMUNICATION CHANGES. In addition to the organically based cognitive, personality, and physical factors that can all have a profound effect on psychosocial functioning, the area of communication disturbances is also of singular importance. Brain injury commonly has impact upon some facets of communicative ability. Humans rely heavily on communication in all aspects of day-to-day functioning; thus the consequence when communicative competence is impaired is potentially quite significant. This certainly appears to be true as it relates to the psychosocial impact of communication disturbance. To a large extent, our sense of value and connection is determined through interpersonal experiences with others. Through these experiences we develop a sense of what is appropriate and inappropriate and learn to both expect and appreciate certain interactional patterns in others. In addition to our highly refined competencies in this area, we possess remarkable sensitivity to even subtle alterations in the stability of these interactional patterns. It is difficult to conceive of a more potentially devastating source of disruption to this process than the effect of brain injury.

At this point let us identify some of the common communication disturbances that have neurologic underpinnings. Wertz (1985) listed five neuropathologies of communication: aphasia, language of confusion, language of generalized intellectual impairment, apraxia of speech, and the dysarthrias (see table 9-1 for descriptions). Other forms of neurogenically based disturbances

Table 9–1. Definitions for five neuropathologies of speech or language or both

Neuropathology	Definitions
Aphasia	Impairment, due to brain damage, of the capacity to interpret and formulate language symbols; a multimodal loss or reduction in decoding conventional meaningful linguistic elements (morphemes and larger syntactic units); disproportionate to impairment of other intellectual functions; not attributable to dementia, sensory loss, or motor dysfunction; manifested in reduced availability of vocabulary, reduced efficiency in applying syntactic rules, reduced auditory retention span, and impaired efficiency in input and output channel selection.
Language of confusion	Impairment of language accompanying neurologic conditions; often traumatically induced; characterized by reduced recognition and understanding of and responsiveness to the environment, faulty memory, unclear thinking, and disorientation in time and space. Structured language events are usually normal and responses utilize correct syntax; open-ended language situations elicit irrelevance, confabulation.
Language of generalized intellectual impairment	Deterioration of performance on more difficult language tasks; reduced efficiency in all modes; greater impairment evident in language tasks requiring better retention, closer attention, and powers of abstraction and generalization; degree of language impairment roughly proportionate to deterioration of other mental functions.
Apraxia of speech	An articulatory disorder resulting from impairment, as a result of brain damage, of the capacity to program the positioning of speech muscles and the sequencing of muscle movements for the volitional production of phonemes. No significant weakness, slowness, or incoordination of these muscles in reflex and automatic acts. Prosodic alterations may be associated with the articulatory problem, perhaps in compensation for it.
Dysarthrias	A group of speech disorders resulting from disturbances in muscular control—weakness, slowness, or incoordination—of the speech mechanism due to damage to the central or peripheral nervous system or both. The term encompasses coexisting neurogenic disorders of several or all the basic processes of speech: respiration, phonation, resonance, articulation, and prosody.

Source: Adapted from F. L. Darley, Aphasia: Input and output disturbances in speech and language processing. Presented in dual session on aphasia to the American Speech and Hearing Association, Chicago, Ill., 1969.

specific to the underlying neurologic condition (i.e., right hemisphere damage [Myers, 1984] or head injury [Hagen, 1984; Sarno, 1984; Levin et al., 1982]) have been described by other authors. These disturbances highlight the unique role of the right hemisphere in processing affectual markers in speech or the impact of cognitive impairment (i.e., mnestic, attentional, or executive functions) on communicative performance.

Communication disturbances can also be described from the perspective of general localization (Wertz, 1985). For instance, language of confusion, language of generalized intellectual impairment, and communicative performance characteristic of cognitive impairment, all occur with bilateral lesions of the cerebral hemispheres. Focal left hemisphere damage typically results in aphasia and/or apraxia of speech, and focal right hemisphere injury produces the "dysprosodias" (Ross & Mesulaum, 1978). Dysarthric syndromes can occur with damage to the upper or lower motor neuron systems, the cerebellum, or the extrapyramidal system.

The psychosocial impact of communication problems in general is likely to be closely associated with the degree to which other people can observe something is "obviously wrong." Also, there are relatively common reactions to any situation in which someone is perceived as being different. It is certainly not unusual to find varying degrees of withdrawal, isolation, shame and embarrassment, heightened sensitivity, frustration,and difficulties with acceptance of limitations among individuals with communication disturbance. These reactions often are closely linked to individuals' "awareness" of the impact of their deficit. In cases in which awareness is lacking or compensatory skill not refined, patients may not understand or may misperceive the reactions of others. This can lead to increased irritability, suspicion, and withdrawal and isolation.

Certainly, those who interact with the communicatively impaired are quite sensitive to the presence of difficulties in skill or style. This awareness may contribute to a general level of awkwardness, discomfort, or avoidance of interaction with individuals who are communicatively impaired. Family members, who may not have the luxury of avoidance, may initially be quite supportive and patient. However, we are well acquainted with numerous situations in which, over time, families become much less tolerant and more frustrated, irritable, and blaming as they react to the communication impairment.

In addition to the more general psychosocial responses already mentioned, certain unique situations may face patients with specific communication deficits. For example, in our experience with patients who have dysarthria, two common issues are encountered. First is a common misperception that dysarthric individuals are "mentally retarded." A second commonly encountered scenario is the dysarthric speaker who is accused of being "drunk" or "on drugs." This situation at times is made worse, particularly in ambulatory patients whose persistent balance and coordination difficulties accompany the dysarthria. The legal implications in such cases are often as significant (if not more so) than the psychosocial impact. Certainly, the acute acoustic characteristics of some dysarthrias can quite easily be mistaken. These patients need opportunities to learn appropriate means of explaining their condition and managing listener reactions in a way that can minimize the initially negative response and convey a sense of comfort and self-acceptance.

Other areas of communication disturbances that have gained considerable attention as they relate to psychosocial impact are those linked to cognitive impairment. Common, particularly to the closed head–injured patient, are disturbances in arousal/attention, thinking/reasoning, and the so-called executive functions. These problem areas typically have little impact on specific language or speech competencies, but rather have significant impact on a speaker's ability to convey a sense of spontaneity, intelligence, appropriateness (especially social appropriateness), sensitivity (particularly to the matrix of subtle, and at times not so subtle, nuances of communication), and attentiveness or interest.

These issues, as they relate to the act of communication, represent a unique feature of our overall linguistic competence known as pragmatic knowledge. Pragmatics, according to Levinson (1983) refers to the role of context in communication, the identities of the participants who are interacting, and the beliefs, knowledge, and intentions of participants. We will not deal extensively with pragmatic theory, but of particular interest as a subcomponent of pragmatics is the concept of conversational maxims (Grice, 1975, 1978). These maxims quite simply establish a logical set of rules governing conversation. Examples of these conversational maxims include (1) conversation should proceed in an orderly and polite way, (2) quality of content is truthful and well substantiated, (3) quantity of information should be no more nor less than necessary to convey intentions, (4) information that is shared should be relevant to this situation/topic, and (5) the manner of presentation should lead to a clear understanding between participants.

In normal circumstances, individuals develop varying degrees of skill in these areas, and certainly we can learn to exercise purposeful control over one or more of them. For example, a speaker may choose to be overly verbose in order to monopolize a discussion or may intentionally be vague or imprecise to avoid commitment or to confuse.

Disruption of cognitive functions can have quite a significant impact on pragmatic competencies. We have encountered a number of symptoms of cognitive impairment in our patients that have seriously impacted overall psychosocial adjustment for this reason. Some of these are (1) a tendency to be hyperverbal and to monopolize; (2) difficulty with topic maintenance or tangentiality; (3) difficulty being clear, concise, and organized in narrative; (4) difficulty with sustained attention or easy distractibility, which may convey a sense of disinterest or lack of spontaneity; (5) reduced ability to gauge one's impact on others, which may be perceived as rude or insensitive behavior; and (6) concrete thinking, mnestic disturbance, or reduced speed of information processing, which may leave the impression of being dull, slow, or confused. In all of these behaviors, the underlying cognitive dysfunction negatively impacts pragmatic competence and the subgroup of conversational maxims. To the extent brain-injured patients or those they communicate with are aware of these violations of interactional expectation, the common and predictable psychosocial reactions will be present.

Factor III: Reaction to Difficulties

Returning for a moment to the pie diagram in figure 9–1, we reviewed preinjury assets and liabilities and the brain injury (organic) factors that contribute to overall levels of psychosocial adjustment. We also made some mention of the emotional reactions that people commonly have to any kind of personal catastrophe (e.g., anger, despair, depression, sadness, grief, shame). Individuals confronting brain injury must generally be helped through the phases of these emotional reactions to this profound life change.

A six-phase model of recovery will be outlined in more detail later. Suffice it to say at this point that helping brain-injured persons learn what is and is not "wrong" or "right" about them, helping them come to accept that reality, and assisting them in making realistic choices vis-à-vis that reality is the bread and butter of rehabilitation. Acceptance and realism do not mean the loss of hope that life can become better. They do mean acknowledging the need for compensatory strategies and the need to take personal responsibility for a set of changes that they did not wish on themselves. It is our feeling that brain-injured persons ultimately show, by their implementation *behaviorally* of the strategies and ideas taught and practiced, whether they have or have not made a successful recovery.

There are a variety of issues that can make this transition a challenge, as noted in factors I, II, and III. If there is one theme that we consistently try to develop with our patients, it is the idea that over time the impact of brain injury has devastating effects on the two major areas of importance to us as individuals: our ability to initiate, develop, and sustain meaningful satisfying relationships, and our ability to economically sustain self and family through work.

Derived from our clinical experience, we have considered a six-phase model of recovery from brain injury (see figure 9-2). Utilizing this conceptual framework, it is possible to pinpoint critical stages during the recovery process and the underlying neurobehavioral or reactionary issues and to begin to track or predict probable outcome, particularly as it relates to patient/family adjustment and work.

Phases I and II describe the period of onset and early adjusting. In some cases (approximately one-third, according to Gilchrist and Wilkinson) patients may return to some form of productive existence following acute medical and rehabilitative intervention. For those patients who do not, a period of decline in functioning is likely.[2] This decline is specific to psychosocial aspects of functioning rather than cognitive, as overall thinking ability quite typically is improved or improving as is overall level of awareness. Other reports support this position, especially as it impacts family (i.e., McKinlay et al., 1981; Brooks & McKinlay, 1983; Rosenbaum & Najenson, 1976).

Phase III marks the beginning of perhaps the most challenging period for families and patients. This is a time of facing up to the realities of what is often a tragic situation. Families have often seen loved ones who were near death survive and regain lost physical functions only to now present major disturbances in personality and emotional functioning. In particular, a rapid rate of early physical recovery may lead families to expect rapid and excellent

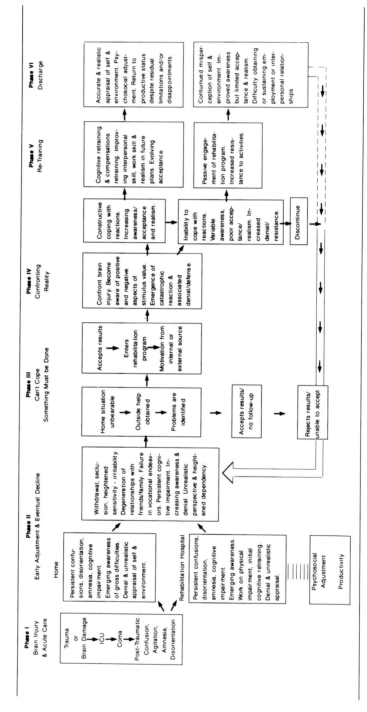

Figure 9–2. Six-phase model of recovery: Neuropsychological Rehabilitation Program HCA-Presbyterian Hospital, Oklahoma City, OK.

cognitive and personality recovery. Patients and families who may have had less appreciation for the long-term implications of brain injury or who had hoped for "complete recovery" must now face a rather harsh reality, relying on an already taxed coping system. This is a period when intensive postacute rehabilitation is often indicated. The decision to engage this help is often difficult. Our typical experience is that families are desperate for some kind of help and patients often don't understand (unaware) or don't acknowledge (deny) the need for further help. For those who reject help, a return to the pattern of decline that precipitated seeking outside consultation is common.

For those that pursue further help, either through self-acknowledged need or through the leverage of others, a difficult process of "confronting reality" begins. The demands of Phase IV are such that varying patterns of outcome emerge. Success during this phase seems less dependent on nature/severity of brain injury and more dependent on constructive coping, not only in patients but in their support systems as well (Pepping & Epler, 1988).

Degree of acceptance of reality determines the effectiveness of retraining efforts during phase V for those who remain in the rehabilitation setting. This "retraining" is directed toward capitalizing on existing strengths, improving or compensating for areas of deficit, and facilitating acceptance and realism. The desired effect of retraining is to reduce or minimize the impact of those issues that contributed to decline in functioning during phases II and III.

The discharge phase is a period during which skills are generalized to a real-world setting. Establishment, reestablishment, and maintenance of important interpersonal relationships is ongoing, and appropriate realistic vocational/avocational interests are pursued. For those who have experienced greater difficulty in sustaining a commitment to the rehabilitation themes of phases IV and V, the likelihood of regression during phase VI is increased. The impact of continued misperception, limited acceptance, and unrealistic judgments outside the shelter of a rehabilitation setting leads to a reemergence of the issues related to psychosocial decline.

The importance of the general themes of awareness, acceptance, and realism, particularly in the postacute phases of recovery, is paramount in facilitating successful psychosocial adjustment. To the extent the varying perspectives of staff, patient, family, and employer can be closely aligned along these themes, succcessful reintegration becomes more likely.

Persistent discrepancies in perspective lead to significant disturbance in interpersonal relationships. In our early investigations of perspective difference via the Patient Competency Rating Scale (Roueche & Fordyce, 1983; Fordyce & Roueche, 1986), we found greatest family turmoil in situations in which rating patterns reflected divergent views of performance. For example, in figure 9–3 patients B and C demonstrate increasing disparity in ratings at posttest. In both cases, family perspective became more closely aligned with staff but grew more distant from patient ratings. In one case, the marriage dissolved and in the other the young man had persistent verbal and physical

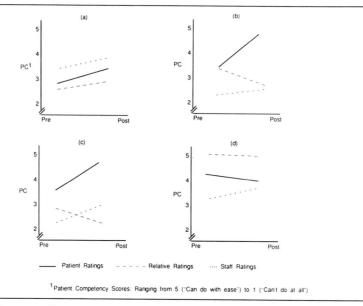

Figure 9–3. Average staff, patient and relative ratings of behavioral competency (PC) before and after rehabilitation.

confrontations with parents. In patients A and D, though there is not perfect agreement, a trend toward similar perspectives is noted. Patient A was able to find appropriate employment postrehabilitation while residing at home with both parents. His mother's tendency to view him as "more impaired" continued to contribute to occasional friction, but overall stability of the relationship was improved. Patient D demonstrated closer alignment with staff at posttest than did his relative, although both acknowledged a more accurate performance appraisal via lower posttest scores. Difficulties in the mother-son relationship persisted at follow-up, though this young man was able to seek and sustain appropriate employment. He eventually moved from his mother's home to an apartment because of the continuing conflicts, in this case some related to the mother's denial of her son's difficulties.

With respect to the stability of marital relationships following brain injury, reports vary. Panting and Merry (1972) reported a 40% rate of divorce in their group. Walker (1972) suggested an 11% rate in his group of World War II veterans. In our own group of 76 brain-injured patients who had completed an intensive neuropsychologically oriented rehabilitation program, 42 were married at the time of injury. Of these, 22 (52%) are now divorced. Of the 22, 27% were divorced prior to the rehabilitation program, 27% divorced during the rehabilitation program, and 45% divorced after rehabilitation. Three of the 76 patients were engaged to be married at the time of injury and did not go on to marry. If these cases are added to our divorced group, the overall statistic increases to a 59% divorce rate. The dissolution of many of these relationships occurred following a number of years of stable, satisfying marriage preinjury.

Successful reintegration into productivity following brain injury is obviously no small task. The capacity of patient and family to strike a reasonable and fair balance between remaining strengths and weaknesses in multiple areas impacting quality of life seems critical to this process. In fact, of all the potential changes in functioning following brain injury that have been outlined thus far, of central importance is the concept of coping. Successful coping for both patient and family involves similarity in perspectives, acceptance of reality without intense emotional response, and realistic planning.

This concept was quite evident as we looked at outcome in the 71 patients who are at least six months postcompletion of our intensive day treatment program (Pepping & Epler, 1988). Of these, 32 (45%) have successfully returned to productive employment. No patient returned to exactly the same level of responsibility that had been achieved preinjury. Twenty-seven patients (38%) were considered intermediate, with improved psychosocial adjustment and productive avocational interests. Our failure group was comprised of 12 patients (17%) who presented with persistent psychosocial maladjustment and nonproductive vocational or avocational status. In reviewing the Patient Competency Rating's of these groups, a predictable pattern of pre/postprogram

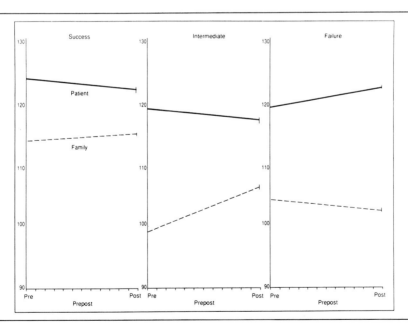

Figure 9–4. Patient Competency Scale: Pre–Post program ratings of patients' behavior by the patients' and their families. (Divided into outcome groups—S, I and F).

appraisal is noted for the success, intermediate, and failure groups (figure 9–4). Clearly, the successes share similar views with family, intermediates reduce the disparity in perspective, and failures widen the gap. These patterns are quite similar, and have similar outcomes, as those of our individual cases described previously.

Additional observation of performance among brain-injured patients in the work setting has been provided by work trial supervisors. For those patients in our group who were placed on a work trial, both patient and supervisor completed performance appraisals through the Work Skill Evaluation (Pepping et al., 1987). This scale asks raters to assess performance in various areas of basic work competency (i.e., attendance, productivity, judgment, ability to get along with co-workers). Patients who were considered successes at 6 months postprogram tended to rate themselves higher than intermediates or failures, and intermediates were rated above failures. Supervisors tended to view successes as more capable than the successes themselves were acknowledging; intermediates and failures, in contrast, were found to overestimate their own performance compared to supervisors' ratings (see figure 9–5). Again, it appears from this work that discrepancy in appraisal, as reflected by patients' overestimates of performance relative to supervisors', occurs more often in patient groups who have less than successful outcome. It is also

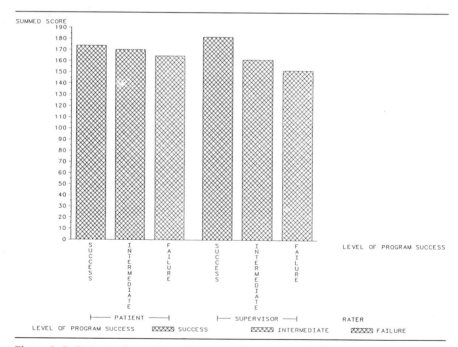

Figure 9–5. Patient and supervisor ratings of work skill evaluation by outcome group

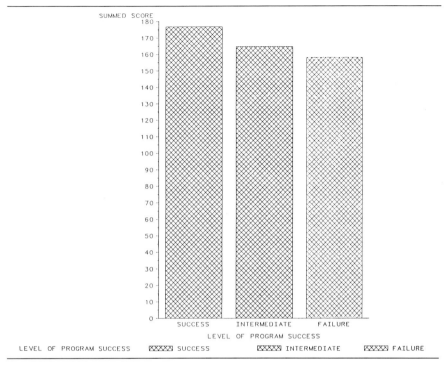

Figure 9–6. Work skill evaluation by outcome group

interesting to note that there is supervisor-patient agreement in ranking the three outcome groups based upon the summed scores, with successes receiving the highest performance ratings, intermediates the middle rating, and failures the lowest rating (see figure 9–6).

What is becoming increasingly clear as it relates to managing the combined effects of brain injury related changes in functioning is the importance of clear and consistent views of capabilities and liabilities among brain-injured patients and their support network. Conflicts are far more likely when different perspectives and expectations exist in the network. As we have seen, the potential impact on the stability of relationships and work success is such that careful attention must be paid to these issues.

IMPLICATIONS FOR EFFECTIVE BRAIN INJURY REHABILITATION

Given that the spectrum of issues believed to be related to eventual psychosocial outcome is a rather broad one, how can clinicians, families, and patients begin to approach these in an effective fashion? While there are many reasonable approaches to the process of recovery and rehabilitation, it is our feeling that the most effective methods tend to have the following tools and ideas in common.

A careful history, with the brain-injured person present for as much of this data gathering as possible, is clearly of utmost importance. Although no single 30- or 45-minute interview will allow gathering of all pertinent data, a family gathering not only allows the transfer of important factual dates and happenings but also underscores the very early importance of family dynamics and interplay. In addition, both the patient and family are receiving a strong message early on from the clinician that all members of this system will play an important role in the eventual outcome. Whenever possible, no one who can reasonably participate is excluded. Obviously, with patients in extremely agitated, obtunded, or severe behavioral states, initial data gathering will be done with the family, friends, and possibly work contacts. As soon as the brain-injured individual can participate, even in a moderate way, she or he should be included.

We have been impressed over time with the honest discrepancies between what family and patients might report about school records and levels of academic achievement and what those actual records may reveal. Even if academic placement per se is not an issue, old school records, with achievement test scores, grades in subjects, conduct, and the like, along with teacher comments, can be extremely interesting.

It is also important to have access to the original records of early medical care, particularly the acute hospital admission and discharge summaries, as well as any operative reports. When available, acute care rehabilitation notes, especially the admitting and discharge summaries or monthly summary notes, are also of tremendous benefit. Often, professionals unfortunately find themselves in the position of trying to evaluate or meet with people about whom they may have received little information. Sometimes this situation cannot be prevented, and evaluation should proceed, with the understanding that eventual access to these records will be important to the final reports and treatment recommendations.

In addition to a careful history that includes contact with the patient and family and review of all pertinent medical and academic records, a thorough evaluation including formal neuropsychological assessment, speech and language assessment, and OT and PT examinations is strongly recommended. In many settings, one or more of these kinds of assessments may be stressed, on occasion at the expense of others. It is our opinion that even in an outpatient setting, most patients would benefit from a full review.

Sometimes, a second opinion on any given issue can be eye-opening, and the evaluation process is a great initial opportunity to see the person and begin to discover his or her presentation style. For example, is the patient able to establish contact with the therapist, and vice versa? How does the patient handle stressful task demands? How does he or she react to success or failure experiences? To what degree is this person aware, to what degree anxious, withdrawn, depressed, inappropriate, defensive, overwhelmed, minimizing, suspicious, and so on? All of these "interstitial" behaviors that form such an important part of the fabric of who this person is, are as important as the actual nature of their objective test performances.

If possible, feedback should be provided to the person and family at the end of the assessment day, even if it is a several-day process. A complete report may not be available at that time, but letting the person and family know a few of the more salient strengths and difficulties that the therapists have noticed can be extremely supportive. Usually, most patients have already been through an extensive series of tests, medical and otherwise, treatments, examinations, and so on, and far too frequently have been given very little direct feedback. In addition to the verbal comments, a full written report should also be provided, not only to the referral sources and to the family, but directly to the patient as well. Perhaps it also goes without saying that nothing should be written in a report that one would not be willing to have the patient read about himself or herself.

Beyond the assessment stages, once therapy per se has been recommended, the importance of healthy family involvement cannot be emphasized enough. In acute settings, staff may find that families feel they have not been informed enough about what is happening, or what is going to happen, and want to be as involved as possible. In the postacute setting, some months or years postinjury therapists may find that families are not always eager to be involved. Frequently, they are in desperate need of some kind of "break" from the strain and may react by not showing up beyond the first one or two appointments required to get their relative started on a new course of treatment. We have struggled with the issue of guidelines, "rules" and recommendations to try to improve the level of family involvement, and we still have not arrived at a very comfortable solution. In successful drug rehabilitation programs, for example, family involvement is a major requirement of admission. Patients whose families do not wish to be involved are not accepted into the program. To some degree, this philosophy appears justifiable. Those individuals who struggle with drugs or alcohol will find it difficult to maintain their gains in a home environment if the family has not also been educated, supported, and worked with toward a common set of goals.

In the brain injury rehabilitation setting, denying an individual treatment because his or her family has refused, politely or otherwise, to be involved is an action we are not ready to take. At the same time, we have to say that those patients with poor family support tend to do poorly, and those with good family support tend to do well. There are clearly exceptions on both sides of this spectrum: those with great families who may do poorly, those with unsupportive families who still manage to get better and maintain their goals.

Part of the dilemma for us as a staff is the frustration inherent in seeing a family refuse to come in and discuss their perspectives, yet realizing that these families continue to exert considerable influence on the patient. In this instance, the patient can be very much caught between two often disparate messages about what is or is not in his or her best interest. How to reach out, support, and eventually engage families who have already reached the end of their personal coping ability remains a major concern for us as therapists and as fellow humans.

We try to resolve this issue to some extent by keeping the family informed, via monthly reports, periodic calls, and invitations to events of interest. At that point, we simply hope that if the time comes when these family members feel they are able to come forward, some degree of support will have been extended and will be perceived by them as positive, not critical. The article written some years ago by Jerome Gans (1983, "Hate in the Rehabilitation Setting") also addresses some of these issues.

Assuming that one has access to a good set of historical information, the results of current and thorough evaluations, and willing family participation, the next optimal ingredient in these brain injury rehabilitation recommendations would include the presence of a milieu or community setting for many aspects of therapy. The power of the group, even for those patients who initially are critical of the idea that *other* brain-injured patients might have something to offer in terms of insight and help, can be an incredible force for positive change. Simply having brain-injured patients spend time together in a group on a weekly basis for "socialization" in and of itself will not provide the kind of power, support, and confrontation we are describing. The confrontational approach, which at times we jokingly call "lapel therapy," encourages both staff and patients alike to be extremely forthright and respectful about what they see and don't see. Issues that concern staff and patients, and the behaviors and outlook they consider to be the most serious obstacles in the patient's road to improved psychosocial adjustment, are all critical issues. They are developed in milieu, in individual treatment time, are part of the long-term rehabilitation focus, and are a critical part of ultimate change.

In the process, those patients providing this type of feedback have a tremendous opportunity to learn how to be tactful, kind, and supportive while telling the truth as they see it. Those receiving the feedback have the opportunity to hear the unvarnished version of what the man or woman on the street is not likely to tell them directly about the problematic aspects of their behavior. Dignity and respect can be found in the truth as each person sees it and struggles to reconcile their feelings and perspectives with those of others.

In this process, the conscious development by staff of therapeutic alliances with the people they are attempting to guide and help in recovery is critical. The therapeutic alliance as we are defining it here means a number of things. For one, it means that a degree of relationship between patient and therapist can develop, so that the patient begins to feel some trust and faith in the therapist. It also means that the patient can come to see and believe that the therapist has the patient's best interest at heart. In this alliance, patients can expect the therapist to work for them and with them in a respectful, committed way to help them address the problems that stand in the way of a successful return, or improvement, of their work and love life.

The other side of this equation, implicitly stated before but explicitly stated now, is that the therapist works extremely hard to remain as fair, open, and honest with self and patient and other staff as possible. The therapist is careful to keep the patient's needs foremost, even if the rate or nature of those needs does not always fit an ideal timetable that the therapist would like to achieve. The therapist is the patient's ally, in the healthiest sense of the word. The therapist is there to teach, to protect, to nurture, and to set limits in ways that maximize the patient's potential and opportunities for long-term happiness.

These latter concepts and tasks (to teach, to protect, to nurture, and to set limits) are the basics of good parenting (Wienecke, 1980, personal communication). It can provide the basis of a therapeutic alliance and a continuing corrective emotional experience for people whose thinking and emotional functions have been altered.

In this entire process, it is also critically important for therapists to continue to address the question of why it is important for them to be in the helping professions. What do they derive from this process? Can they discuss openly and honestly the issues of power, influence, control, transference, and counter-transference that can all be a part of "helping others." The degree to which therapists are helping themselves in the process of their own work is important to acknowledge. Ways in which our own values impinge on the patients with whom we work, for better or worse, need to be made as explicit and current as possible.

Effective brain injury rehabilitation carries with it daily staff meetings to address not only the needs of the patients per se but the ways in which the staff interact with each other, the patients, and the families. Discussions generally focus on patient care, yet reactions to patients, to each other, and to the rehabilitation process are all critical components of what needs to be discussed and integrated.

In addition to these process issues already noted, one of the most important parts of effective rehabilitation is the development, orchestration, and consistency of themes/issues for each patient. For example, if a patient has major problems with impulsivity, this difficulty is monitored and addressed throughout the course of his or her rehabilitation day. It may appear in cognitive retraining tasks, or in practice of ADLs, in interpersonal behaviors, or in the physical therapy setting. The staff take a consistent approach to this kind of behavior, helping the patient identify it and over time accept that it is true and helping the patient bring these episodes up for further group discussion, particularly milieu. This latter meeting involves all staff and all patients in the full-time program and meets once a day. A list of compensatory strategies, developed with the patient and primary therapist, is made a matter of public record. Charts are maintained, monitoring the times, places, and situations where impulsivity may be likely to occur. Various types of compensations will be attempted. Progress is also a matter of public record and discussion.

Comments on behavior and interpersonal skills are not only the purvue of psychologists in this type of format—all staff members, including physical therapists, are oriented to the psychosocial impact of all assets and deficits shown by each patient. These same themes and issues are developed with the family, in individual meetings with them, and in the weekly relatives group meeting. Ability to get along with others, and to become more cognizant of impact on others, is also monitored via the work trial. The supervisors there, in cooperation with program staff, are sensitized to these issues over time, secondary to the patient's behavior while at work. Weekly discussions are also held with the work supervisors to monitor progress, and they complete work skill evaluation forms, as do the patients.

The previously mentioned focus on both strengths and weaknesses is extremely important in the rehabilitation process. Our experience has been that many patients are so demoralized by what has happened to them, their sensitivities to errors or evidence of difficulty may be quite heightened. Another way to say this is, the patient may not initially realize exactly what is causing him or her problems, but over time notices the lack of friends, lack of job, and so on. When the reasons for some of these difficulties in adjustment begin to be pointed out, it can be overwhelming. At that point in time many patients do not appreciate the extent and nature of their strengths. As part of an overall catastrophic reaction to the change in their functioning (which is understandable), they may have a tendency to minimize, overlook, or downplay their true assets. We routinely develop a list of strengths and difficulties with each patient, have it typed up, and made a part of their "personal record." It is displayed prominently for easy reference in the notebook each carries throughout the day. The strengths and weaknesses are typically divided into four areas: cognitive, interpersonal/personality, physical/occupation (gross/fine motor), and vocational/prevocational.

All this information is collected, refined, and developed over a 10- to 12-week period of time. At this point, the patient is placed on a work trial designed to make use of his or her strengths and also to provide important feedback about basic work skills (attendance, punctuality, dress, speed, efficiency, ability to get along with co-workers and supervisors, ability to learn and perform tasks accurately, judgment in getting help when needed, or in taking breaks, etc.). The work trial has proven invaluable to us in assessment and treatment of brain injury (and preinjury) issues. The same difficulties and strengths seen in the full-time program invariably emerge on the work trial and provide a real-world perspective and further grist for the therapuetic mill (and milieu!).

These work trials can be incorporated into a full-time program, or into a modified part-time program for a patient who may have had a moderate injury. In most instances, these work trials are most effective when all the reports about progress, and problems, can be interwoven into the groups and milieu that are such a critical part of the full-time NRP. Themes and issues can also be orchestrated with the part-time patients, but with less therapeutic leverage or power. These latter patients have only one group meeting a week, and no milieu session. In many cases, the part-time program serves as an entry to the full-time program, so it is the rare individual who has only part-time rehabilitation and a work trial combined.

Ideally, the spectrum of care, from acute rehabilitation, through the early stages of residential postacute, into day treatment programs and vocational/work trial placements and community reintegration would all occur within a consistent treatment philosophy framework. Although many institutions and programs advertise "well-orchestrated" or "interdisciplinary" team approaches, it has been our experience that most of these programs provide good care but not in the way as described here. It requires consistent and fair confrontation, in an environment of support, respect, and education, to help most brain-injured patients come to grips with their changes in functioning. This is a long-term process and a difficult one for all concerned: the patient, the family, and staff. Yet improving psychosocial functioning after severe brain injury requires this type of effort. Outcome statistics thus far suggest that for those individuals who have not been able to make it back to a productive life on their own following acute rehabilitation, this kind of approach may be essential.

NOTES

1. We wish to thank Ms. Joy D. Dirham, R. P. T., for her invaluable input regarding physical functioning in the postacute brain-injured population.
2. Certainly in our experience, this decline may also occur in the family or work relationships of some of those who do return to work early in this course, as they begin to experience real-life consequences of their brain injury and/or family and employers become less tolerant of behavioral/cognitive changes (also see Brooks, 1984, p. 2).

REFERENCES

Adams, K. M., Sawyer, J. D., & Kvale, P. A. (1980). Cerebral oxygenation and neuropsychological adaptation. *Journal of Clinical Neuropsychology* 2, 189–208.

Adams, R. D., & Victor, M. (1977). *Principles of neurology.* New York: McGraw-Hill.

Akiskal, H. S., & McKinney, W. T. (1974). Overview of recent research in depression. *Archives of General Psychiatry* 32, 285–305.

Baker, G. (1982). (Personal communication)

Barth, J. T., Macciocchi, S. N., Giordani, B., Rimel, R., Jane, J. A., & Boll, T. J. (1983). Neuropsychological sequelae of minor head injury. *Neurosurgery* 13 (5), 529–533.

Ben-Yishay, Y. (1982). *Rehabilitation monograph no. 64: Working approaches to remediation of cognitive deficits in brain damaged persons.* New York: Institute of Rehabilitation Medicine.

Ben-Yishay, Y., Rattok, J., & Diller, L. (1979). *Working approaches to remediation of cognitive deficits in brain damage,* Supplement to Seventh Annual Workshop for Rehabilitation Professionals, New York University, Institute of Rehabilitation Medicine.

Blackwood, W. (1958). Vascular disease of the central nervous system. In J. G. Greenfield, W. Blackwood, W. H. McMenemey, A. Meyer, & R. M. Norman, *Neuropathology* (pp. 67–131). London: Edward Arnold.

Bond, M. R. (1975). Assessment of the psychosocial outcome after severe head injury. CIBA 34, Elsever Excerpta Medica, 141–157.

Brennon, M. A. (1981). Resumption of work following discharge from a hospital. *Irish Medical Journal* 74 (1), 5–7.

Broe, G. A. (1982). The concept of head injury rehabilitation. In G. A. Broe & R. L. Tate (Eds.),

Brain impairment. Proceedings of the Fifth Annual Brain Impairment Conference. Sydney: Postgraduate Committee in Medicine of the University of Sydney.

Brooks, N. (1984). *Closed head injury: Psychological, social, and family consequences.* New York: Oxford University Press.

Brooks, D. N., & McKinlay, W. (1983). Personality and behavioural change after severe blunt head injury—A relative's view. *Journal of Neurology, Neurosurgery, and Psychiatry* (1972). 46, 336–344.

Bruckner, F. E., & Randle, A. P. H. (1972). Return to work after severe head injuries. *Rheumatology and Physical Medicine* 11 (7), 344–348.

Crosson, B. (1987). Treatment of interpersonal deficits for head-trauma patients in inpatient rehabilitation settings. *Clinical Neuropsychologist* 1 (4), 335–352.

Dennerll, R. D., Rodin, E. A., Gonzalez, S., Schwartz, M. L., & Lin, Y. (1966). Neuropsychological and psychological factors related to employability of persons with epilepsy. *Epilepsia* 7, 318–329.

Dikmen, S., & Morgan, S. F. (1980). Neuropsychological factors related to employability and occupational status in persons with epilepsy. *Journal of Nervous and Mental Disease* 168 (4), 236–240.

Fieschi, C., Battistini, N., Beduschi, A., Boselli, L., & Rossanda, M. (1974). Regional cerebral blood flow and intraventricular pressure in acute head injuries. *Journal of Neurology, Neurosurgery, and Psychiatry,* 37, 1378–1388.

Finger, S. (1978). *Recovery from brain damage.* New York: Plenum Press.

Fordyce, D. J., & Roueche, J. R. (1986). Changes in perspectives of disability among patients, staff and relatives during rehabilitation of brain injury. *Rehabilitation Psychology* 41 (4), 217–229.

Fordyce, D. J., Roueche, J. R., & Prigatano, G. P. (1983). Enhanced emotional reactions in chronic head trauma patients. *Journal of Neurology, Neurosurgery, and Psychiatry* 46, 620–624.

Gans, J. S. (1983). Hate in the rehabilitation setting. *Archives of Physical Medicine and Rehabilitation,* 64, 176–179.

Gilchrist, E., & Wilkinson, M. (1979). Some factors determining prognosis in young people with severe head injuries. *Archives of Neurology* 36, 355–359.

Gjone, R., Kristiansen, K., & Sponheim, N. (1972). Rehabilitation in severe head injuries. *Scandinavian Journal of Rehabilitation Medicine* 4, 2–4.

Goldstein, K. (1942). *Aftereffects of brain injury in war.* New York: Grune & Stratton.

Goldstein, K. (1952). The effect of brain damage on the personality. *Psychiatry* 15, 245–260.

Greenfield, J. G. (Ed.), (1958). *Neuropathology.* Baltimore: Williams & Wilkins.

Grice, H. P. (1975). Logic and conversation. In P. Cole & J. Morgan (Eds.), *Syntax and semantics: Vol. 3, Speech acts* (pp. 41–58). New York: Seminar Press.

Grice, H. P. (1978). Further notes on logic and conversation. In P. Cole (Ed.), *Pragmatics* (pp. 113–127). New York: Academic Press.

Grubb, R. L., & Cox, W. S. (1978). Trauma to the central nervous system. In S. G. Eliasson, A. L. Prensky, & W. B. Hardin, Jr. (Eds.), *Neurological pathophysiology.* New York: Oxford University Press.

Hagen, C. (1984). Language disorders in head trauma. In A. L. Holland (Ed.), *Language disorders in adults.* San Diego: College-Hill.

Heaton, R. K., & Pendleton, M. G. (1981). Use of neuropsychological tests to predict adult patients' everyday functioning. *Journal of Consulting and Clinical Psychology* 49 (6), 807–821.

Johnston, I. H., & Rowan, J. O. (1974). Effect of rising intracranial pressure (ICP) on cerebral blood flow (CBF). *Journal of Neurology, Neurosurgery, and Psychiary* 37, 585–592.

Kreutzer, J. S. (1988). *Family issues in brain injury: A review of the research and its implication for clinical practice.* Paper presented at the Fourth Annual Houston Conference on Neurotrauma, Houston, Texas, February.

Labaw, W. (1969). Denial inside out: Subjective experiences with anosognosia in closed head injury. *Psychiatry,* 32, 174–191.

LeVere, T. E., Davis, N., & Gonder, L. (1979). Recovery of function after brain damage: Toward understanding the deficit. *Physiological Psychology* 7, 317–326.

Levin, H. S., Benton, A. L., & Grossman, R. G. (1982). *Neurobehavioral consequences of closed head injury.* New York: Oxford University Press.

Levin, H. S., & Grossman, R. G. (1978). Behavioral sequelae of closed head injury. *Archives of Neurology* 35, 720–727.

Levin, H. S., Grossman, R. G., Rose, J. E., & Teasdale, G. (1979). Long-term neuropsychological outcome of closed head injury. *Journal of Neurosurgery* 50, 412–422.

Levinson, S. C. (1983). *Pragmatics*. Cambridge: Cambridge University Press.

Lezak, M. D. (1978). Living with the characterologically altered brain-injured patient. *Journal of Clinical Psychiatry* 39 (7), 592–598.

Lezak, M. D. (1983). *Neuropsychological assessment* (2nd ed., pp. 164–203). New York: Oxford University Press.

Lishman, W. A. (1968). Brain damage in relation to psychiatric disability after head injury. *British Journal of Psychiatry* 114, 373–410.

Lishman, W. A. (1973). The psychiatric sequelae of head injury: A review. *Psychological Medicine* 3, 304–318.

Lishman, W. A. (1978). *Organic psychiatry*. Oxford: Blackwell Scientific Publications.

Luria, A. R. (1965). Neuropsychological analysis of focal brain lesions. In B. B. Wolman (Ed.), *Handbook of clinical psychology*. New York: McGraw-Hill.

McKinlay, W. W., Brooks, D. N., Bond, M. R., Martinage, D. P.; & Marshall, M. M. (1981). The short-term outcome of severe blunt head injury as reported by relatives of the injured persons. *Journal of Neurology, Neurosurgery, and Psychiatry* 44, 527–533.

Miller, D., & Adams, H. (1972). Physiopathology and management of increased intracranial pressure. In M. Critchley, J. L. O'Leary, & B. Jennett (Eds.), *Scientific foundations of neurology*. London: Heineman.

Miller, J. D. (1983). Early evaluation and management. In M. Rosenthal, E. Griffith, M. Bond, & J. D. Miller (Eds.), *Rehabilitation of the head injured adult* (pp. 37–58). Philadelphia: F. A. Davis.

Myers, P. S. (1984). Right hemisphere impairment. In A. L. Holland (Ed.), *language disorders in adults*. San Diego: College-Hill.

Newcombe, F. (1969). *Missile wounds of the brain*. London: Oxford University Press.

Newcombe, F., & Radcliff, G. (1979). Long-term psychological consequences of cerebral lesions. In M. S. Gazzaniga (Ed.), *Handbook of behavioral neurobiology* (Vol. 2). New York: Plenum Press.

Oddy, M. J.; Humphrey, M. E.; & Uttley, D. (1978). Subjective impairment and social recovery after closed head injury. *Journal of Neurology, Neurosurgery, and Psychiatry* 41, 611–616.

Oddy, M., & Humphrey, M. (1980). Social recovery during the year following severe head injury. *Journal of Neurology, Neurosurgery, and Psychiatry* 43, 798–802.

Ommaya, A. K., Grubb, R. L., & Naumann, R. A. (1971). Coup and contre-coup injury: Observations on the mechanics of visible brain injuries in the rhesus monkey. *Journal of Neurosurgery* 35, 503–516.

Overgaard, J., & Tweed, W. A. (1974). Cerebral circulation after head injury. Part 1: Cerebral blood flow and its autoregulation after closed head injury with emphasis on clinical correlations. *Journal of Neurosurgery* 41, 531–541.

Panting, A., & Merry, P. H. (1972). The long-term rehabilitation of severe head injuries with particular reference to need for social and medical support for the patient's family. *Rehabilitation* 38, 33–37.

Pepping, M.,& Epler, E. (1988). *Long-term follow-up after neuropsychological rehabilitation for severe brain injury: who benefits, who doesn't, and why?* Presented at the Fourth Annual Houston Conference on Neurotrauma, Houston, Texas, February.

Pepping, M., Roueche, J. R., Zeiner, H. K., Dirham, J. D., Meyer, R., Heilbronner, R. L., & Ayers, M. R. (1987). *Brain injury service models: Learning from outcome data—Phase II*. Presented at the Annual Meeting of the American Congress of Rehabilitation Medicine, Orlando, Florida, October.

Prigatano, G. P. (1986a). Higher cerebral deficits: The history of methods of assessment and approaches to rehabilitation: Part I. *BNI Quarterly* 2 (3), 15–26.

Prigatano, G. P. (1986b). Higher cerebral deficits: History of methods of assessment and approaches to rehabilitation: Part II. *BNI Quarterly* 2 (4), 9–17.

Prigatano, G. P. (1986c). *Neuropsychological rehabilitation after brain injury*, Baltimore: Johns Hopkins University Press.

Prigatano, G. P., Fordyce, D. J. (1986). Cognitive and psychosocial adjustment after brain injury. In G. P. Prigatano, *Neuropsychological rehabilitation after brain injury*. Baltimore: Johns Hopkins University Press.

Rimel, R. W., Giordani, B., Barth, J. T., & Jane, J. A. (1982). Moderate head injury: Completing the clinical spectrum of brain trauma. *Neurosurgery* 11 (3), 344–350.

Rimel, R. W., Giordani, B., Barth, J. T., Boll, T. J., & Jane, J. A. (1981). Disability caused by minor head injury. *Neurosurgery* 9 (3), 221–228.

Rimel, R. W., & Jane, J. A. (1983). Characteristics of the head-injured patient. In M. Rosenthal, E. Griffith, M. Bond, & J. D. Miller (Eds.), *Rehabilitation of the head injured adult* (pp. 9–21). Philadelphia: F. A. Davis.

Rosenbaum, M., & Najenson, T. (1976). Changes in life patterns and symptoms of low mood as reported by wives of severely brain-injured soldiers. *Journal of Consulting & Clinical Psychology* 44, 881–888.

Rosenthal, M., Griffith, E. R., Bond, M. R., & Miller, J. D. (Eds.), (1983). *Rehabilitation of the head injured adult*. Philadelphia: F. A. Davis.

Ross, E. D., & Mesulam, M. M. (1978). Dominant language functions of the right hemisphere. *Archives of Neurology* 36, 144–148.

Roueche, J. R., & Fordyce, D. J. (1983). Perceptions of deficits following brain injury and their impact on psychosocial adjustment. *Cognitive Rehabilitation* 1, 4–7.

Sarno, M. T. (1984). Verbal impairment after closed head injury. *The Journal of Nervous and Mental Disease* 172 (8), 475–479.

Semmes, J., Weinstein, S., Ghent, L., & Teuber, H.-L. (1960). *Somatosensory changes after penetrating brain wounds in man*. Cambridge, MA: Harvard University Press.

Semmes, J., Weinstein, S., Ghent, L., & Teuber, H.-L. (1963). Correlates of impaired orientation in personal and extrapersonal space. *Brain* 86, 747–772.

Smith, E. (1974). Influence of site of impact on cognitive impairment persisting long after severe closed head injury. *Journal of Neurology, Neurosurgery, and Psychiatry*, 37, 719–726.

Teasdale, G., & Mendelow, D. (1984). Pathophysiology of head injuries. In N. Brooks (Ed.), *Closed head injury*. New York: Oxford University Press.

Teuber, H.-L. (1962). Effects of brain wounds implicating right or left hemisphere in man. Discussion. In V. B. Mountcastle (Ed.), *Interhemispheric relations and cerebral dominance*, Baltimore: John Hopkins Press.

Teuber, H.-L. (1964). The riddle of frontal lobe function in man. In J. M. Warren & K. Akert (Eds.), *The frontal granular cortex and behavior*. New York: McGraw-Hill.

Thomsen, I. V. (1974). The patient with severe head injury and his family. *Scandinavian Journal of Rehabilitation Medicine* 6, 180–183.

Walker, A. E. (1972). Long-term evaluation of the social and family adjustment of head injuries. *Scandinavian Journal of Rehabilitation Medicine* 4, 5.

Walker, A. E., & Jablon, S. A. (1961). *A follow-up study of head wounds in World War II*. Washington, D.C.: Veterans Administration Medical Monograph.

Weddell, R., Oddy, M., & Jenkins, D. (1980). Social adjustment after rehabilitation: A two-year follow-up of patients with severe head injury. *Psychological Medicine* 10, 257–263.

Wertz, R. T. (1985). Neuropathologies of speech and language: An introduction to patient management. In D. F. Johns (Ed.), *Clinical management of neurogenic communicative disorders* (pp. 1–96). Boston: Little, Brown.

Wienecke, R. (1980). (Personal communication)

Wienecke, R. (1986) (Personal communication)

Zimmerman, R. A., Bilaniuk, L. T., Bruce, D., Dolinskas, C., Obirst, W., & Kuhl, D. (1978). Computed tomography of pediatric head trauma: Acute general cerebral swelling. *Radiology* 126, 403.

10. WORKING: THE KEY TO NORMALIZATION AFTER BRAIN INJURY

PATRICIA L. PRICE AND WILLIAM L. BAUMANN

INTRODUCTION

Working is among the most familiar of adult activities, yet it requires the highest degree of physical, cognitive, and behavioral integration of skills to be successful. The identification of a career goal or path is an intricate interplay of personal experience, familial and societal expectations, economic need, and opportunity. Following a brain injury, the delicate fabric of work potential, once solid and strong and made of the fibers of skill, social and personal acceptance, and economic viability, is tattered and torn, its useful potential in question. Mending the fabric takes time, special skill, and expertise, but the key determinant is the quality of the fabric itself, what it was before, and what it is now. Regardless of the skill of the tailor, delicate fabric will always show some flaws or irregularities, but the skill of the tailor can make the difference in the purpose and usability of the cloth.

The purpose of this chapter is to examine some of the unique ways in which cognitive, physical, behavioral, personal, psychological, and societal factors affect the vocational rehabilitation process of the adult with a brain injury. The purpose is not so much to map out the process of vocational rehabilitation with this group but rather to bring into focus those aspects of brain injury that are commonly known, but rarely incorporated, into the overall rehabilitation plan. It is with some reservation that the authors chose not to address issues of funding, legislation, public service systems, and professional personal investment in the overall outcome of persons with brain injury. Suffice it to say that the influence of each of these issues has a tremendous bearing on every case, and the scope of this chapter could not do justice to any of them. These issues also must be dealt with on a state-by-state, facility-by-facility, and case-by-case basis in order to effect real and viable change.

In many cases the individual with a brain injury, the family, and the professional approach the end stages of rehabilitation with the feeling that a vocational future for the person might be possible. These ideas stem from the knowledge of how far an individual has come in their rehabilitation program (essentially comparing what the person was on admission and what he or she is now), the identification and acknowledgment of "splintered skills" that appear to have vocational application, and the understanding of the individual's motivation and desire to work. It is not uncommon for these expectations to go unrealized in any one setting, as present systems and constraints on reimbursement structures prevent the continuous provision of the gamut of services. For this reason it is likely that professionals at any level of the rehabilitation process—i.e., hospital to community—may find themselves in the position to provide vocational services. This chapter attempts to bridge the gap between the clinical knowledge of brain injury and the vocational expectation held by an industrial society.

MEANING OF WORK

The meaning of work in society is a concept that most of us are aware of to some degree. For most the understanding of work's personal relevancy is at an unconscious level, perhaps because of its subtle pervasive influence in our every day life. Work is a key determinant of the kinds of experiences we have in our lives: educational, social, economical, and recreational. As we grow and develop as children and adults, our future plans and work experiences contribute significantly to our individual feelings of self-acceptance, self-respect, and self-worth. American society places a great value on the contributions that individuals make as workers. Consequently, the value of an individual in the community often is measured by the work he or she performs (Price & Schmidt, 1987). Applying the "Who I am = What I do" (Price, 1987, p. 1) principle to the rehabilitation of individuals with a brain injury provides a context or framework from which to understand and approach the vocational adjustment and rehabilitation process.

Unlike developmentally disabled individuals, those with a brain injury bring to the rehabilitation process a normal career development past. Although there are numerous theories of career development, Ginzberg and colleagues (1951) summarized the concept by postulating: "Occupational choice is a developmental process: it is not a single decision, but a series of decisions made over a period of years. Beginning in childhood, each step in the process has a meaningful relation to those which precede and follow it" (p. 185). In light of the career development concept, it can be assumed that, prior to incurring a brain injury, these individual's career development began many years ago. These adults have already made an identity investment in a particular career direction. Those who are traumatically brain injured as young adults were in the process of establishing themselves more firmly within the identified occupational group by developing common realms of education or training, social-interpersonal relationships, personal economics, and leisure interests. It is this dimension of normal personal and career development, the establishment of life dreams, that separates the person with a brain injury in a significant way from some other disability groups.

VOCATIONAL REHABILITATION AND ITS IMPACT ON PSYCHOSOCIAL ADJUSTMENT

Persons with a brain injury and their family generally enter into the vocational rehabilitation process with great hopes and dreams for the future. In spite of the catastrophic losses that have occurred, hope of attaining the dreams has been reinforced by predictions made by the doctors and therapists that have not come true (e.g., remaining in a coma or being unable to walk, etc.). By the time the vocational rehabilitation process begins the person with a brain injury and his family distrust professionals whose job it is to make predictions regarding functional outcome. Sometimes they are unable to consider the vocational options that are available to them, because engaging in vocational rehabilitation also signals the decline in restorative therapies. Even though this change in the emphasis of rehabilitation is seemingly positive, it can be confrontative to individuals due to the recognition that 100% of their preinjury status cannot be reached. It is also likely that individuals will "experience confusion and anxiety as they look toward their vocational future. Not only has their career development been abruptly interrupted, but awareness of changed abilities and skills becomes more apparent" (Price, 1986, p. 118). Emotional responses to these realizations are often characterized by anxiety/catastrophic reaction to failure experience, denial of deficits or minimizing their effects, depression or withdrawal, and aggression or defensiveness (Prigatano, 1986). These characterizations of intrapsychic conflict, though not unusual reactions for those who experience a traumatic injury, do impede the vocational adjustment of the person with a brain injury. As a result of their unawareness of the vocational options available to them (e.g., vocational naiveté and their current level of ability), these individuals may cling to their preinjury career goals because they do not see that they have viable vocational alternatives or substitutes. Consequently, the dreams they have preinjury compete against the messages given in the rehabilitation process postinjury and present yet another opportunity to challenge the professionals and reinforce the distrust that has developed.

Another barrier to vocational counseling with an individual with traumatic brain injury will be "judgment and lack of insight deficits that lead him to equate hospital discharge with recovery and the belief he will automatically re-enter society at his pre-onset level" (Smith, 1983, p. 2026). If individual problem-solving abilities are such that this attitude is maintained, it is likely the person will meet with failure. Making the transition from patient to worker can cause confusion due to the large discrepancy in the demands of the environments, stress due to an inability to accommodate the increased demands, and ultimately even failure to achieve vocational expectations.

Familial influence and it's impact on the vocational rehabilitation of the brain-injured individual is a significant aspect to consider in the counseling process. Families have an investment in the individual's career development. Prior to injury the family has been the major source of encouragement and support. It is not uncommon for them to continue in this role postinjury, and in doing so they may reinforce unrealistic goals and plans. Though they may be more insightful than the individual who is brain injured, they are nevertheless in the process of grieving "what was" and "what could have been." "In order to reach a stage where they can accept the loss that has occurred, grief must be experienced" (Barry, 1984, p. 1). According to Barry this grief process experiences four stages in some combination throughout the recovery process: shock, anxiety, anger, and depression. "It [the grieving process] hurts, and it's natural, and a necessary part of the adjustment process" (Barry, 1984, p. 1). The familiar cliché "timing is everything" most certainly applies as much in the vocational rehabilitation process as in any other stage of rehabilitation. Rosenthal and Muir (1983) wrote, "Since each person's recovery pattern is unique, as is the ability of family members to understand and accept the disability, it is vital that a given intervention not be initiated before a patient or family is ready" (p. 413).

VOCATIONAL OPTIONS

The concept of vocational rehabilitation has traditionally focused on returning a disabled individual to gainful employment. However, the changes experienced by many people with brain injuries will limit them from working competitively. Although 50–60% of these individuals may find placement in full-time, part-time, or sheltered work situations, less than half (20–25%) maintain employment for longer than 6 to 12 months. This grim statistic does not mean, however, that the importance or necessity of working is in any way minimized in the view of the person with a brain injury. Despite repeated attempts and failures, the need to obtain the personal relevancy that work provides still persists. Another less benevolent reason exists for investigating more realistic vocational goals with this group: maintenance of skills regained through rehabilitation. The functional abilities recovered or acquired through rehabilitation need to be utilized in order to be maintained. The essence of work provides the vehicle and purpose for needing and demonstrating the recovered abilities on a regular basis. Super (1976) defined work as

the systematic pursuit of an objective valued by oneself and desired by others; directed and consecutive, it requires the expenditure of effort. It may be compensated (paid work) or uncompensated (volunteer work or an avocation). The objective may be intrinsic enjoyment of work itself, the structure given to life by the work role, the economic support it makes possible, or the type of leisure which it facilitates. (p. 20)

Given Super's definition of work, it is possible and useful to expand the traditionally accepted definition of work to accommodate the vocational needs of those with a brain injury. As a worthwhile contribution to one's community, either in the community at large, in the neighborhood, or in the home, work can occur in any of the following types of placements: competitive employment, full or part-time; self-employment; supported employment; volunteer work; sheltered employment; extended employment; work activity programming; and adult day programming.

Extending the definition of work to include these options presents issues such as who can be considered for these options, what are the typical demands of the position, and what is expected. To determine the level of "productive contribution" individuals can make to their living environment, the professional must compare and contrast the demands of the workplace to the individuals' ability. Each site or placement option should, of course, be considered individually for its degree of compatibility in the following areas: productivity level, quality of work, environmental and social demands, and the focus goals of the individual.

Super's definition of work suggests that many types and levels of work are available to the individual with a brain injury. In each situation, environment is a key determinant of the individual's success. Environmental factors include how the work tasks are taught, how instructions are given and/or expectations communicated, presence of office politics, and degree of cooperation needed to work with supervisors/co-workers. The evaluation process for any job should include an assessment of both the job skills and work behaviors required as well as the nonproduction-related expectations that the work environment presents. The environment to a large extent dictates how one should react to the situational demands. The individual's present ability to manage those environmental expectations appropriately is a key determinant of vocational success. Assisting the individual to identify not just a job or vocational situation but one that is a strong match is a critical element that should be provided by a professional.

In comparing the same job and job responsibilities at two different work sites, environmental demands can differ significantly. Job matching then is not as simple as identifying a job title, as this difference may dictate whether the person with a brain injury will succeed in a placement. Even though the individual may have a good mastery of the work skills required to perform the job tasks, environmental demands need to be kept in mind when reviewing any of the following vocational placement options.

In a competitive employment situation, the productivity, quality, expectations, and environmental influences are not usually modified to any significant degree for the person with a brain injury. The standards for the individual are the same as for the other nondisabled employees. A person with a brain injury, with a certain combination of strengths and limitations may be able to function independently in a job where the demands complement his or her abilities. In general this is the goal of the vocational rehabilitation process: to identify placements that minimize limitations and utilize strengths and remaining work skills in the work setting.

Self-employment for the brain-injured population has a number of positive and negative factors to consider. A high level of quality in work is expected, although work quantity can be flexible. There is generally good ability to control the work environment, allowing modification of the demands to complement an individual's abilities. Individuals can work at their own pace, allowing flexibility in accommodating endurance issues if necessary. This type of placement allows persons to feel productive, although self-employment usually does not permit the same level of socialization opportunities as a competitive work setting. Many times a friend or family member is needed to assist in the management of a self-employment situation.

Supported employment allows for some modification of the work environment and provides on-site skill development toward the goal of a competitive job. Production and quality expectations can be modified depending on the nature of the work tasks, generally with the expectation that with time less assistance and fewer modifications will be necessary. In most cases support is provided by the rehabilitation community in the form of job coaches, individuals on-site to assist in the mainstreaming of the disabled. This assistance includes job restructuring, job counseling, orientation to site and job tasks, providing feedback regarding work behaviors, and employer education.

Volunteer work often can provide the benefits of socialization and the feeling that one is making a contribution. The person works within the community at large, and generally is performing modified tasks with the production/quality rates at a below-entry level depending on the task being completed. The individual is generally expected to demonstrate acceptable social skills/work behaviors. Job coaching in this situation is unavailable because of funding restrictions due to the fact that the brain-injured person is not on a competitive employment (wage-earning) track. The goal of a volunteer placement may be to move into a supported work program or may be considered a long-term placement.

Sheltered employment programming is delivered in a modified environment with reduced production and quality expectations. The focus of treatment is to upgrade work behaviors and skill levels to allow the individual to enter a supported work program within the community. Benefits include being involved in a work program whose goal is to enable community integration with the modification of designated behaviors. It provides an income for the work performed and, as with all of the programs to follow, social opportunities.

Extended employment is dissimilar to sheltered employment only in that the the goals are more long-term in nature. In extended employment, persons with a brain injury are viewed as regular employees. Usually they can participate at a work task, although due to cognitive/physical/behavioral factors production rates and work behaviors restrict their options. Persons are paid for what they produce (piece rate), and the renumeration is generally minimal.

Work activity and adult day care (day enrichment) programming are similar to one another except through the means of intervention. The focus of each program is on upgrading of personal and community activities of daily living, improving socialization, prevocational training, and recreational programming. In work activity programming these areas are developed through prevocational and work tasks and some classroom and individual teaching. An adult day care program utilizes avocational training, social skills groups, individualized therapy programs, and activities of daily living instruction to address these areas. Both settings involve the individual in modified activities within a controlled environment. These types of programs are usually long term in nature. Renumeration for work performed is usually provided.

The vocational rehabilitation programs already discussed are readily available for other disability groups. Serving the individual who has a brain injury in those programs that include mixed disabilities is usually unsuccessful and not therapeutic. The reasons for this lack of success include differing programming needs, a staff not trained in brain injury rehabilitation, and identity issues whereby the brain-injured person does not want to be viewed as developmentally disabled or emotionally disturbed. There are a few programs that are designed specifically for persons with a brain injury in this country, but there is a growing need for that number to increase to meet demand.

With the inclusive rather than exclusive definition of vocational rehabilitation, many of the benefits received through gainful employment (full-time competitive employment) become available to the person with a brain injury. Individuals can participate in a productive life-style, while continuing to maintain and integrate the individual rehabilitation goals at a community level. The process of, and the placement in, such alternative settings serves to maintain and upgrade functional skills and develop social relationships, while providing individuals with an opportunity to make a worthwhile contribution to their community.

CRITICAL BEHAVIORS NECESSARY FOR WORK

Extending the definition of work to include options like those mentioned previously brings another question to bear on the topic of vocational rehabilitation: "Who can be considered?" Every person must be evaluated individually through the tools and guidelines of vocational evaluation but it is helpful to examine the work of experts to get a sense of the qualifications of acceptable candidates.

Herr (1975, p. 15) outlined the survival skills needed to succeed in a job:

1. Knowledge of one's personal strengths and weaknesses, preferences, values, and the skill to relate these to available educational and occupational options; the ability to make realistic self-estimates
2. Ability to use existing exploratory resources—that is, educational opportunities, part-time works, books, audio-visual resources, and so on—to reality-test personal characteristics and choices
3. Knowledge of educational, occupational, social, life-style options and the skills to determine the interaction among them
4. Ability to choose—to understand and apply the decision-making process purposefully and rationally
5. Skill in interpersonal relationships—the ability to work cooperatively with others; understanding of worker-supervisory relations; adaptability to different persons and conditions
6. Employability and job-seeking skills—understanding of applications and interviewing behavior
7. Understanding of personal roles as an employee, a customer, a client, a manager, and an entrepreneur
8. Understanding of the interdependence of the educational and occupational structures—the pathways between them, the relationship of subject matter to its application in professional, technical, and vocational settings
9. Knowledge of how to organize one's time and energy to get work done, to set priorities, and to plan
10. Ability to see onself as some one, as a person of worth and dignity, as a basis for seeing oneself as something

It should be noted that these skills do not exclude the importance of basic academic and actual job performance behaviors.

Krantz (1971) listed critical work behaviors in the areas of (1) job objective behaviors, (2) job-getting behaviors, and (3) job-keeping behaviors, which are similar in a number of areas to Herr's list. In addition, Krantz emphasized that an individual must have the ability to meet production rates at an appropriate level of quality. In general, one can consider the industrial norm as the standard against which both quantity and quality are measured, and 60% as the acceptable level of performance for both quality and quantity at the competitive level.

These basic abilities considered necessary to succeed in competitive employment can be grouped into several key areas. Persons must be able to produce work at a specified level of quality and quantity. They must have certain functional skills in the cognitive, interpersonal, and intrapersonal areas. They must be able to evaluate their strengths and limitations in order to choose and guide their job/career development. They must be able to demonstrate the ability to deal with others and have an understanding of how to relate to the business' patrons, co-workers, and supervisors. A worker must be able to initiate and organize work to meet deadlines. Both Krantz and Herr considered it important that workers have realistic vocational objectives; that is, they should be able to evaluate and adjust their work expectations according to abilities and limitations.

There are additional criteria that are generally required for persons with a brain injury to participate in any of the vocational options described earlier. These include their being medically stable and out of the acute stage of medical care. Adequate medical care must be available to them. They must be continent of bowel and bladder. They must be able to maintain a level of awareness during programming and demonstrate the physical abilities that will allow them to consistently interact with their environment in a meaningful manner. Individuals must be able to manage their own behavior so as not to inflict physical harm to self or others. The assistance required to meet these criteria should be in the form of counseling and behavioral techniques at most and should not require the physical presence of another person to be reliable.

VOCATIONALLY RELATED DIFFICULTIES FOR PERSONS WITH A BRAIN INJURY

Literature in the field of brain injury rehabilitation speaks to the likelihood of clients exhibiting one or a combination of physical, cognitive, and behavioral sequelae following a brain injury. Frequently cited deficits include difficulty in arousal; difficulty in maintaining and sustaining attention; mental flexibility; memory loss affecting old and/or new learning; difficulty in processing information, verbal and/or nonverbal; difficulty with visual, auditory, and/or sensory perception; motor disturbances involving loss of power, loss of balance, and/or disorders of muscle tone; altered control and expression of emotions due to medical, cognitive, and/or psychological phenomena; difficulties in social and/or safety judgment; difficulties in reasoning and problem solving; slowed thinking process; and inconsistency in repeated performances of the same activity.

Though this list certainly speaks to the complex nature of brain injury, its primary usefulness is in the education of others to the general dynamics of the disability. In considering the development of a vocational program or plan, it is necessary for the vocational rehabilitation professional to gain insight into (1) the possibility of there being certain deficits that are more frequently possessed by this group, (2) which of these deficit areas tend to cause the most difficulty relevant to vocational adjustment and rehabilitation, (3) the specific difficulties that are experienced within an area of cognition, (4) the cause or etiology underlying the deficit work behaviors, and (5) whether the problems are different from those experienced by other disability groups and if so in what way(s).

Most workers, disabled and nondisabled, lose jobs due to problems in interpersonal relationships and in demonstrating adequate work-related behavior rather than because of lack of skill (Pruitt, 1977). The logical point in examining employability of persons with brain injury should begin in the area of critical work behaviors, rather than the area of aptitudes and skills. Such a study was undertaken by Price (1987), which involved a retrospective study of work behavior data collected on 27 persons with a diagnosis of brain injury.

METHODOLOGY

Using the Work Personality Profile (Bolten & Roessler, 1986), a behaviorally oriented work assessment instrument, 27 brain-injured persons receiving vocational services were evaluated. The evaluation team was composed of a neuropsychologist, occupational therapist, physical therapist, special educator, speech and language pathologist, recreational therapist, social worker, and vocational counselor. Composite scores were obtained by averaging individual ratings on each of the 58 items on the Work Personality Profile.

The data were first analyzed to ascertain each subject's performance on each of five broad dimensions of work behavior: task orientation, social skills, work motivation, work conformance, and personal presentation. The data were further analyzed to determine subject performance on 11 primary scales: acceptance of work role, ability to profit from instruction or correction, work persistence, work tolerance, amount of supervision required, extent trainee seeks help from supervisor, degree of comfort or anxiety with supervisor, appropriateness of relations with supervisor, teamwork, ability to socialize with co-workers, and communication skills. Items in each primary scale were identified for their contribution to the overall scale total.

The data analysis showed that for this group of subjects there were in fact some areas of deficit that were more prevalent. The prevalent problem areas were also different from those found in the norm group used by Bolten and Roessler. The norm group was described as a general rehabilitation population comprised of three major disabling conditions: physical (26%), intellectual (31%), emotional (43%).

The major dimension of work behavior found to be problematic was work conformance; Bolten and Roessler (1986) defined this dimension as "understanding the rules of work etiquette" (p. 145). Specifically, work conformance includes such behaviors as exercising good judgment in the expression of negative behaviors, even-temperedness, and controlled self-presentation. Over 51% of the subjects in this study were rated as having definite problems in work conformance severe enough to limit their chances for employment. The primary scales and particular items that contributed to poor performance include the following dimensions:

Acceptance of worker role: 53.8% did not carry out assigned tasks without prompting, 42% displayed poor judgment in the use of obscenities, 30.7% displayed poor judgment in playing practical jokes, and 30.7% were temperamental.
Degree of comfort or anxiety with supervisor: 46% became upset when corrected.

Appropriateness of personal relations with supervisor: 34.6% discussed personal problems that were not work related.

Social communication skills: 84.6% expressed likes and dislikes inappropriately, 61.5% expressed negative feelings inappropriately (e.g., anger, fear, sadness), and 46% interrupted others while they were speaking.

The second dimension of work behavior found to be problematic was task orientation. This dimension was defined by the authors as adaptable and responsible, possessing good learning ability on the job, with capability for self-direction. Task orientation encompasses both cognitive skills and good work habits and includes the ability to learn quickly, initiate activity, perform independently, and ask questions only when necessary (Bolten & Roessler, 1986). A total of 40.7% of the subjects were rated as having the greatest amount of difficulty demonstrating behaviors in this dimension. In all cases, for those who experienced their greatest difficulty in this area, the ratings again indicated that the problems were severe enough to definitely limit the chances for employment. The following primary scales and particular items contributed to poor performance on task orientation:

Work persistence: 51.6% were not able to maintain work pace when distractions occurred.

Amount of supervision required: 57.6% did not recognize their own mistakes, 46% needed more than the average amount of supervision, and 46% required frequent help with problems.

Work tolerance: 38% performed unsatisfactorily in tasks that required variety, and 34.6% did not accept changes in work assignments.

Less than 10% of the subjects studied demonstrated definite problems in the remaining dimensions of work behavior, with most performing in the adequate range. Personal presentation and work motivation dimensions were particular strength areas. Specific items in which the subjects were rated as having either adequate performance or performance that could be considered a definite strength were accepting assignments without arguing, conforming to rules and regulations, maintaining satisfactory personal hygiene habits, arriving appropriately dressed for work, expressing pleasure in accomplishment, approaching supervisory personnel with confidence, demonstrating stable performance in supervisor's presence, showing an interest in what others are doing, seeking out co-workers to be friends with, and joining social groups when they are available.

The results of this study, though limited, provide some clues as to the kinds of problems that a person with a brain injury is most likely to experience vocationally. It is clear that even though this population is likely to present with a varied and complex combination of physical, cognitive, and behavioral sequelae following a brain injury, all deficits do not impact on the critical demonstration of work behavior equally. Particular cognitive problems seem to impact performance more than others. Problems in demonstrating behaviors in the work conformance dimension seem to be more affected by difficulties of poor social judgment, processing and expressing verbal information, and altered control of emotion. Difficulties in maintaining and sustaining attention, organization, reasoning and problem solving, mental flexibility, and processing of verbal and/or nonverbal information toward new learning seemed to be the underlying problems affecting the dimension of task orientation.

CONCLUSION

The American society has become one of the most complex, mobile, and affluent of any in the world. From the days when people lived in the same community as their grandparents and worked to provide the essentials, the society has changed immensely. Work no longer meets only the economic needs of adults; American workers expect that their broad social and psychological needs will be satisfied as well. Most adults rarely consider the personal relevancy of their work, but with the onset of a disability an awareness and reexamination of these issues becomes a necessary part of the rehabilitation process. The vocational rehabilitation of the adult with a brain injury begins at this premise and culminates with a mutual and satisfactory resolution between the individual and the community or employer. The steps in between are preparation for the ensuing negotiation. They include clarifying the needs and values one has related to work, understanding of the principles of supply and demand (what one has to give and what is needed in the work situation) both at the basic and specific level, obtaining the necessary requirements, and, finally, some adjustment to what is desired and what is possible.

For those with an incurred brain injury, the process is complicated by combined and complex physical, cognitive, and behavioral sequelae. These sequelae can impair the individual's ability to reconstruct a fragmented self-concept, access and acquire relevant information, and carry out or demonstrate desired behaviors or tasks. Rehabilitation professionals can be instrumental in assisting individuals to achieve and maximize their functional and work skills. It is important that professionals communicate their willingness to support and collaborate with individuals toward the goals they have for themselves. Although most often the preinjury status will not be achieved, many times an acceptable alternative can be identified. Almost always individuals will need to adjust to an altered vocational future, one that may be slightly or significantly different from their lifelong dream. Though identification and placement into some level of productive activity (paid or nonpaid) is the desired outcome of vocational rehabilitation, it is the degree to which the individual is able to acknowledge and adjust to the altered vocational future that determines the ultimate vocational rehabilitation success.

REFERENCES

Barry, P. (1984). *Family adjustment to head injury*. Framingham, MA: National Head Injury Foundation.

Bolten, B., & Roessler, R. (1985). *The Work Personality Profile*. Arkansas Research and Training Center, University of Arkansas.

Bolten, B., & Roessler, R. (1986). The Work Personality Profile: Factor scales, reliability, validity and norms. *Vocational Evaluation and Work Adjustment Bulletin* 19(4), 143–149.

Ginzberg, E., Ginsburg, S. W., Axelrad, S., & Herma, J. R. (1951). *Occupational choice: An approach to a general theory*. New York: Columbia University Press.

Herr, E. L. (1975). Testimony on the career guidance and counseling act. *Proceedings of the U.S. House of Representatives, Committee on Education and Labor, Subcommittee on Elementary, Secondary and Vocational Education*. Washington, D.C., April 10.

Krantz, G. (1971). Critical vocational behaviors. *Journal of Rehabilitation*, July/August, pp. 14–16.

Price, P. L. (1986). Facilitating client-directed vocational planning in head injured adults. *Vocational Evaluation and Work Adjustment Bulletin* 19(3), 117–119.

Price, P. L. (1987). *A study of critical work behaviors demonstrated by persons with severe head injury*. Boston, MA: Greenery Skilled Nursing and Rehabilitation Center. (unpublished)

Price, P. L., & Schmidt, N. D. (1987). *The vocational readiness manual for families: A home program for a person with a head injury*. Cambridge, MA: Carolyn Jenks Literary Agency.

Prigatano, George R. (1986). *Neuropsychological rehabilitation after brain injury*. Baltimore, MD: John Hopkins University Press.

Pruitt, W. A. (1977). *Vocational work evaluation*. Menonmonie, WI: Walt Pruitt Associates.

Rosenthal, M., & Muir, C. A., (1983). Methods of family intervention. In M. Rosenthal, E. R. Griffith, M. R. Bond, J. D. Miller (Eds.), *Rehabilitation of the head injured adult* (pp. 407–420). Philadelphia, PA.: F. A. Davis.

Smith, R. K. (1983). Prevocational programming in the rehabilitation of the head-injured patient. *Physical Therapy* 63(12), 2026–2029.

Super, D. E. (1976). Career education and the meaning of work. *Monograph on Career Education*. Washington D.C.: U.S. Office of Education.

11. NEUROPSYCHOLOGICAL REHABILITATION: TREATMENT OF ERRORS IN EVERYDAY FUNCTIONING

KEITH D. CICERONE AND DAVID E. TUPPER

When new turns in behavior cease to appear in the life of the individual its behavior ceases to be intelligent.

G. E. COGHILL, *ANATOMY AND THE PROBLEM OF BEHAVIOR* (NEW YORK: CAMBRIDGE UNIVERSITY PRESS, 1929), P. 79.

INTRODUCTION

It is perhaps a truism that the goal of rehabilitation after brain injury is the improvement of functioning in real-life contexts. In practice, this goal requires the training of new behaviors to replace the impaired functions and the learning of new ways to perform a wide range of daily activities in a variety of situations. Unfortunately, the cognitive processes underlying the acquisition, maintenance, and production of those new behaviors are the very ones that are impaired. Cognitive deficits not only interfere with the ability to profit from traditional rehabilitative therapies, but they often represent the major obstacle to successful everyday functioning. Thus there have been increasing efforts to develop specific remedial interventions for cognitive disability after brain injury and, more recently, concern that these interventions are relevant to patients' lives beyond therapy.

Interventions for cognitive deficits after brain injury appear to vary along several principal dimensions (Kirsch et al., 1987). Therapies may focus on modification of neurocognitive structure and capacity or on the external environmental conditions that affect performance. Therapies may also emphasize retraining of multiple, basic neurocognitive components or the retraining

Table 11-1. Models of neuropsychological remediation

Model	Focus	Emphasis	Mechanism	Approach
Process	Internal	Neurocognitive Components	Restitution	Bottom-up
Functional	External	Functional skills	Compensation based on task-specific learning	Bottom-up
Noetic	Internal	Functional	Compensation based on awareness	Top-down

of more integrative abilities and functional skills. The mechanism purported to underlie change can be based on practice and restoration of deficient skills or on the development of compensatory strategies. Finally, the therapeutic approach can be "bottom-up," based on the sequential building from elementary to complex skills, or "top-down" via the application of superordinate controls over subordinate processes. Most intervention can be described within three models of cognitive remediation based on four dimensions (table 11-1).

Process models of cognitive remediation assume that specific interventions can impact differentially on component neurocognitive deficits. For example, Gordon and colleagues (1985) combined specific well-controlled training procedures in basic scanning, somatosensory stimulation and size estimation, and visual-spatial organization into a comprehensive perceptual remediation program. The training program was effective in promoting improvement on psychometric measures closely related to the training areas. Limited generalization of improvements to measures not specifically related to the training tasks occurred, although the investigators noted more time spent in recreational reading after treatment. Sohlberg and Mateer (1987) utilized a hierarchy of training tasks within the domain of attention. Four brain-injured patients who received the training showed significant improvement on a psychometric measure of attention. Attention training was not associated with a generalized improvement in other cognitive abilities (e.g., visual processing), which was interpreted as supporting a model of therapy directed at remediation of underlying neurocognitive deficit processes. Although some general functional gains occurred with these four subjects, it was difficult to attribute these gains to the attention training.

Functional skills training concentrates on the patient's ability in domain-specific, context-specific areas of functioning and the retraining of "competencies of daily life" (Mayer, Keating, & Rapp, 1986). Mayer et al. suggested several approaches to training, such as (1) repetition of a whole skill in a natural context (e.g., drinking from a cup during breakfast), (2) training of component parts (e.g., looking for the cup, reaching, grasping, etc). followed by whole-skill training, and (3) various attempts to substitute new procedures to perform the desired activity. Although conceptualizing behavior and presumable interventions according to a hierarchy of preskills, individual skills, and routine and activity patterns, Mayer et al. did not consider the cognitive task attributes distinct from the functional skills being trained. Following Tsvetkova's (1972) notion of retraining within the context of a broader function, they gave the example that

one should not address an individual's inability to visually recognize letters except when this deficit manifests itself within the function of reading which includes the movement of the eyes, auditory analyses and synthesis of reading material, reading comprehension, etc. Extending this concept to our approach, it would, for example, appear necessary to address visual scanning as it relates to locating items upon a grocery shelf within the context of a shopping trip. . . . We feel strongly that training exercises in memory, attention, logical reasoning and so on are not the most practical way to deal with the rehabilitation objective of adaptiveness. . . . The rehabilitation objective in this situation is not to improve the patient's memory in some abstract or general way but, in fact, to accomplish the goal of shopping. (p. 221)

Though the work of Schacter and Glisky (1986) is derived from neuro-cognitive-oriented work on spared memory abilities after brain injury, their training approach is very functionally oriented in its emphasis on the acquisition of domain-specific knowledge by memory-impaired patients. They utilized a method of "vanishing cues" to teach four brain-injured amnestic patients 30 new computer-related vocabulary words. Consistent with a functional approach, the training was intended to provide the patients with specific knowledge in an area important to the patients' everyday lives (computer terms) rather than produce general improvements in memory function. Schacter and Glisky (1986) suggested that the same procedure might be applied toward the acquisition of complex forms of knowledge by brain-injured patients, as well as the possibility of training patients to become expert in specific, defined content areas.

Kirsh and co-workers (1987) utilized a conceptual framework in which complex activities were (hierarchically) analyzed into tasks, stages, and behavioral options. They developed a computerized task guidance system that enabled their patient to perform a complex functional activity (baking cookies and preparing icing) that the patient could not otherwise perform. By developing highly structured and individualized task guidance systems for a large number of tasks, it should be possible for the patient to compensate throughout an entire day's activities. In each of these functional approaches the patient is trained on the same task that he or she is expected to perform in the context of daily activities, and training is specific to that situation. Generalization to other related situations is not expected as a consequence of the initial training. Thus the necessity of training a wide range and number of specialized, context-specific skills and routines is characteristic of the functional model.

One other model, which we refer to as a noetic approach, places its major emphasis on training at the level of the patient's capacity for self-regulation (Cicerone & Wood, 1987) and self-awareness (Crosson et al., 1989). Cicerone and Wood (1987) used self-instructional training with a single head-injured patient who exhibited an executive planning dysfunction. The self-instructional training was intended to provide the patient with a cognitive mediation strategy to control his impulsive behavior. Over the course of training the patient showed a significant reduction in off-task behaviors and improvement on posttraining measures that reflected the focus of training. Generalization of improvements to real-life situations was not observed during this period but was apparent during subsequent treatment that included self-monitoring of behaviors outside the treatment setting. Sohlberg, Sprunk, and Metzelaar (1988) used an external cueing procedure to promote self-monitoring of initiation and socially appropriate responses with a head-injured patient with bilateral frontal damage. The intervention produced increases in both behaviors, presumably due to the reactive effects of self-monitoring (Kazdin, 1974). These desirable behaviors decreased but persisted after the external cueing was eliminated. They also noted anecdotal generalization to community settings and suggested continued, gradually diminishing cueing "until appropriate behaviors became automatic"[1] (p. 39). At a practical level, self-management techniques can be applied to a wide range of cognitive and functional deficit areas (Malec, 1984): The underlying assumption that patients will be able to *internalize* the effects of training, and can develop sufficient awareness and insight to apply strategies in a variety of situations, is a distinctive aspect of the noetic approach. Prigatano and Fordyce (1986) described aspects of training designed to increase patient awareness of deficits and acceptance of strategy use. The awareness training included extensive use of objective, impartial feedback, graphing of progress with and without strategy usage, patient self-monitoring and comparisons of performance, and intensive reinforcement of insight and compensatory behaviors. Crosson et al. (1989) further identified intellectual, emergent, and anticipatory levels of awareness after brain injury. Different degrees of compensation may be available to patients, depending on their degree of awareness deficit; these patients with marked deficits of intellectual awareness may require external, task-specific compensation whereas patients with minimal awareness deficits may compensate by recognition or anticipation of problems while moving from one environment to another several times in the course of their daily functioning.

In addition to the theoretical and practical distinctions among the process, functional, and noetic models, there are common concerns as well. These concerns, which appear essential to any neuropsychological therapy attempting to remediate patients' everyday behavior, include (1) the impact of patients' emotional, psychological, and interpersonal status (including the therapeutic relationship) on their daily functioning; (2) the relation between neuropsychological deficits and abilities and real-life cognitive and functional disability, especially in relation to the selection of appropriate levels and breadth of skill training; and (3) the maintenance and application of training in ways that improve the patient's real-life functioning.

COMMON CONCERNS OF NEUROPSYCHOLOGICAL THERAPIES

Psychosocial Factors and the Therapeutic Alliance

Neuropsychological abilities exhibit a fairly consistent though modest relation to patients' everyday functioning (Heaton & Pendleton, 1981; Klonoff, Costa, & Snow, 1986; McSweeney et al., 1985), but personality and emotional factors exert significant influence, at least on patients' subjective disability. Chelune, Heaton, and Lehman (1986) found that patients' complaints of cognitive, memory, communication, and sensorimotor impairment were much more strongly related to their MMPI results than to their neuropsychological test performance. In particular, patients' levels of emotional distress discriminated between those who "exaggerated" and those who "minimized" their disability, irrespective of actual neuropsychological impairment based on test results. Changes in levels of emotional distress over the course of neuropsychological rehabilitation appear to vary according to patients' subjective reports of disability and relate to rehabilitation outcome (employment) status, independent of changes in neuropsychological impairment (Fordyce & Roueche, 1986). On the basis of these studies, it is likely that patients' emotional and personality status influence their ability to function in everyday life (irrespective of neuropsychological impairments) and may therefore exert a significant influence on the process and outcome of neuropsychological rehabilitation. It appears reasonable to assert that these factors need to be addressed within the context of any therapeutic approach.

The role of the "therapeutic alliance" has been recognized as a crucial key to change in diverse forms of therapy (Bordin, 1979), but it has been given remarkably little attention in neuropsychological rehabilitation. The therapeutic alliance has three basic characteristics: *patient-therapist expectancies* and belief in the helping relationship, *patient commitment* especially as expressed through defensiveness and resistance to therapy (Gaston et al., 1988), and the *patient-therapist collaboration* on the goals and tasks of therapy (Frieswyck et al., 1986).

The establishment of a common expectation is an essential aspect of the initial rehabilitation process. Patients and therapists alike bring with them into treatment attributions regarding past performance and treatment possibilities; patients may tend to underestimate their deficits (Fordyce & Roueche, 1986), whereas clinicians may tend to overdiagnose pathology (Faust et al., 1988). The rehabilitation process may generate additional attributions regarding patient change. Rehabilitation therapists appear to attribute patient improvement to therapy, and lack of progress to patients' lack of motivation or unrealistic expectations; patients are more likely to attribute gains to their own motivation and family support, and to cite lack of appropriate therapy and insufficient social support as reasons for their lack of improvement (Cicerone,

1987). The assumptions of both patient and therapist contribute to the therapeutic alliance and to expectations regarding patients' real-life functioning.

Patients' lack of awareness regarding the existence or severity of deficits after brain injury represents a particular area of significance and is often a central concern for neuropsychological intervention. Patients who are unable to recognize or acknowledge their limitations are likely to be difficult to engage in therapy, not surprisingly. Based on patient, family, and staff ratings of competency prior to treatment, Fordyce and Roueche (1986) identified two groups of head-injured patients. One group rated themselves similar to the ratings of staff, whereas the other exhibited a pronounced tendency to underestimate their level of impairment as compared to staff members' estimates. The latter group could be further divided on the basis of change in patients' ratings in relation to staff's ratings over the course of rehabilitation. In one group patient and staff ratings converged, whereas for the final group differences in perspective actually increased. Among the patients who showed increased awareness of deficits 78% were engaged in productive activity following their rehabilitation, but among the patients with persistent lack of awareness of deficits only 25% were engaged in productive activity. Clinically, the findings suggest that for patients unable to engage in treatment due to their unawareness of deficits, priority needs to address patients' awareness deficits and resistance in therapy. One of the most common and costly errors of treatment may be the failure to confront the patient's unawareness. The success of such confrontations requires the establishment of a stable and supportive treatment relationship so that the patient's defensiveness can be addressed in the "safety of a therapeutic environment."

Within the context of a therapeutic alliance, patients' awareness of deficits can be effectively addressed by providing them with specific, objective feedback. Rather than relying on normative or dichotomous neuropsychological statements about deficits or the therapist's performance expectancies, patients can be asked to predict their own performance capabilities. This tack would allow the therapist to address the discrepancies between the patient's perceived and actual competencies. The possible relations and implications of the patients' deficits to their everyday functioning, including any difficulty in accurately assessing their own performance, can be interpreted with them regularly. In general, we agree with Deaton's (1986) suggestion that "all treatments should involve a balance between positive (supportive) and negative (confrontative) elements" (p. 235).

The formation of an effective patient-therapist collaboration relies on therapist's ability to create a shared understanding and conceptualization of therapy and the negotiation of common goals and treatment objectives. In a general rehabilitation setting, the practice of patient and therapist sharing decisions about treatment was more important than interpersonal or affective dimensions of the therapy relationship for achievement of rehabilitation goals (Lobitz & Shephard, 1983). Galano (1977) compared neuropsychiatric patients who had treatment goals determined by therapists and patients who actively collaborated with therapists on their treatment goals. Active collaboration increased achievement of treatment goals, and this increase was not due to differences in goal difficulty or real-life usefulness.

In working with patients after brain injury, the ability to form a collaboration will depend on several patient characteristics, for example, organic bases for awareness, levels of psychological distress, defensiveness and need to exert control, severity of cognitive impairments, and capacity to actively participate in therapy. Therapist actions that can facilitate collaboration need to be considered in neuropsychological remediation (cf. Foreman & Marmor, 1985); schema like Crosson and co-workers' (1989) distinction among types of awareness deficits represent a valuable start in this direction. The collaborative aspect of the patient–therapist interaction requires careful attention from all clinicians providing cognitive remediation and may be the most important ingredient to creating a functionally meaningful therapy.

Neuropsychological Deficits and Real-Life Abilities

Understanding the relation between neuropsychological constructs and everyday functioning is limited by the lack of adequate measures of the latter. Though global constructs of functioning ("employed") or criterion-referenced measures ("dresses by self in morning") have some applicability, they are not sufficient for understanding the nature of real-life cognitive abilities and errors, much less for refining ecologically valid cognitive remediations. Recent efforts to describe and understand everyday cognition have emphasized the social-dialectical aspects of practical thinking and the embedding of cognition within activities and environments (Rogoff & Lave, 1984; Cole & Griffin, 1983). For example, Scribner (1984, 1986) conducted a series of naturalistic analyses of cognition in everyday (work) settings. Practical thinking appeared to involve the acquisition and use of setting-specific knowledge, fine-tuning to the environment, and refinement of general cognitive strategies so that specific task demands were incorporated into problem solutions. Variability was the hallmark of skilled performance in all of the tasks studied. This variability of performance was neither random (in which case it might be considered error) nor arbitrary but an adaptation to the ever-changing conditions of the task environment. This perspective is similar to Neisser's (1976) view that cognition directs activity in the environment and is continually modified as a result of that interaction (figure 11–1), as the environment is a source of variability necessitating renewed adaptation.

Willis and Schaie (1986) also discussed the variability between superficially similar tasks and older adults' application of previously acquired cognitive operations in new contexts. These authors utilized Cattell's (1971) distinction between fluid and crystallized abilities to examine the relation between psychometric ability predictors and tasks characterizing real-life activities (e.g., understanding labels, filling out forms) in community living. Although

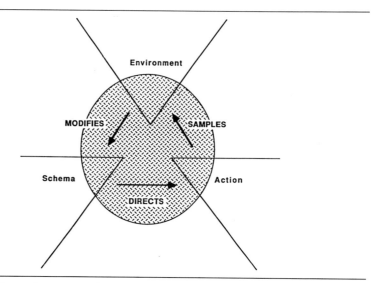

Figure 11–1. Interaction among schema, actions, and available information from the environment. Adapted from Neisser, 1976 with permission.

the real-life tasks were of a practical nature and appeared to require familiar knowledge and skills, and therefore expected to require crystallized ability, the fluid ability predictors were found to be more strongly related to real-life task performance. Willis and Schaie (1986) suggested that although the content of the real-life tasks was familiar, the problems could not be solved by the automatic use of previously acquired knowledge; rather, their solution required the recognition and application of "novel" relationships in the context of seemingly familiar tasks.

Sternberg (1981) distinguished between automatic tasks, in which knowledge is assumed to be content-specific and applied in a routine manner, and "nonentrenched" tasks, which involve a degree of novelty or organization of information into new relationships. The distinction between *automatic* versus *effortful* or *controlled* processing has been applied to cognitive activities of attention (Schneider & Shiffrin, 1977; Shiffrin & Schneider, 1977) and memory (Hasher & Zacks, 1979), and the possible neurologic correlates of these processes have been explored (Pribram & McGuinness, 1975). Memory-impaired brain-injured patients demonstrate impairment on "effortful" recall tasks but also perform poorly on tasks that are ordinarily processed automatically such as the encoding of context (Hirst & Volpe, 1984) and frequency (Levin et al., 1988). Cognitive processes that are usually automatic appear to become effortful for the amnesic subjects. When these patients can remember, they may have difficulty relating the results of learning to the appropriate context or source, a phenomenon borne out by clinical and experimental observation (Schacter, 1983).

Shallice (1981, 1982; Norman & Shallice, 1986) elaborated on the automatic-controlled processing dimension in his neuropsychological model of cognitive processes. The model proposes two levels of processing structures and two levels of regulation or executive control. The first level of processing consists of special-purpose cognitive subsystems such as object recognition, semantic comprehension, spatial orientation, and so on. These subsystems can, of course, be selectively damaged by focal brain lesions, and these deficits can be analyzed by fractionation of the subsystems into the involved components. Another level of processing structure is the schema, which consists of the organization of cognitive subsystems into relatively invariant routines, for example, eating breakfast or driving home from work. Schemata may be activated by the products of the cognitive subsystem or other schemata, and because they are relatively automatic, several schemata may be active at any time. *Routine* control of schemata is accomplished through a process referred to as contention scheduling, based on the strength of various overlearned triggers that allow for the rapid and efficient selection of schemata and the inhibition of weaker competing schemata.

However, an additional level of *nonroutine* control over schemata is required to account for the *variability* apparent in skilled performance. The supervisory attentional system represents a level of voluntary, strategic control that is necessary when planning is required, when the correction of unexpected errors is required, when the required response is novel or not well learned, or when habitual responses need to be inhibited. The activity of the supervisory attentional system thus represents a form of regulation of the higher cognitive functions, which is typically attributed to the frontal lobes (Shallice, 1981), a suggestion that has received some neuropsychological (Shallice, 1982) and neurological (Roland, 1982) support.

Norman (1981) and Reason (1977) utilized a similar framework to describe a variety of errors of everyday functioning. Reason (1977) considered two general categories of cognitive error. In the first category the supervisory plan of action is inadequate, although specific actions go as planned; in the second category the plan is adequate, but the actions do not go as planned. Within the second category, four types of actions-not-as-planned seem to account for most everyday lapses. *Selection failures* occur when an inappropriate action is substituted for the intended one (e.g., turning on the light switch when leaving a room in daylight). *Storage failures* involve either the forgetting of an intention (e.g., forgetting to mail a letter while out shopping) or forgetting a preceding action (not being able to locate an item that was just put down). *Discrimination failures* occur when a stimulus is incorrectly identified during an ongoing action, leading to an erroneous response (e.g., taking out your own door key on arriving at a friend's house). Finally, there are verification or *test failures* in which a planned action is terminated too early (e.g., leaving the dressing room without getting fully dressed) or continued too far (e.g., putting on one's hat and overcoat on the way to the kitchen for breakfast). Both storage failures (particularly intentional forgetting) and selection failures were common among normal subjects, occurred during the conduct of routine or habitual tasks without conscious attention, and were somehow related to the existing plan or one closely associated with it.

Norman (1981) also distinguished between failures resulting from errors in the formation of a plan or intention, and failures resulting from faulty activation of schemas. Faulty activation of schemas result in *capture errors*, in which familiar habits are substituted in an intended action (similar to Reason's selection errors), or *loss of activation* of a schema (similar to Reason's storage errors).

Breakdowns in the process of nonroutine selection (i.e., the supervisory attentional system) can result in errors in the formation of an intention or plan, errors due to the inappropriate activation of habitual sequences of behavior, or errors due to loss of activation and inertia. When the distribution and allocation of attention is reduced, the result is an increase in the rate of cognitive failures and a greater degree of routinization of cognitive and functional activities (Reason, 1984). Lapses of attention and cognitive failures are more frequent among normal subjects who are distracted or otherwise occupied (Reason, 1984). Subjects who report higher frequencies of everyday cognitive lapses also have greater difficulty performing two tasks at the same time, although isolated task performance is intact (Baddeley, 1981).

Clinically, patients with even relatively minor brain injury often experience their greatest difficulty when they need to attend to two things at once. More severe damage, especially to the frontal lobes, may result in marked dependencies on the social or physical environment (Lhermitte, Pillon & Serdaru, 1986), apparently due to the faulty activation or release of stereotypical, automatic behaviors. Similar deficits may appear only in relation to complex social behaviors (Lhermitte, 1986). Eslinger and Damasio (1985) described a patient with bilateral frontal lobe injury who had normal neurological and neuropsychological findings, yet he exhibited little volitional behavior in real-life activities and responded only when the environment triggered the expected actions.

Although these failures of everyday behavior in brain-injured patients may appear extreme, they are understandable in light of the type and mechanism of errors described. It would be important to recognize that brain-injured patients might differ only in the rate and severity of real-life errors, but not necessarily in the kind of mistakes they make. However, the cognitive lapses reported by subjects in the studies of Reason (1977) and Norman (1981) were necessarily recognized by them; thus it is possible that brain injury does not cause a qualitative change in the type of errors that occur but does decrease the likelihood of error recognition and error correction (Konow & Pribram, 1970). Norman (1981) emphasized the importance of feedback mechanisms and error monitoring in detecting cognitive failures, by evaluating discrepancies between what is expected and what occurs. Reason (1984) proposed a similar process operating during the early stage of skill acquisition (i.e., learning), which may also account for the variability required for skilled performance. It is fascinating, therefore, to consider that this same process may represent the general operation of the cerebral cortex.

The operation that is of overwhelming importance for all higher neural functions is the detection of associations. *What is needed in order to build up more elaborate behavior on a set of fixed reflex responses to fixed classes of stimuli is the ability to recognize that in one set of circumstances one response to a stimulus is appropriate, whereas in another set of circumstances a different response to the same stimulus is required:* and for this it is necessary to detect, not just the occurrence of the stimulus, but its occurrence in association with another event or events signifying that the circumstances have changed. The words hitherto used to describe the role of the cortex are all unconscionably vague and undefined—"the seat of intelligence," its "unifying action," the "source of the will," and so on—but surely this detection of associations is an operation without which none of these higher functions would be remotely possible. The kind of association that we think the brain needs especially to detect is that described in detective stories as a "suspicious coincidence"—an unexpected combination of occurrences that seems to require a causal explanation because it would be unlikely to occur by chance. We think that nerve cells use the same inductive logic as the detective, and that statistically significant coincidences are the informational fodder that they grab hold of and devour to build higher perceptual concepts and more complex forms of organized behavior. (Phillips, Zeki, and Barlow, 1984). (italics added)

Phillips and colleagues (1984) go on to discuss the cortical organization of "coincidence detectors" according to known anatomy. Primary and secondary coincidences would be those related to changes in the sensory projection areas. Higher-order coincidences would include those between second-order and polymodal coincidences, between sensory and affective events, and between expected and actual events.

What is the significance of this for neuropsychological rehabilitation, beyond an understanding of the nature of real-life cognitive errors and cerebral functioning? The operation of the supervisory system must reciprocate with the cognitive subsystems and schemata, receiving information from them, generating expectancies based on past associations and modifying and fine-tuning the processing structures to future events (cf. Neisser, 1976). We believe that this hierarchical and reciprocal model of neuropsychological organizations provides a framework for the cognitive analysis of errors in everyday functioning and for the design of remedial interventions (table 11–2). For example, brain injury that produces a fractionation of one or more cognitive subsystems will result in relatively focal *processing deficits* characterized by errors of stimulus recognition and discrimination. Remediation might then be directed toward specific cognitive operations or reorganization of the cognitive subsystem to utilize intact operations, for example.

Deficits at the level of the schema would be likely to produce problems with the *integration* of cognitive operations into complex behavioral routines. Inter-

Table 11–2. Effect of brain injury and possible
remedial strategies at different levels of "everyday cognitive functioning"

Component	Effect of injury	Remedial strategies
Cognitive subsystem	Processing deficits	– Basic skill training – Intrasystem reorganization – Train functional activities – Self-monitoring and error correction
Schema	Integrative deficits	– Whole-skill training – Train functional activites – Self-monitoring and error correction
Supervisory attentional system	Regulatory deficits	– Self-monitoring and error correction – Train "deviation from routine" – Environmental modification

ventions directed at this level would probably utilize whole-skill training or the development of alternative procedures to accomplish the complex functional routine. Since lower-level processing deficits might also be expected to alter the schema in which they are integrated, the use of whole-task training using functional activities would also be appropriate for remediation of deficits at that level.

Finally, breakdown at the level of the supervisory system would produce decreased variability in response to changing task demands, reduced volitional control over action, and release of environmentally dependent behaviors. We assume that the influence of the supervisory attentional system is exerted over not only the selection of schemas but also on the composition of the schema and probably the momentary organization of the cognitive subsystems. Thus intervention at the level of reestablishing voluntary control—for example, through the use of overt verbalization and formal self-monitoring—would be appropriate not only for treatment of regulatory deficits (Cicerone & Wood, 1987) but also for integration deficits (Stanton et al., 1983) and processing deficits (Glasgow et al., 1977; Webster & Scott, 1983). There is particular challenge to intervention at this level in increasing patients' flexibility and ability to respond to novel or changing situations. It might be possible to include training of "deviations from routine" into a patient's functional routine or to teach a "novelty routine" triggered by detection of confusion. For example, with a client who has successfully learned to perform his morning care routine, we have replaced his toothpaste with a tube of shaving gel, thus forcing him (at either the visual or gustatory level of processing!) to recognize and adapt to this discrepancy from what he expected.

In principle, we believe that therapy should be initiated at the highest level of deficit exhibited by the patient. This premise is based in part on the view that the higher cognitive functions regulate the lower levels and govern the expression of symptoms (Luria, 1980), and in part on the difficulties encountered in attempting to transfer training of isolated cognitive skills to functional activities (Kavale & Mattson, 1983). In practice, treatment is likely to require that the *therapist* exhibit significant variability in the design and implementation of therapies. In most effective interventions, therapists need to attend to several levels of intervention simultaneously. The cognitive activities of the clinician will be discussed further in a later section.

Generalization of Remediation After Brain Injury

If variability is the hallmark of skilled performance, the application of skilled performance across a range of relevant, real-life situations should be characteristic of effective everyday functioning and therefore a goal of neuropsychological remediation. Unfortunately, the failure to observe generalization of treatment effects to ecologically valid areas of patients' lives is frequently a limiting factor of remediation. The absence of transfer of therapeutic gains is not unique to neuro-rehabilitation, however; it is a pervasive characteristic of most methods of psychotherapy and behavior change (Brown, 1978; Goldstein & Kanfer, 1979). The major basis for the failure to observe generalization may be the assumption that it will occur automatically from skill-specific training, sometimes referred to as the "train and hope" technique (Stokes & Baer, 1977). The assumption of automatic generalization is clearly not supported by clinical or empirical evidence. People do not automatically transfer solutions to logically isomorphic problems that differ in content unless they first detect the underlying similarities ("suspicious coincidences") between problems, at which point transfer is relatively simple (Gick & Holyoak, 1980). Rogoff and Gardner (1984) identified guidance in transfer as a major characteristic of formal and informal instruction and noted that generalization required "searching for similarities between new problems and old ones, guided by previous experience with similar problems and instruction in how to interpret and solve such problems" (p. 96).

The observation that patients frequently *do not* transfer the effects of training to everyday situations is sometimes taken as evidence that patients with brain injury *cannot* generalize. This interpretation treats generalization as an outcome rather than an eventual goal of intervention. If the goal of remediation is to enable patients to apply improved abilities to their everyday functioning, such applications must be planned for and included in patients' treatments. Interventions promoting generalization typically need to consider two dimensions: (1) the changes in cues between the therapy and real-life setting, or among different real life settings; (2) the need to vary responses as situational demands change. The following list of therapeutic techniques to enhance generalization is derived largely from the work of Stokes and Baer (1977) and Goldstein and Kanfer (1979); the reader is referred to those sources for more detailed descriptions.

1. *Train Identical Elements.* This technique involves bringing elements of the natural environment into the therapy situation in order to maximize the carryover from one setting to another—for example, teaching meal pre-

paration skills in a natural kitchen setting rather than a clinic, which might furthermore be made to resemble the patient's own kitchen. Training family members as caretakers or behavioral managers in order to establish consistent stimulus control is another use of this technique.

2. *Train in the Natural Environment.*   This technique represents an extension of the training of common elements, in that treatment is delivered in the actual surroundings in which the target behavior is required. The use of a "place and train" model in which the patient is taught specific job-related skills at the actual job site (Fawber & Wachter, 1987) is one example.

The techniques of training identical elements and training in the natural environment attempt to strengthen associations between eliciting stimuli and cognitive schema or functional routines by minimizing the variability between the treatment and real-life settings. Reliance on context-specific training appears effective in ensuring treatment effects in the desired setting, yet it may also function to actually reduce skill generalization to other environments (White, Leber, & Phifer, 1985).

3. *Train General Principles.*   This procedure also attempts to capitalize on similarities between training and transfer environments, but it also provides a general procedure that applies across settings. For example, a patient may be provided with a "script" to follow on all of her job interviews; this approach may overcome failures of stimulus generalization but does not allow for response variability in different situations. Teaching general problem-solving skills is another example of this approach. For example, Foxx, Martella, and Marchand-Martella (1989) identified verbal analogs of real-life problem situations related to the areas of community skills, medication and substance use, stating one's rights, and emergency-safety procedures and taught three head-injured patients a general problem-solving strategy. Generalization of verbal problem-solving skills to simulated problem situations was observed, including those with novel content. Unfortunately, these authors did not evaluate actual problem-solving behaviors aside from verbal reports. We have observed similar competencies in our patients' verbal solutions to "real-life" problems— for example, "What could you do if you arrived at a friend's house and found the lights out and door locked and nobody home?" Yet when the door to their treatment-conference room was found locked the next morning, none of eight patients exhibited an appropriate attempt to solve this "problem."

4. *Train Sufficient Examples.*   This procedure involves training patients in a "sufficient" number of situations to ensure that they can apply the skill independently. For example, a patient being taught to fill vending machines was trained on a number of different types of machines until he demonstrated that he could fill a new machine without the therapist's intervention. This procedure attempts to avoid the dilemma of training the patient in all potential situations where the skill may be required by training in a *sufficient* number of different yet related situations to establish skill transfer.

Training sufficient examples is the most frequent method of generalization reported in the general literature (aside from the train-and-hope method) (Stokes & Baer, 1977). Its incidental application in brain injury rehabilitation may account for some reports of "spontaneous" or fortuitous generalization after training. In its planned application, it may be useful in extending the range of patients' competence and, when applied in a controlled manner, preparing patients for deviations from routine.

5. *Train Mediation.* In the preceding section, we proposed that the supervisory attentional system was responsible for the adaptive variability of human skilled performance. It is therefore not surprising that self-regulatory behaviors, such as self-instruction and self-monitoring, are assumed to have broad, transituational applicability that facilitates generalization. Cicerone and Wood (1987) reported that self-instructional training did not automatically generalize beyond the treatment setting but that continued training in interpersonal contexts improved everyday behavior. Lira, Carne, and Masri (1983) found self-instructional training effective in reducing anger outbursts and impulsivity across interpersonal settings. These and other relevant studies (Sohlberg et al., 1988; Webster & Scott, 1983) suggest that training in self-regulation combined with programmed application to real-life situations may be effective. More generally, there is some evidence to suggest that adequate executive functioning is necessary for successful transfer of cognitive remediation to community settings, with other patients requiring context-specific functional training (Fryer & Haffey, 1987).

6. *Train Generalization.* Generalization might be considered a higher-level cognitive skill and therefore might be amenable to training. Patients might be taught to recognize and "search for similarities" between areas of training and application through practice or instruction. The systematic use of instructions to generalize can be readily combined with other skill-specific training; for example, having been trained to scan to the left of a page, the patient would be instructed to apply the "same" procedure when looking for grocery items on the kitchen shelf. Using the earlier "locked door" example, after explicit instructions on the relation between the verbal and situational problems and potential application of one to the other, those patients subsequently showed improved transfer from verbal to real-life behavioral solutions.

Training for generalization does not preclude context-specific learning, although strictly context-specific training may preclude generalization. The generalization of remediation to everyday functioning appears to be enhanced when training is prolonged, the patient is given increasing cognitive involvement and responsibility for task performance, and feedback about the application and utility of the skilled behavior is provided. Finally, generalization is not an all-or-none phenomena, and patients will exhibit varying ability to apply training outside of treatment; the patients' characteristics, the environmental attributes, and the therapeutic interventions that support generalization require further attention.

ACTIVITY OF THE THERAPIST IN NEUROPSYCHOLOGICAL REMEDIATION
Neuropsychological rehabilitation requires the adequate assessment of the patient's subjective complaints, cognitive strengths and weaknesses, ability to benefit from instruction, emotional status, and functional behavior. The initial conceptualization of therapy requires a shared understanding of the nature of the patient's cognitive and functional disability and collaboration on the goals and direction of treatment. The therapist must analyze the patient's deficits in a functional context and create a task–situation that replicates those deficits within treatment. Intervention provides the patient and therapist with the opportunity to increase awareness of deficit areas, explore discrepancies between presumed and actual abilities, and develop and practice remedial strategies within the controlled therapeutic environment (whether this is the clinic or a real-life setting). The therapist needs to make explicit the relation between the therapeutic and real-life environments and foster the real-life application of the intervention. This process establishes the flow of therapy from the real-life environment into the therapeutic situation and back out to the real-life environment.

This process may characterize both the microstructure of the treatment session and more general course of treatment. Through the course of therapy the patient assumes increasing cognitive responsibility for successful perform-ance and monitoring of task demands, and social responsibility for the applica-tion of acquired skills in real-life contexts.

Whereas most descriptions of cognitive remediation seem to concentrate on the treatment task or exercise, models of everyday skills acquisition and instruction emphasize the activity of the teacher or the interaction between teacher and learner (Greenfield, 1984). We identified three classes of therapist activities, based primarily on our clinical and conceptual approach to neuro-psychological rehabilitation but relying upon pedagogic principles from instructional (Greenfield, 1984; Rogoff & Gardner, 1984; 1976) and psycho-therapy (Hoyt et al., 1981; Vallis, Shaw, & Dobson, 1986) process research. These three classes are facilitative, instrumental, and metacognitive therapeutic actions (table 11–3).

Facilitative activities establish the functional learning environment in which therapy occurs. The setting of a therapeutic agenda makes treatment compre-hensible to the patient by providing a rationale for the task—and more gener-ally the treating relationship. The therapist ensures that the task demands are compatible with the patient's existing level of skill, thus defining the "region of sensitivity to instruction" (Wood, Wood, & Middleton, 1978, p. 133). Facilitation of the patient's engagement, and participation and success in therapy, is also accomplished by reinforcement of appropriate behaviors, which helps to maintain adequate frustration tolerance and acknowledges the patient's emotional reactions to the task.

Collaboration between the therapist and patient is nurtured by encouraging the patient's active participation and responsibility for treatment. The patient's

Table 11–3. Activities of the therapist in neuropsychological remediation

---

I. FACILITATIVE ACTIVITY

Setting an agenda: providing rationale and instructions for the task, relating session to past or future sessions
Reinforcement: providing specific feedback regarding the accuracy or quality of performance related to specific task characteristics
Support: more general comments intended to provide assurance, maintain adequate frustration tolerance, or acknowledge and address client's emotional reaction to the task
Collaboration: attempts to actively engage client in shared goal setting or negotiation of an activity; attempts to establish a therapeutic alliance, including attempts to address client's feelings about therapy or resistance to treatment
Query: questions intended to clarify what the client was doing or confirm a therapist observation

II. INSTRUMENTAL ACTIVITY

Task Monitoring: providing or maintaining continuity within session, pacing of session, redirecting client to the task
Modeling: direct demonstration of appropriate steps or solution by the therapist, or general modeling of a skill, behavior, or technique
Instruction: telling the client what to do in order to alter client's performance or cognitive activity
Explanation: attempts to point out discrepancies between client's performance and appropriate steps or solutions; emphasis on behaviors primarily or exclusively *within* the session; similar to instructional technique of "marking critical features"
Scaffolding: modulation of task demands by increasing or decreasing therapist's assistance while holding the actual task constant, usually to increase client's success or create a better "fit" between client capabilities and task demands
Exploration: pointing out or developing strategies, especially in terms applicable beyond single task; remains at nonpersonal or intratherapy level

III. METACOGNITIVE ACTIVITY

Confrontation: any intervention (not hostile) intended to increase task complexity or difficulty or otherwise manipulate performance so that client directly *experiences* a discrepancy between expected and actual performance capability
Questioning: use of relatively open-ended questions intended to foster awareness of performance capabilities or induce self-evaluation ("Are you sure?")
Interpretation: attempts to make overt the relation of specific deficits or behaviors occurring *within* therapy session to activities or situations *outside of treatment*. Relies on use of relevant, "real-life" activities of the client. Relates from the task to the environment
Replication: attempts to identify real-life activities where client experiences deficits, especially with the intent of introducing or recreating them in the context of the within-session treatment activity. Relates from the environment to the task
Instigation: prescriptive attempts to foster the application and/or use of behaviors or strategies occurring within session to real-life, functional activities of the client

---

expectations regarding treatment should be explored, including attempts to address the patient's feelings about therapy or resistance to treatment. Goals and tasks of therapy need to be negotiated between therapist and patient, often including the broader social systems of each.

Instrumental activities comprise the principle didactic interactions of therapy. For example, therapists need to variously point out the relevant features of the task, interpret discrepancies between the patient's attempts at solution and acceptable performance, explore possible strategies, and demonstrate their relevance. Emphasis is placed on the patient's active participation in the activity and graduated assumption of responsibility for task accomplishment (Rogoff & Gardner, 1984).

Wood, Bruner, and Ross (1976) developed the concept of the "scaffold" as a central metaphor for the instructional process in natural contexts. The scaffold functions as a tool to extend the ability of the patient by providing support for those aspects of the task the patient cannot do. The use of scaffolding consists of the therapist "controlling those elements of the task that are initially beyond the learner's capacity, thus permitting him to concentrate upon and complete only those elements that are within his range of competence" (Wood, Bruner, & Ross, 1976, p. 90). The scaffold initially provides maximal support, but it does not assure errorless performance. Errors are expected to occur as the therapist transfers responsibility for the task to the patient, and these occurrences provide the principal basis for determining the patient's competence and adjusting the level of intervention. Wood et al. (1978, p. 133) described an elegant "contingency rule" that is readily adapted to the therapy setting: If the patient succeeds, the next intervention should provide less assistance; if the patient fails, the next intervention should assume more control. Because some errors are inevitable, the patient is able to practice the recognition and correction of errors; the therapist might also shift the emphasis to anticipation of errors as a means of increasing the patient's cognitive responsibility for the task (Greenfield, 1984).

Scaffolding differs from the behavioral procedure of shaping through successive approximations and the use of cognitive exercises of graduated task difficulty, both of which rely on simplified versions of the desired response, in that it holds the task constant while modulating the patient's requirements through the graded intervention of the therapist. Basic skills are embedded within basic activities (Cole & Griffin, 1983). In terms of neuropsychological remediation, the patient's neurocognitive deficits (e.g., scanning) are addressed in the context of an integrative functional activity (e.g., reading a newspaper), with the therapist supporting other abilities necessary for task completion.

Finally, the *metacognitive* activities of the therapist are intended to foster patients' awareness of their performance and application of treatment to their actual real-life activities. We have made liberal use of a treatment paradigm requiring the patient to predict the outcome of the treatment task, which seems to induce a set to self-monitor. Applied to the patients' predictions of their own performance, the therapist may confront any limitations in the patients' awareness, as noted earlier. We consider such confrontation, defined as any therapeutic manipulation through which the patient experiences a discrepancy between expected and actual performance capabilities, as an essential aspect of brain injury remediation.

Similarly, it is beneficial to make frequent interpretations of intratherapy results in terms of possible implications outside of therapy. The use of formal self-monitoring procedures, behavior rehearsal, homework assignments, and other instigative techniques helps to facilitate change between sessions. The goal of all these procedures, of course, is to maximize the likelihood of treatment gains and functional improvements in patients' everyday lives.

CONCLUSION

We have attempted to describe some intratherapy characteristics of neuropsychological intervention that are basic to, and perhaps necessary for, producing improvements in patients' real-life functioning after brain injury. These include the nature of the therapeutic relationship, a description of the relation between neuropsychological constructs and everyday functioning that emphasizes the nature of real-life errors and the variability of skilled human performance, the planned generalization of therapeutic gains to the natural environment, and the real-life activities of the therapist.

We have not discussed other, extra-therapy factors such as the patient's general psychosocial functioning, the influence of the family and social systems, and the assessment of the actual environment. All these factors contribute heavily to the ecological functioning of the patient.

Considerable work is required in this area—in the language of our chapter, the gap between our existing and desired knowledge is too great to be bridged by a single intervention. At the present time, the neuropsychological remediation of everyday functioning requires sensitivity to the patient's subjective experience, careful observation of the patient's condition, and diligence in helping the patient find ways to mend, bridge, or circumvent the rifts in the patient's quotidian reality.

NOTE

1. Interestingly, Sohlberg et al. base this latter conclusion on the same evidence (Cohen & Squire, 1980) that served as one basis for Schacter & Glisky's study.

REFERENCES

Baddeley, A. (1981). The cognitive psychology of everyday life. *British Journal of Psychology* 72, 257–269.

Bordin, E. S. (1979). The generalizability of the psychoanalytic concept of the working alliance. *Psychotherapy: Theory, Research and Practice* 16 (3), 252–260.

Brown, A. L. (1978). Knowing when, where and how to remember: A problem in metacognition. In R. Glaser (Ed.), *Advances in instructional psychology*. Hillsdale, NJ: Erlbaum.

Cattell, R. B. (1971). *Abilities: Their structure, growth and action*. Boston: Houghton Mifflin.

Chelune, G. J., Heaton, R. K., & Lehman, R. A. W. (1986). Neuropsychological and personality correlates of patients' complaints of disability. In G. Goldstein (Ed.), *Advances in clinical neuropsychology* (Vol. 3). New York: Plenum.

Cicerone, K. D. (1987). *Overcoming obstacles to change*. Workshop presented at National Head Injury Sixth Annual Symposium, San Diego, CA.

Cicerone, K. D., & Wood, J. (1987). Planning disorder after closed head injury: A case study. *Archives of Physical Medicine and Rehabilitation* 68, 111–115.

Cole, M., & Griffin, P. (1983). A socio-historical approach to remediation. *The Quarterly Newsletter of the Laboratory of Comparative Human Cognition* 5 (4), 69–74.

Crosson, B., Barco, P. P., Velozo, C. A., Bolesta, M. M., Cooper, P. V., Werts, D., & Brobeck,

T. C. (1989). Awareness and compensation in post-acute head injury rehabilitation. *Journal of Head Trauma Rehabilitation* 4(3), 46–54.

Deaton A. V. (1986). Denial in the aftermath of traumatic head injury: Its manifestations, measurement and treatment. *Rehabilitation Psychology* 31(4), 231–240.

Eslinger, P. J., & Damasio, A. R. (1985). Severe disturbance of higher cognition after bilateral frontal lobe ablation: Patient EVR. *Neurology* 35, 1731–1741.

Faust, P., Guilmette, T. J., Hart, K., Arkes, H. R., Fishburne, F. J., & Davey, L. (1988). Neuropsychologists training, experience and judgment accuracy. *Archives of Clinical Neuropsychology* 3, 145–163.

Fawber, H. L., & Wachter, J. F. (1987). Job placement as a treatment component of the vocational rehabilitation process. *Journal of Head Trauma Rehabilitation* 2 (1), 27–33.

Fordyce, D. J., & Roueche, J. R. (1986). Changes in perspectives of disability among patients, staff and relatives during rehabilitation of brain injury. *Rehabilitation Psychology* 31 (4), 217–229.

Foreman, S. A., & Marmar, C. R. (1985). Therapist actions that address initially poor therapeutic alliances in psychotherapy. *American Journal of Psychiatry* 142 (8), 922–926.

Foxx, R. M., Martella, R. C., & Marchand-Martella, N. E. (1989). The acquisition, maintenance and generalization of problem-solving skills by closed head injured adults. *Behavior Therapy* 20, 61–76.

Frieswyck, S. H., Allen, J. C., Colson, D. B., Coyne, L., Gabbard, G. O., Horwitz, L., & Newsom, G. (1986). Therapeutic alliance: Its place as a process and outcome variable in dynamic psychotherapy research. *Journal of Consulting and Clinical Psychology* 54 (1), 32–38.

Fryer, J. L., & Haffey, W. J. (1987). Cognitive rehabilitation and community adaptation: Outcomes from two program models. *Journal of Head Trauma Rehabilitation* 2 (3), 51–63.

Galano, J. (1977). Treatment effectiveness as a function of client involvement in goal-setting and goal planning. *Goal Attainment Review* 3, 1–16.

Gaston, L., Marmar, C. R., Thompson, L. W., & Gallagher, D. (1988). Relation of patient pretreatment characteristics of the therapeutic alliance in diverse psychotherapies. *Journal of Consulting and Clinical Psychology* 56 (4), 483–489.

Gick, M. L., & Holyoak, K. J. (1980). Analogical problem solving. *Cognitive Psychology* 12, 306–355.

Glasgow, R. E., Zeiss, R. A., Barrera, M., & Lewinsohn, P. (1977). Case studies on remediating memory deficits in brain damaged individuals. *Journal of Clinical Psychology* 33, 1049–1054.

Goldstein, A. P., & Kanfer, F. H. (Eds.), (1979). *Maximizing treatment gains: Transfer enhancement in psychotherapy*. New York: Academic Press.

Gordon, W. A., Hibbard, M. R., Egelko, S., Diller, L., Shaver, M. S., Lieberman, A., & Ragnarsson, K. (1985). Perceptual remediation in patients with right brain damage: A comprehensive program. *Archives of Physical Medicine and Rehabilitation* 66, 353–359.

Greenfield, P. M. (1984). A theory of the teacher in the learning activities of everyday life. In B. Rogoff & J. Lave (Eds), *Everyday cognition: Its development in social context*. Cambridge, MA: Harvard University Press.

Hasher, L., & Zacks, R. T. (1979). Automatic and effortful processes in memory. *Journal of Experimental Psychology: General* 108, 356–388.

Heaton, R. K., & Pendleton, M. G. (1981). Use of neuropsychological tests to predict adult patients' everyday functioning. *Journal of Consulting and Clinical Psychology* 49 (6), 807–821.

Hirst, W., & Volpe, B. T. (1984). Automatic and effortful coding in amnesia. *Neuroscience*.

Hoyt, M. F., Marmar, C. R., Horowitz, M. J., & Alvarez, W. F. (1981). The therapist action scale and the patient action scale: Instruments for the assessment of activities during dynamic psychotherapy. *Psychotherapy: Theory, Research and Practice* 18 (1), 109–116.

Kavale, K., & Mattson, D. (1983). "One jumped off the balance beam": Meta-analysis of perceptual-motor training. *Journal of Learning Disabilities* 16 (3), 165–173.

Kazdin, A. (1974). Reactive self-monitoring: The effects of response desirability, goal setting and feedback. *Journal of Consulting and Clinical Psychology* 42 (5), 704–716.

Kirsch, N. L., Levine, S. P., Fallon-Krueger, M., & Jaros, L. A. (1987). The microcomputer as an orthotic device for patients with cognitive deficits. *Journal of Head Trauma Rehabilitation* 2 (4), 77–86.

Klonoff, P. S., Costa, L. D., & Snow, W. G. (1986). Predictors and indicators of quality of life in patients with closed head injury. *Journal of Clinical and Experimental Neuropsychology* 8 (5), 469–485.

Konow, A., & Pribram, K. H. (1970). Error recognition and utilization produced by injury to the frontal cortex in man. *Neuropsychologia* 8, 489–491.

Levin, H. S., Goldstein, F. C., High, W. M., & Williams, D. (1988). Automatic and effortful processing after severe closed head injury. *Brain and Cognition* 7, 283–297.

Lhermitte, F. (1986). Human autonomy and the frontal lobes. Part II: Patient behavior in complex and social situations: The "environmental dependency syndrome." *Annals of Neurology* 19, 326–334.

Lhermitte, F., Pillon, B., & Serdaru, M. (1986). Human autonomy and the frontal lobes; Part I: Imitation and utilization behavior: A neuropsychological study of 75 patients. *Annals of neurology*, 19, 326–334.

Lira, F. T., Carne, W., & Masri, A. M. (1983). Treatment of anger and impulsivity in a brain damaged patient: A case study applying stress inoculation. *Clinical Neuropsychology* 5, 159–160.

Lobitz, C., & Shepard, K. (1983). Effect of compatibility on goal achievement in patient-physical therapist dyads. *Physical Therapy* 63, 319–324.

Luria, A. R. (1980). *Higher cortical functions in man* (2nd ed.). New York: Basic Books.

Malec, J. (1984). Training the brain-injured client in behavioral self-management skills. In B. A. Edelstein & E. T. Couture (Eds.), *Behavioral assessment and rehabilitation of the traumatically brain damaged.* New York: Plenum Press.

Mayer, N. H., Keating, D. J., & Rapp, D. (1986). Skills, routines and activity patterns of daily living: A functional nested approach. In B. Uzzell & Y. Gross (Eds.), *Clinical neuropsychology of intervention.* Boston: Martinus Nijhoff.

McSweeney, A. J., Grant, I., Heaton, R. K., Prigatano, G. P., & Adams, K. M. (1985). Relationship of neuropsychological status to everyday functioning in healthy and chronically ill persons. *Journal of Clinical and Experimental Neuropsychology* 7 (3), 281–291.

Neisser, U. (1976). *Cognition and reality.* San Francisco: W. H. Freeman.

Norman, D. A. (1981). Categorization of action slips. *Psychological Review* 88 (1), 1–15.

Norman, D. A., & Shallice, T. (1986). Attention to action: Willed and automatic control of behavior. In R. J. Davidson, G. E. Schwartz, & D. Shapiro (Eds.), *Consciousness and self-regulation* (Vol. 4), New York: Plenum Press.

Phillips, C. G., Zeki, S., & Barlow, H. B. (1984). Localization of function in the cerebral cortex: Past, present and future. *Brain* 107, 327–361.

Pribram, K. H., & McGuinness, D. (1975). Arousal, activation and effort in the control of attention. *Psychological Review* 82, 116–149.

Prigatano, G. P., & Fordyce, D. J. (1986). The neuropsychological rehabilitation program at Presbyterian Hospital, Oklahoma City. In G. P. Prigatano et al., *Neuropsychological rehabilitation after brain injury.* Baltimore and London: John Hopkins University Press.

Reason, J. T. (1977). Skill and error in everyday life. In M. J. A. Howe (Ed.), *Adult learning.* New York: John Wiley.

Reason, J. (1984). Absent-mindedness and cognitive control. In J. E. Harris & P. E. Morris (Eds.), *Everyday memory, actions and absent-mindedness.* London: Academic Press.

Rogoff, B., & Gardner, W. (1984). Adult guidance of cognitive development. In B. Rogoff & J. Lave (Eds.). *Everyday cognition: Its development in social context.* Cambridge, MA: Harvard University Press.

Rogoff, B., & Lave, J. (Eds.), (1984). *Everyday cognition: Its development in social context.* Cambridge, MA: Harvard University Press.

Roland, P. E. (1982). Cortical regulation of selective attention in man: A regional cerebral blood flow study. *Journal of Neurophysiology* 48, 1059–1078.

Schacter, D. L. (1983). Amnesia observed: Remembering and forgetting in a natural environment. *Journal of Abnormal Psychology* 92, 236–242.

Schacter, D. L., & Glisky, E. L. (1986). Memory remediation: Restoration, alleviation and the acquisition of domain-specific knowledge. In B. Uzzell & Y. Gross (Eds.), *Clinical neuropsychology of intervention.* Boston: Martinus Nijhoff.

Schneider, W., & Shiffrin, R. M. (1977). Controlled and automatic human information processing: I. Detection, search and attention. *Psychological Review* 84, 1–66.

Scribner, S. (1984). Studying working intelligence. In B. Rogoff & J. Lave (Eds.), *Everyday cognition: Its development in social context.* Cambridge, MA: Harvard University Press.

Scribner, S. (1986). Thinking in action: Some characteristics of practical thought. In R. J. Sternberg & R. K. Wagner (Eds.), *Practical intelligence: Nature and origins of competence in the everyday world.*

Cambridge: Cambridge University Press.

Shallice, T. (1981). Neurologic impairment of cognitive processes. *British Medical Bulletin* 37 (2), 187–192.

Shallice, T. (1982). Specific impairments of planning. *Philosophic Transactions of the Royal Society of London, B.,* 298, 199–209.

Shiffrin, R. M., & Schneider, W. (1977). Controlled and automatic human information processing: II. Perceptual learning, automatic attending and a general theory. *Psychological Review* 84, 127–190.

Sohlberg, M. M., & Mateer, C. A. (1987). Effectiveness of an attention-training program. *Journal of Clinical and Experimental Neuropsychology* 9, 117–130.

Sohlberg, M. M., Sprunk, H., & Metzelaar, K. (1988). Efficacy of an external cuing system in an individual with severe frontal lobe damage. *Cognitive Rehabilitation* 6, 36–41.

Stanton, K. M., Pepping, M., Brockway, J. A., Bliss, L., Frankel, D., & Waggener, S. (1983). Wheelchair transfer training for right cerebral dysfunctions: An interdisciplinary approach. *Archives of Physical Medicine and Rehabilitation* 64, 276–280.

Sternberg, R. J. (1981). Intelligence and nonentrenchment. *Journal of Educational Psychology* 73, 1–16.

Stokes, T. F., & Baer, D. M. (1977). An implicit technology of generalization. *Journal of Applied Behavior Analysis* 10, 349–367.

Tsvetkova, L. S. (1972). Basic principles of a theory of reeducation of brain-injured patients. *Journal of Special Education* 6, 135–144.

Vallis, T. M., Shaw, B. F., & Dobson, K. S. (1986). The cognitive therapy scale: Psychometric properties. *Journal of Consulting and Clinical Psychology* 54 (3), 381–385.

Webster, J. S., & Scott, R. R. (1983). The effects of self-instructional training on attentional deficits following head injury. *Clinical Neuropsychology* 5, 69–74.

White, O. R., Leber, B. D., & Phifer, C. E. (1985). Training in the natural environment and skill generalization: It doesn't always come naturally. In N. Haring, K. Liberty, F. Billingsley, O. White, V. Lynch, J. Kayser, & F. McCarty (Eds.), *Investigating the problem of skill generalization* (3rd edition). Seattle: University of Washington Research Organization.

Willis, S. L., & Schaie, K. W. (1986). Practical intelligence in later adulthood. In R. J. Sternberg & R. K. Wagner (Eds.) *Practical intelligence: Nature and origins of competence in the everyday world.* Cambridge: Cambridge University Press.

Wood, D., Bruner, J. S., & Ross, G. (1976). The role of tutoring in problem solving. *Journal of Child Psychology and Psychiatry* 17, 89–100.

Wood, D., Wood, H., & Middleton, D. (1978). An experimental evaluation of four face-to-face teaching strategies. *International Journal of Behavioral Development* 1, 131–147.

12. LONG-TERM ADJUSTMENT TO TRAUMATIC BRAIN INJURY

INGER VIBEKE THOMSEN

INTRODUCTION

The earliest references in the Western literature to sequelae after traumatic brain injury are presumably those of Valerius Maximus (ca. A.D. 30) and Pliny (A.D. 23–79). They described how a learned man of Athens with the stroke of a stone forgot his letters and could read no more, but that his memory otherwise served him well. Pliny also referred to the case of a man who, with a fall from the roof of a high house, lost his remembrance of his own mother, friends, and neighbors (Benton, 1960). It may be supposed that the two patients represent different types of traumatic brain injury, the former a focal lesion and the latter severe diffuse neuronal damage.

Since the First World War innumerable studies on defects following focal cerebral lesions, such as f. inst. aphasia, have been published. A similar interest in the sequelae of blunt head trauma—that is, of diffuse neuronal damage—has not been present until the last 20 years or so, when it has become fully recognized that the main burden of disablement falls on the younger working population, whose youth enables them to survive injuries that kill their seniors and who, furthermore, retain a normal expectation of life (London, 1967). The majority of survivors are under 30 years and may have 50 or more years of disability ahead of them. It is estimated that there are 150 markedly disabled persons per 100,000 in the United Kingdom (Research Aspects, 1982). In many parts of the United States the frequency of severe cerebral trauma is much higher than in Britain, and there are 40 times as many head injuries each year as spinal cord injuries (Kalsbeek et al., 1980). The quality of life of the patients and their relatives is seriously impaired, and the financial burdens to the families and the communities are enormous.

Diffuse neuronal damage, produced at the moment of impact, is the primary mechanism of brain injury in blunt head trauma; its severity is a deciding factor in duration of unconsciousness and in degree of recovery. Posttraumatic amnesia (PTA), defined as the interval between injury and regaining continuous day-to-day memory, has for many years been accepted as the most useful guide to severity of brain damage (Russell, 1932; Russell & Nathan, 1946). The present chapter deals with the long-term adaption in cases of severe and mainly very severe cases of blunt head trauma with a PTA of days, weeks, or months.

LONG-TERM FOLLOW-UP STUDIES
Blunt head trauma causes physical, cognitive, and psychosocial (including behavioral, emotional, and social) disturbances. There are few studies of consecutive, long-term follow-up, and comparison of investigations is difficult because of inconsistency in data. Typically, studies use a variety of criteria for admission policy, including severity of brain injury, age, type of assessment, intervals, and methods of follow-up.

In 1965 Miller and Stern reported the results of a long-term follow-up of nearly 100 head injury cases, half of them blunt head injuries. They concluded that the long-term outcome had proved much more favorable than was expected or predicted. More detailed studies 2 years later expressed more cautious views. Fahy, Irving, and Millac (1967) mentioned that remarkable improvement could take place with the passage of time but that few survivors escaped permanent sequelae. London (1967) gave many examples of behavioral problems and emphasized that one of the most distressing effects of severe cerebral injury was on the patient's personality and that this laid a much heavier burden on the family than on the community. Studies in the following two decades have confirmed that the severest late effects of head trauma are the psychosocial sequelae and their lifelong consequences for the patient and relatives.

During recent years three long-term studies of patients with severe blunt head trauma were published in Europe, and in all of them information was obtained from patients and relatives. In Glasgow 42 patients (36 male), aged 17 to 59 years when injured, were seen 3, 6, and 12 months and then 5 years after injury (McKinlay et al., 1981, Brooks et al., 1986). No one had a PTA of less than 2 days, and 60% had a PTA of 15 days or more. The lower classes were overrepresented, and some patients had criminal records before the accident. The patients were included in a follow-up of up to 7 years of 134 patients (Brooks et al., 1987a). Weddell, Oddy, and Jenkins (1980) and Oddy et al. (1985) examined social adjustment in 44 patients (27 male), aged 16 to 39 years when injured, 2 years after the trauma and reexamined 34 of the sample 7 years after injury. All had a PTA of more than 7 days. The subjects lived within London or adjacent counties. In a Danish study (Thomsen, 1974, 1984) 40 patients (28 male), aged 15 to 44 years when injured, were primarily seen at an average of 4.5 months after the accident and treated during the following months or years. No one had a PTA of less than one month and two-thirds had a PTA of more than 3 months. It is thus a sample of very severely injured patients. About 40% had signs of brain stem involvement, and another 40% had focal lesions verified by surgery. A follow-up took place 2.5 years on average after the trauma and a second one 10 to 15 years after injury. On both occasions patients and relatives were visited in their homes. The patients came from all over Denmark, and in contrast to many series, no grossly maladjusted or obvious alcoholics were included in the material.

LONG-TERM SEQUELAE

Physical Deficits

Since Miller and Stern (1965) reported unexpected good, late recovery in head-injured patients with spastic pareses, many investigations have confirmed at least a tendency for motor impairment to diminish in time. Bond and Brooks (1976) found that the greater part of recovery of physical defects occurred within 6 months after injury. Grosswasser and colleagues (1977) had similar results. They examined a group of severely head-injured patients 6 and 30 months after the trauma and found that definitive motor results were obtained in most patients by the end of the first 6 months, but that few of them showed further progress later on. In the present author's sample (Thomsen, 1974, 1984) a third were severely disabled 2.5 years after injury and the results were the same 10 to 15 years after the accident. Many patients, also among those with moderate motor impairment, had cerebellar ataxia. Gilchrist and Wilkinson (1979) reported similar findings in their long-term follow-up of 72 severely head-injured patients. The fact that very few patients and relatives in my series complained of even severe motor disability is in agreement with Bond's (1975) conclusion that family cohesion appears to be resistant to physical defects. In the Glasgow studies (McKinlay et al., 1981; Brooks et al., 1986) the degree of severe motor impairment was low both 1 and 5 years after injury, but nearly half the patients had continuing problems of balance.

Dysarthria, the motor impairment of oral communication, was present in more than a third of the Danish sample initially and at both follow-up examinations and no one recovered. Monotony and slow speed were the severest defects. A further complication was reduced facial expression seen in some patients with damage to deep cerebral structures. Severe traumatic dysarthria constitutes a distressing social impairment for the patient, and it is disappointing that even long-term treatment usually has limited effect.

Among other neurological dysfunctions, permanent visual defects often turn out to be a greater social handicap than motor impairment, and anosmia, or loss of smell, can be a life-threatening danger (Miller and Stern, 1965; Fahy, Irving, & Millac, 1967). Epilepsy, the only physical complication that can occur months or years after the trauma, is much more common in severe cases than in moderate ones; its chance of occurrence is increased by the presence of a hematoma or a depressed fracture. Fits may occur for the first time after a substantial delay. In a 10- to 25-year follow-up of 300 head-injured patients, late epilepsy thus began more than 5 years after injury in 13% (Roberts, 1976).

Cognitive Deficits

Attention and concentration, perception, learning and memory, speed, persistence, and language are the cognitive functions commonly affected by head trauma. Many of the dysfunctions were described in 1938 by Conkey. The most obvious long-term defects are in learning and memory and in mental speed. General slowness was thus the most frequent impairment reported by relatives in the 7-year follow-up by Brooks et al. (1987a), and poor concentration and poor memory were described in three-quarters of their patients. The same percentage of memory defects was reported in my material at both follow-up examinations. In the severest cases, patients were not always oriented to the time of the day; when sad, they forgot why in a few minutes. Several lost track of what was said or forgot what was mentioned a moment ago. In more moderate cases, patients had problems in remembering names and appointments and in misplacing things. Four of the forty patients and their relatives denied any memory impairment in daily life both 2.5 years and 10 to 15 years after injury. In contrast to the vast majority, three of them returned to work and the fourth became an independent home-minder.

Regarding language, 27 of the 40 patients in my investigation presented aphasic symptoms when first seen, on average, 4 months after injury (table 12–1). The table shows that four had recovered from aphasia at the follow-up 2.5 years after the accident. The most common symptoms at that time were

Table 12–1. Defects of communication at first examination and at follow-up in 27 head-injured patients

Defects	Patients (no.)	
	4 months	2.5 years
Impaired auditory analysis	21	12
Impaired analysis of reading	21	12
Amnestic aphasia	23	20
Verbal paraphasia	22	15
Literal paraphasia	10	5
Paragrammatism	8	8
Agraphia	21	9
Dysarthria in combination with aphasia	6	6
Perseveration	21	21
No symptoms	6	4

impaired analysis of speech and reading, amnestic aphasia, verbal paraphasia, agraphia, and perseveration. The problems were observed in ˙patients with diffuse neuronal damage (Thomsen, 1975) and in those with a combination of diffuse neuronal damage and focal lesion in the dominant hemisphere (Thomsen, 1976). The frequency and severity were highest in the latter group. Ten to fifteen years after injury, subnormal rate of speaking, amnestic problems, and perseveration were the dominant features in the sample. The discrepancy between the initially aphasic and nonaphasic patients had diminished, and the linguistic defects could often be looked on as instances of general cognitive impairment (Thomsen, 1984). Similar results have been reported by Levin et al. (1979). Anomia was the most prominent expressive disturbance in their patients. Slowed speech and movements were frequent, with conversation often drifting to irrelevant topics. Brooks et al. (1986) found that late language/speech problems appeared relatively often, in 33% at 5 years, but, in contrast to the results in the present author's study, they thought that the impairment had little impact on the patients' communication abilities. In the 7-year follow-up (1987a) these authors also concluded that it often was difficult to know if the impairment of communication represented a language problem or a more general cognitive disturbance involving slowness in information processing of a concentration or memory disturbance.

Disorders of language related to personality changes are not uncommon. Verbal expansiveness or overtalkativeness—"talking too much, too loud, and with too little regard for logical continuity"—was a main complaint of relatives in a one-year follow-up study of patients with closed head injury (Oddy, Humphrey, & Uttley, 1978). Prigatano (1986) found a correlation between verbal expansiveness and neuropsychological and psychosocial impairment and suggested that the problem might be related to frontal lobe dysfunction. In the present author's sample, extreme verbal expansiveness was reported during many years in a young patient with severe bilateral fronto-orbital lesions and severe changes in personality and emotion (case 2, p. 299).

Improvement in communication can take place during many years, even in

Table 12–2. Defects of communication 2 and 12 years after severe head trauma (case 1)

Defects	2 years	12 years
Impaired semantic analysis	+++	+
Impaired phonemic discrimination	+	
Dyslexia	+	
Amnestic aphasia	+++	++
Verbal paraphasia	+++	(+)
Neologisms	++	
Paragrammatism	+++	+
Dysgraphia	++	+
Rigidity/perseveration	+++	++

+++ = severe; ++ = moderate; + = mild

aphasic patients with very severe initial cognitive impairment. The following case, illustrated in table 12–2 and described in detail in a former publication (Thomsen, 1981), illustrates this finding:

Case 1. A 44-year-old right-handed man, a teacher, sustained a severe blunt head trauma with multiple left posterior skull fractures. An epidural hematoma, extending over the greater part of the left hemisphere, was removed six days after admission to hospital. Eye-contact was not possible until more than 3 months after injury. PTA was at least 6 months. During the first 2 years very slow, gradual improvement from automatic to intellectual language occurred concurrently with improvement in the initially extremely severely impaired mental functions. About two years after the trauma the patient started sheltered work in a library. He has done well and has for many years had the responsibility of half a million index cards. He has a good social life.

A follow-up examination took place when the intensive treatment was stopped 2 years after injury and a second one was done 12 years after the accident. At the former the WAIS Performance IQ was 91. No verbal score could be given because of the aphasia. At the latter examination the Verbal IQ was 114 and the Performance IQ 108. In all but one test improvement was registered in competence and not in speed. Table 12–2 shows the great improvement in tests of language. It is also worth mentioning that the rate of silent reading had become normal and that the ability of verbal learning in delayed story recall, which was extremely bad at first follow-up, had become normal. The long-term outcome was thus much more favorable than expected in the first two posttraumatic years. The spouse's patience and support and the return to an active life were no doubt attributable causes to the great improvement during the years.

Psychosocial Deficits

General changes

The psychosocial dysfunctions, including poor memory, personality, emotional, social, and subjective problems, as reported by patients and relatives 2.5 years and 10–15 years after injury, are shown in table 12–3.

At the first follow-up the spontaneous complaints of the patients were few. Panting and Merry (1972) reported similar results. The relatives in my investigation declared that cognitive impairment, particularly poor memory, presented difficulties, but that changes in personality and emotion ("another person") created the severest troubles in daily life. In 1967 Fahy, Irving, and Millac concluded that temperamental changes distressed the relatives most of all but that the patients seldom acknowledged the difference in behavior, and London (1967) emphasized, as mentioned before, the negative posttraumatic changes and the consequences for the family. Many studies have confirmed these findings (Jennett, 1972; Panting & Merry, 1972, Thomsen, 1974, 1984; Rosenbaum & Najenson, 1976; McKinlay et al., 1981; Brooks & McKinlay, 1983; Brooks et al., 1986, 1987a). At second follow-up some relatives described gradual improvement in personality and emotion, yet two-thirds of the patients had permanent changes (table 12–3). The percentage was presumably an underestimate, since information from relatives could not be obtained in

Table 12–3. Problems in 40 patients at first and second follow-up

Domain	Problems	No. of patients with problems 2.5 years	10–15 years
Memory	Poor memory	32	30
Personality	"Another person"	32	26
	Childishness	24	10
	Aspontaneity	17	21
	Restlessness	11	15
	Disturbed behaviour	10	9
Emotional	Irritability	15	19
	Emotional blunting	2	10
	Emotional lability	16	13
Social	Lack of contact	23	29
	Lack of interests	8	23
Subjective	Poor concentration	30	21
	Tiredness	11	20
	Slowness	26	22
	Sensitivity to distress	10	26

all cases because of divorces and deaths. Brooks et al. (1986) reported an increase in personality changes from 1 to 5 years after injury (60% and 74%, respectively).

Childishness was the most frequent personality problem in the Danish study at first follow-up, and the regressive features were outstanding in some patients, as the following case illustrates:

Case 2. A 17-year-old woman was involved in a traffic accident in which both her parents were killed. The patient sustained a severe blunt head trauma with multiple skull fractures, especially in the anterior base and in the fronto-orbital regions. She developed severe hydrocephalus. Four months after the accident she had no pareses, but hypertonia. In bed she spontaneously placed herself in presentation. There were grasping, sucking, and yawning movements. She spoke almost constantly, often with echolalia and palilalia. When alone she wailed terribly. Her pattern of sleep was abnormal and she was incontinent with urine in a very demonstrative way. Five months after injury she was orientated in time, but she did not become continent with urine until one year after the trauma. At that time it was not possible to establish a genuine emotional contact with her.

The patient stayed in nursing homes during the next eleven years. The head of the nursing home, where she lived the last seven years of the period, reported severe behavioral and emotional problems with lack of sexual inhibition, aspontaneity, and severe untidiness. She often talked so much that people avoided her company. Her memory was poor and it had not been possible to teach her anything. All attempts of establishing emotional contact with her had been fruitless. Three years later, when she had been living with a partner the age of her father for about two years, an unexpected improvement in functional state had taken place and the emotional contact was much better than before.

At the first follow-up, emotional lability was frequent. Loss of emotional control with rapid changes among apathy, irritability, and hot temper was a main complaint of seven spouses, who declared that their husbands or wives had become complete strangers. "One moment she caresses the boy and the next she beats him, and I cannot see any reason at all," a husband complained. Ten to fifteen years after injury, emotional changes were most frequently reported in single patients who lived with their parents. Emotional blunting was then an even greater burden than lability.

The most serious behavioral disorders are aggressiveness and lack of sexual inhibition. In the Glasgow series (McKinlay et al., 1981) threats of violence and inappropriate behavior were present in about a fifth of patients during the first year after injury. The same percentage of disturbed behavior was registered in my material 2.5 years after injury (table 12–3). The frequency was almost the same at second follow-up. Contingency tables showed that four patients had acquired problems after the first follow-up and that five patients had recovered during the interval between the examinations, four from verbal aggressiveness and one, a woman of 37 years when injured, from extreme lack of sexual inhibition, which persisted during the first five post-traumatic years. Severe increasing behavioral problems were reported in some patients, as seen in cases no. 3 and no. 4:

Case 3. A 19-year-old right-handed man, a skilled laborer, sustained a blunt head trauma. A tardive subdural hematoma over the left parietal region was removed one month after injury. PTA was 4 months. At that time the patient had a right hemiparesis and aphasia. Auditory analysis was only moderately impaired, but severe amnestic aphasia, verbal paraphasia, perseveration, dyslexia, and dysgraphia were present. Motor functions and language improved much during the following months. When seen three years after the accident, the patient and his parents focused on the moderate physical handicap and complained of lack of continuous treatment. The parents reported memory impairment and behavioral problems with severe aspontaneity, hot temper and rapid emotional changes. The patient had lost contact with premorbid friends and had not been able to establish new friendships.

Fourteen years after injury the parents described improvement in physical state during the first 5 posttraumatic years, but increasing behavioral problems. The patient was on bad terms with everybody and the family had become totally isolated. His mother was afraid of touching him, because he got sexually excited and he had knocked down his father three times because of jealousy. The patient had for several years had a sexual relationship with a woman much older than this mother. When she died, he did not seem to care. He was often depressed, but had violent and rapid changes of mood. The patient spontaneously declared that he would be all right in a few months.

Case 4. A 20-year-old right-handed woman, a student at a kindergarten college, sustained a blunt head trauma with comminuted skull fractures and severe cerebral oedema. The patient reacted to speech 3 weeks after injury. There were severe confusion, agitation, and disinhibited sexual behavior in the following months. Six months after the accident mild right hemiparesis and aphasia were present. The auditory analysis was rather severely impaired and the patient's facial expression revealed her confusion. Speech was slow, mainly because of amnestic problems. The patient was very restless, untidy and often childish. According to her parents she had become "a total stranger." When visited in her home (she lived by herself) 2.6 years after the trauma the patient was pregnant. She walked the streets. She complained bitterly of her total isolation; the relationship to her parents was bad and she had no friends. After an abortion she spent some months at a school for grown-ups. She was not accepted by the other students. The head of the school said that the patient now and then asked some good questions, but at other times her comments were totally irrelevant. The WAIS Performance IQ was 97.

When seen 14 years after injury she still lived alone. She had failed in all types of unskilled work and had at last accepted a disablement pension. She had frequent fits of rage and revealed hypomania and dementia. The patient still walked the streets and lived a dangerous life because of her contact with criminals. She had never had any epileptic fits.

Levin and Grossman (1978) found that early agitation frequently was associated with aggressiveness and sexually explicit behavior during the course of recovery from head injury. The case presented here indicates that the changes can be lifelong. In the 5-year follow-up from Scotland (Brooks et al., 1986) the great increase in disturbed behavior, including bizarre, puzzling, violent, and inappropriate behavior, was the most negative finding. Threats or gestures of violence were reported in 54% (against 15% at one year). Twenty percent of the relatives said that the patient had exhibited physical violence, involving an actual assault on the relative (10% at one year), and several family members were afraid of the patient. A third of the patients had been in some trouble with the law since the accident, but, in contrast to the subjects in the Danish sample, more than half had had some brush with the law prior to injury.

Regarding subjective symptoms (table 12–3), a significant reduction was described in impaired concentration. However, very few patients involved themselves in intellectual tasks, such as reading a book. A significant increase was found in tiredness and sensitivity to distress. When severe, the last mentioned dysfunction resulted in an extremely compulsive way of life, as the following case illustrates:

Case 5. A 16-year-old man, the son of a medical practitioner, sustained a blunt head trauma in an accident in which his brother was killed. A subdural hematoma over most of the left hemisphere was removed a few hours after admission to the neurosurgical department. The brain was severely concussed. PTA was 7 months. During the first posttraumatic year aspontaneity was outstanding. At the first follow-up the patient had no motor impairment, but mild amnestic aphasia. The WAIS Performance IQ was 82 (premorbidly the patient was above average intelligence) and the changes in personality, including apathy, childishness, and emotional blunting, were severe. The parents tried hard to reeducate their son.

When seen again 11 years after injury the patient lived in his own flat. Attempts of rehabilitation had finally been stopped after 9 years, in which the patient, despite his great efforts, had failed in all types of sheltered work. He was extremely slow, aspontaneous, and unable to learn anything new. Except for his parents, who kept in touch, the patient's social isolation was total. He did exactly the same things at the same hours day by day. He took the same walk every day and had to do so in exactly the same number of minutes. He much resented meeting people he knew on his route because he then had to run to keep time. He thought it might be nice to have a girlfriend, but preferred not in case his daily system might be broken.

Specific Changes

DEPENDENCE. Twenty-four of the forty patients (60%) in the present author's sample were dependent at first follow-up. Nine needed help with washing, dressing, and eating, and the rest could not be left alone. At second follow-up half the 24 patients were able to take care of themselves, and the 12 patients who remained dependent had difficulties in self-care. Two had no motor impairment and a further two had only mild motor problems. PTA was significantly longer in those with permanent dependence than in those with transitory dependence. The relationship between severity of cerebral damage, as judged by length of posttraumatic amnesia, and late dependence was also present in the 5-year follow-up by Brooks et al. (1986), in which dependence was the only category of seven in which a positive correlation was found. In the great series examined up to 7 years after injury (Brooks et al., 1987a), only 7% were thought to be in the very high dependence category, but 36% needed "looking after" and about a quarter of the patients had problems in personal hygiene, more often because of behavioral (unwillingness to wash) than physical (inability to wash) problems.

WORK CAPACITY. In the literature, the proportion of head-injured people who return to work varies enormously in the individual investigations, and it is difficult to find comparable groups. Severity of brain damage, age, previous personality and occupational level, length of follow-up, personality changes, and social conditions are important factors in social recovery, including return to work (Humphrey & Oddy, 1980). In the two year follow-up by Weddell, Oddy, and Jenkins (1980), nearly half the patients were unable to work at all, and among those working, only a few had returned to their premorbid work. Seven years after the trauma those who were unemployed at two years remained so. None of the patients working at a lower capacity at the first follow-up had been able to get back to their original job or a comparable one (Oddy et al., 1985). In some cases in the present author's study (Thomsen, 1974, 1984) the capacity of working either improved in the course of time or was not used until several years postinjury. Eleven of the eighteen patients with some work capacity at second follow-up did not start working until several years after the accident. A woman with PTA of 3 months began unskilled work 6 years after injury, and a man, premorbidly a farmer, was trained as a bookkeeper 5 years after injury. Two women, who had been divorced after the trauma, were able to manage their housekeeping and shopping themselves 3 to 4 years after the accident. A most unexpected late improvement was observed in the following case:

Case 6. A 19-year-old man, a locksmith, sustained a blunt head trauma with brain stem involvement. He did not respond verbally or nonverbally to speech until four months after injury. PTA was 7 months. There was severe hypertonia in both arms and legs. Operations were not successful. One year after the accident the patient was totally dependent with severe dysarthria and severe emotional regression but only moderate cognitive defects. He was in a nursing home for 3 years without much improvement. According to his own explanation, he then started asking himself whether he wanted to spend the rest of his life in this way. A year later he went to a school for grown-ups and stayed there for a year. At second follow-up he lived alone and had taught himself to walk indoors. He hoped to obtain "studentereksamen," that is, admission to university, and had passed in half the subjects, but had taken much longer time than normally. He was content with his lot and had many friends.

In a recent study Brooks and co-workers (1987b) examined return to work within the first 7 years after severe head trauma in 98 patients. The employment rate dropped from 86% before injury to 29% after. The authors found that the presence of cognitive, behavioral, and personality changes was significantly related to failure to return to work, and they were able to give a detailed account of negative features. General memory impairment and attention and communication deficits, such as carrying on and understanding a conversation, were highly significant predictors, and the same was the case concerning self-care (personal hygiene and taking responsibility) and emotional problems (mood and control of anger). There was little evidence that physical impairment was an important predictor of return to work.

SOCIAL AND LEISURE ACTIVITIES. Humphrey and Oddy (1980) pointed out the crudity of returning to work as an index of social recovery at the cost of neglecting personal relationships and leisure activities, which may be even more important to the patient. In the 2-year follow-up by Weddell, Oddy, and Jenkins (1980), the patients had significantly fewer friends, interests, and hobbies than a comparison group of patients who had recently suffered severe head injury. The problems were significantly higher in those with personality change than in those without. Lack of social adjustment is a general problem in head trauma (Oddy et al., 1985; Newton & Johnson, 1985). Lezak (1987) examined a mixed group of head injuries (mild, moderate, and severe cases) up to 5 years after trauma. By the third year postinjury the majority performed well on cognitive tests, but 85% had not resumed normal leisure activities and 90% or more had difficulties with social contact.

The Danish patients' greatest problem 2.5 years after injury was lack of social contact (see table 12–3), which increased in the following years. Very few had been able to keep in touch with premorbid friends and hardly any made other than casual acquaintances ("people I meet on the bus") . Several preferred to make friends with old people because they were kind and patient, an observation also reported by Weddell and colleagues. At least three had or had had sexual relationships with partners the age of their parents, as described in cases 2 and 3. Total social withdrawal was present in some of the most disabled patients. They had often experienced constant failures in coping, as the patient in my material (case 5). Levin and Grossman (1978) found that social withdrawal was positively related to severity of brain damage, as measured by length of coma, and a combination of social withdrawal, emotional blunting, and lack of insight was reported in some of their most severely injured patients.

Lack of interests had increased significantly during the years in the present author's sample (see table 12–3). It is worth mentioning that some patients with motor impairment had more interests than those without physical deficits. The former often joined the associations for the disabled and took part in meetings and travel, whereas the latter, when invited, usually refused to go because "they were not disabled."

THE PATIENT AND THE FAMILY

At second follow-up three patients in my series were in nursing homes and one in a psychiatric ward. The greatest change in place of living during the interval between the two follow-up examinations was the great number of single patients who were able to live alone. Some left their childhood homes by their own choice, the remaining because they lost their parent(s). At the first follow-up most parents thought that their son or daughter was unable to live on their own and the late results were thus promising. Nine patients were married at first follow-up; seven were divorced in the following years. They all had children. The two who remained married had no children. Eight patients were married or started cohabiting with a permanent partner after first follow-up, half the cases with a disabled man or woman.

Relatives' burden in the years after severe head injury was analyzed in Glasgow. By one year (McKinlay et al., 1981) mental and behavioral changes in the patient were associated with significantly increased stress in the relative, whereas physical and language/speech deficits were not. In a later study (Brooks & McKinlay, 1983) "high burden" in the relative was associated with a variety of features in the patient, such as lack of emotional control, reduction in energy, immaturity, emotional coldness, unhappiness, cruelty, meanness, and unreasonableness. However, in addition to the patient's personality changes, the relative's personality was important in the genesis of burden. The significance of the type of family relationship has been discussed by some authors. Panting and Merry (1972) and Thomsen (1974) concluded that the husband-wife relationship was less stable than the parent–grown-up-child relationship. Mothers were generally able to accept or tolerate childlike dependency behavior and might even consider the changes quite gratifying, as mentioned by Rosenbaum and Najenson (1976). Very few spouses managed to do so. Lezak (1978) summarized the spouse's special problems in cases of severe head trauma. The spouse lives in a social limbo, cannot mourn decently, cannot divorce with dignity or in good conscience, and her or his sexual and affectional needs are frustrated, a problem emphasized in Rosenbaum and Najenson's investigation. If the family has young children, the spouse is confronted with the difficulty of divided loyalties. Furthermore, the spouse may not have the possibility of support from other family members or from close friends. Mauss-Clum and Ryan (1981) thus found that nearly three times as many wives as mothers complained of decreased social contacts, and the wives in Rosenbaum and Najenson's sample saw their friends less frequently than before the trauma, but the number of contacts with their husbands' parents had increased. There was often a tense relationship between the wives and the inlaws, who sometimes considered it their duty to protect their son from the possibility of the wife divorcing him. The spouse was up against emotional, social, and practical difficulties so heavy that the situation became chaotic. It was no wonder that nearly all spouses in the present author's 2.5 year follow-up (Thomsen 1974) expressed severe frustration and despair. At that time most parents living with a disabled son or daughter still hoped for further improvement and very few described the situation as unbearable. Ten to fifteen years after injury the situation had changed for the worse in families in which a patient still lived with his parents. Five of the nine single patients, all males, were totally dependent and were nursed or supervised by their mothers. The parents' marriage had suffered greatly, with the father feeling left out of things because his wife devoted all her energy and care to the disabled son. Furthermore, the family had become socially isolated because the siblings and friends had stopped visiting, as described in case 3. The relatives' burden can thus be just as severe in the grown-up-child–parents relationship as in the marital relationship, or even worse, since the relationship first mentioned often remains for life, but the crisis in the families occurs at different times after severe cerebral trauma.

COMMUNICATION BETWEEN RELATIVES AND CLINICIANS

Difficulties in communication between relatives and clinicians, particularly medical staff, have been discussed by several authors. About half the relatives in Panting and Merry's (1972) study felt that they had received too little information, especially about prognosis. Oddy and colleagues (1978) reported that 40% of their relatives had some criticism to make, the most common being dissatisfaction with the level of communication between medical staff and themselves. Some had wanted to hear more about the extent and nature of the brain injury, and some viewed the social services as inadequate. In the present author's investigation 2.5 years after trauma (Thomsen 1974), nearly half the relatives declared that they had received too little information during hospitalization. All relatives who were dissatisfied belonged to the lower social classes, and in some cases the relatives' lack of knowledge and failure to comprehend may have been a contributory cause of the problem. Difficulties may also be due to the defense mechanism of denial described by Romano (1974). Some relatives' comments, such as "I was afraid and did not listen" and "I did not want to hear what the doctor said" are likely to be manifestations of denial. The same was the case regarding a spontaneous comment of a mother to one of my patients, "I do not think my son will ever recover, but if you share this opinion, please do not tell me." Denial is, as Brooks (1984) said, not necessarily "a bad thing." Denial can be highly functional, especially in the early stages after cerebral injury, but when denial is permanent it becomes a hindrance to rehabilitation and increases the family burden. Case 3 in the present author's series is an extreme example of everlasting denial. The fact that the parents supported him in his unrealistic opinion many years after the accident may have been a contributory cause of the patient's total lack of insight.

FACTORS THAT MAY INFLUENCE LONG-TERM OUTCOME

Some factors are positively related to head trauma: male predominance (males are three times more likely to be injured than females), age 15 to 30 years, lower socioeconomic classes, abuse of alcohol, and social maladjustment. Among the investigations most reported in this chapter, the Glasgow series no doubt has the highest percentage of "accident-prone" patients.

Severity of injury, age, premorbid personality, stability of family background, and occupational level are factors mentioned as important predictors of outcome. Regarding severity in blunt head trauma, length of coma or more frequently length of post-traumatic amnesia has been regarded the best yardstick and a PTA of 7 days has been considered a cutoff point between severe and very severe blunt head trauma (Russell, 1932). However, recent investigations, such as the Dutch study by Van Zomeren and Burg (1985) and the 7-year follow-up by Brooks et al. (1987a), have indicated that a PTA of around 13 days is a watershed, with a relatively low frequency of persisting deficits with a PTA of less than 13 days and a high frequency with a PTA above this level. Brooks et al. also found a consistent and significant relationship between increase in PTA and increase in levels of all types of disability, but when the individual patients' scores in the different severity groups were examined, some patients, even in the severest groups (with a PTA of 29 days or more), were entirely symptom-free on each of seven outcome categories. The authors concluded that severity, as judged by PTA, was not a safe enough predictor beyond 2 years after injury. In the present author's sample (Thomsen 1984), in which all patients had a PTA of one month or more, no one was symptom-free, but a quarter of the patients had only two to four symptoms. Tiredness was the most frequent problem, followed by impairment of language and speech and memory defects.

Age is regarded an important factor. No doubt the young have a better survival rate than the old, but what about long-term outcome? Many authors have stressed the importance of young age as a positive prognostic factor. From the results of a 10-year follow-up of a great material, Carlsson, Essen, and Löfgren (1968) even went as far as to declare that the probability of restitution in patients under the age of 20 was totally independent of severity (coma period). Gilchrist and Wilkinson (1979), in contrast, found very little difference in outcome, as judged by return to work in a group of patients up to 40 years when injured, but they pointed out that many of their patients under 20 years were among the most severely disabled in the sample. In the Danish long-term study no significant correlation was found between age when injured and PTA, but a highly significant negative correlation was found between age when injured and number of problems 10–15 years postinjury (i.e., the younger the patient the more permanent or late problems). Further statistical analysis proved that the problems in question were the behavioral and emotional changes (Thomsen, 1989). It is reasonable to assume that the immature personality is particularly vulnerable in severe head trauma. Sensitization by relatives, who as time passed came to identify problems that had been neglected or denied in earlier stages, and reactive changes in the patient (Brooks et al., 1986) may also have played an important role in the long-term outcome in young single patients who lived with their parents for many years after the trauma.

CONCLUDING COMMENTS

The late features of psychosocial disability in severe and very severe blunt head trauma and the consequences for the patient and family have been described. Clinical experience and long-term research have indicated that traditional rehabilitation facilities that focus on physical impairment do not consider the needs of head-injured patients and that a multidisciplinary approach is necessary in dealing with the complex mixture of deficits. In recent years intensive neuropsychologically oriented rehabilitation programs have been developed, mainly in the United States, and data have been published indicating that improvement in late psychosocial adjustment is possible by this type of intervention (Prigatano et al., 1984). This possibility even applies to returning to work. The results from a late American study (Ben Yishay et al., 1987) showed that the majority of 94 head-injured patients who had been considered unemployable were able to work after attending a comprehensive outpatient day program.

The long-term, often life-lasting, psychosocial sequelae of traumatic brain injury alter relatives' as well as the victim's life; rehabilitation efforts therefore should be directed as much toward the family as toward the patient. In addition to professional treatment, the Family Associations, the National Head Injury Foundation in the United States, and HEADWAY (the National Head Injuries Association) in Britain develop volunteer support groups for head trauma families.

REFERENCES

Benton, A. L. (1960). Early descriptions of aphasia. *Archives of Neurology* 3, 205–221.

Ben-Yishay, Y., Silver, S. M., Piasetsky, E., & Rattok, J. (1987). Relationship between employability and vocational outcome after intensive holistic cognitive rehabilitation. *Journal of Head Trauma Rehabilitation* 2, 35–48.

Bond, M. R. (1975). Assessment of the psychosocial outcome after severe head injury. In *Outcome of severe damage to the central nervous system*. CIBA Foundation Symposium 34, pp. 141–158, Amsterdam: Elsevier.

Bond, M. R., & Brooks, D. N. (1976). Understanding the process of recovery as a basis for the investigation of rehabilitation for the brain injured. *Scandinavian Journal of Rehabilitation Medicine* 8, 127–133.

Brooks, N., & McKinlay, W. (1983). Personality and behavioral change after severe blunt head injury—A relative's view. *Journal of Neurology, Neurosurgery, and Psychiatry* 46, 336–344.

Brooks, N. (1984). Head injury and the family. In N. Brooks (Ed.), *Closed head injury. Psychological, social, and family consequences.* New York: Oxford University Press.

Brooks, N., Campsie, L., Symington, C., Beattie, A., & McKinlay, W. (1986). The five year outcome of severe blunt head injury: A relative's view. *Journal of Neurology, Neurosurgery and Psychiatry* 49, 764–770.

Brooks, N., Campsie, L., Symington, C., Beattie, A., Bryden, J., & McKinlay, W. (1987a). The effects of severe head injury upon patient and relative within seven years of injury. *Journal of Head Trauma Rehabilitation*, 2, 1–13.

Brooks, N., McKinlay, W., Symington, C., Beattie, A., & Campsie, L. (1987b). Return to work within the first seven years after severe head injury. *Brain Injury* 1, 5–19.

Carlsson, C. A., von Essen, C., & Löfgren, J. (1968). Factors affecting the clinical course of patients with severe head injuries. *Journal of Neurosurgery* 29, 242–251.

Conkey, R. C. (1938). Psychological changes associated with head injuries. *Archives of Psychology* 232, 1–62.

Fahy, T. J., Irving, M. H., & Millac, P. (1967). Severe head injuries. *Lancet* 2, 475–479.

Gilchrist, E., & Wilkinson, M. (1979). Some factors determining prognosis in young people with severe head injuries. *Archives of Neurology* 36, 355–359.

Grosswasser, Z., Mendelson, L., Stern, M. J., Schechter, I., & Najenson, T. (1977). Re-evaluation of prognostic factors in rehabilitation after severe head injury. *Scandinavian Journal of Rehabilitation Medicine* 9, 147–149.

Humphrey, M., & Oddy, M. (1980). Return to work after head injury: A review of post-war studies. *Injury* 12, 107–114.

Jennett, B. (1972). Late effects of head injuries. In M. Critchley, B. Jennett, & J. O'Leary (Eds.), *Scientific foundations of neurology.* London: Heinemann.

Kalsbeek, W. D., McLaurin, R. L., Harris, B. S. H., & Miller, J. D. (1980). The national head and spinal cord survey: Major findings. *Journal of Neurosurgery* (Suppl), 53.

Levin, H. S., & Grossman, R. G. (1978). Behavioral sequelae of closed head injury. *Archives of Neurology* 35, 720–727.

Levin, H. S., Grossman, R., Rose, J., & Teasdale, G. (1979). Long-term neuropsychological outcome of closed head injury. *Journal of Neurosurgery* 50, 412–422.

Lezak, M. D. (1978). Living with the characterologically altered brain injured patient. *Journal of Clinical Psychiatry* 39, 592–598.

Lezak, M. D. (1987). Relationships between personality disorders, social disturbances, and physical disability following traumatic brain injury. *Journal of Head Trauma Rehabilitation* 2, 57–69.

London, P. S. (1967). Some observations on the course of events after severe injury of the head. *Annals of the Royal College of Surgeons of England* 41, 460–479.

Mauss-Clum, N., & Ryan, M. (1981). Brain injury and the family. *Journal of Neurosurgical Nursing* 13, 165–169.

McKinlay, W., Brooks, N., Bond, M. R., Martinage, D. P., & Marshall, M. (1981). The short-term outcome of severe blunt head injury as reported by relatives of the injured persons. *Journal of Neurology, Neurosurgery, and Psychiatry* 44, 527–533.

Miller, H., & Stern, G. (1965). The long-term prognosis of severe head injuries. *Lancet* 1, 225–229.

Newton, A., & Johnson, D. A. (1985). Social adjustment and interaction after severe head injury. *British Journal of Clinical Psychology*, 24, 225–234.

Oddy, M., Coughlan, T., Tyerman, A., & Jenkins, D. (1985). Social adjustment after closed closed head injury: A further follow-up seven years after injury. *Journal of Neurology, Neurosurgery, and Psychiatry* 48, 564–568.

Oddy M., Humphrey, M., & Uttley, D. (1978). Stresses upon relatives of head-injured patients. *British Journal of Psychiatry* 133, 507–513.

Panting, A., & Merry, P. (1972). The long-term rehabilitation of severe head injuries with particular reference to the need for social and medical support for the patient's family. *Rehabilitation* 38, 33–37.

Prigatano, G. P. (1986). *Neuropsychological rehabilitation after brain injury*. London: John Hopkins University Press.

Prigatano, G. P., Fordyce, D. J., Zeiner, H. K., Roueche, J. R., Pepping, M., & Wood, B. C. (1984). Neuropsychological rehabilitation after closed head injury in young adults. *Journal of Neurology, Neurosurgery, and Psychiatry* 47, 505–513.

Research aspects of rehabilitation after acute brain damage in adults. (1982). Report of a coordination group. *Lancet* 2, 1034–1036.

Roberts, A. H. (1976). Sequelae of closed head injuries. *Proceedings of the Royal Society of Medicine* 69, 137–140.

Romano, M. D. (1974). Family response to traumatic head injury. *Scandinavian Journal of Rehabilitation Medicine* 6, 1–4.

Rosenbaum, M., & Najenson, T. (1976). Changes in life patterns and symptoms of low mood as reported by wives of severely brain-injured soldiers. *Journal of Consulting Clinical Psychology* 44, 881–888.

Russell, W. R. (1932). Cerebral involvement in head injury. *Brain* 35, 549–603.

Russell, W. R. & Nathan, P. W. (1946). Traumatic amnesia. *Brain* 69, 183–187.

Thomsen, I. V. (1974). The patient with severe head injury and his family. *Scandinavian Journal of Rehabilitation Medicine* 6, 180–183.

Thomsen, I. V. (1975). Evaluation and outcome of aphasia in patients with severe closed head trauma. *Journal of Neurology, Neurosurgery, and Psychiatry* 38, 713–718.

Thomsen, I. V. (1976). Evaluation and outcome of traumatic aphasia in patients with severe verified focal lesions. *Folia Phoniatrica* 28, 362–377.

Thomsen, I. V. (1981). Neuropsychological treatment and long-time follow-up in an aphasic patient with very severe head trauma. *Journal of Clinical Neuropsychology* 3, 43–51.

Thomsen, I. V. (1984). Late outcome of very severe blunt head trauma: A 10–15 year second follow-up. *Journal of Neurology, Neurosurgery, and Psychiatry* 47, 260–268.

Thomsen, I. V. (1989). Do young patients have worse outcomes after severe blunt head trauma? *Brain injury* 3, 157–162.

Weddell, R., Oddy, M., & Jenkins, D. (1980). Social adjustment after rehabilitation: A two-year follow-up of patients with severe head injury. *Psychological Medicine* 10, 257–263.

Van Zomeren, A. H., & Van den Burg, W. (1985). Residual complaints of patients two years after severe head injury. *Journal of Neurology, Neurosurgery, and Psychiatry* 48, 21–28.

INDEX

Academic skills
  arithmetic, 38–39, 79
  development of, 38
  disorders of, 45–91 (*see also* Reading
    disorders, Writing disorders,
    Mathematic disorders)
Activities of daily living
  and practical intelligence, 188–190
  instrumental, 144–146
  relation to cognitive processes, 192–194
Adjustment
  and family issues, 204–205
  and reaction to difficulties, 240–241
  and work, 259–260
Agraphia, 71–76
Alexia, 46–69
Amnesia
  in dementia, 139
  in temporal lobe epilepsy, 117–119
Anticonvulsant medication
  behavioral effects, 120–122
Attention
  and school behavior, 34–35
  and television viewing, 94–98, 101–102
  lapses of, 280
  neural mechanisms, 34–35

Attention deficit disorder and frontal lobe
    function, 34–35

Behavioral intervention
  for treatment of seizures, 113–114
Brain activity
  and processing styles, 32–33
  and television viewing, 98–103
  in dyslexia, 61–63
Brain injury
  and cognitive changes, 229–232
  and communication changes, 237–240
  and physical changes, 236–237
  and personality changes, 232–236
  psychosocial model of, 217–218
  secondary effects, 227–228
  vocationally related difficulties, 265–268

Cognitive deficits
  and anticonvulsant treatment, 121
  common after brain injury, 229–232
  impact on pragmatic competencies, 240
  levels of, 281–282
  long term sequelae of head injury,
    296–298

Cognitive rehabilitation, 203
Communication deficits, 297
Competence
    based model of functioning, 2
    behavioral, and everyday functioning,
        140–142
    to perform activities of daily living, 190
Competencies
    of daily life, 272
Corpus callosum
    and development, 19, 37

Dementia
    and problems in everyday functioning,
        145–146
    definitions of, 136–140
Development
    changes in basic mental activities,
        186–188
    changes in tasks of daily living, 188–192
    hemispheric functions in, 25–30
    maturational theory of, 30–32
    neural organization, 18–24
    neuropsychological concerns, 3–6
Dyslexia 50–56
    and functional reading, 63–69
    neuroanatomy and brain activity, 61–63

Ecological perspective
    and neuropsychological functioning,
        2–3, 9–10
Education
    readiness and school behavior, 35–39
Everyday functioning
    and basic mental abilities, 191–192
    and problems of elderly, 145–192
    relationship to neuropsychological task
        performance, 169–179, 192–194,
        277–283
    remedial strategies for, 281–282

Family
    contributions to rehabilitation, 205–207,
        260
    dynamics, 222–224
    involvement, 7, 203–205
Family therapy, 206–208
Frontal lobe
    and attention deficit disorder, 34–35

and personality change, 234
Functional rating scales, 140, 151–153, 178
Functional skills training, 272–273

Generalization, 10
    and remediation after brain injury,
        283–285

Hemispheric functions
    and cognitive abilities, 25–30
Hemispheric specialization
    and dendritic organization, 20
    neurophysiologic measures of, 22–23
Hormones
    influences on development, 23

Individual differences
    in development, 194
    in television viewing, 97
Information processing
    automatic vs. controlled, 278–279
    dimensions and task demands, 9
    styles, 32–34
Intelligence
    fluid-crystallized, 186–187
    mechanics of 184, 195
    multiple, 184
    pragmatics, 184, 195
Intervention
    and diagnosis, 6–7
    for cognitive deficits, 271–274
    for seizures, 113–114, 119–122

Leisure activity, 303–305
    and everyday problem solving, 193

Mathematic disorders, 79–84
Maturational theory, 30–32
    and critical periods, 31
    and spatial performance, 30
    neurophysiology, 27
Metacognition
    and learning strategies, 119

Neural development, 18–21
Neurolinguistic
    deficits after brain injury, 237–240

Neuropsychological remediation, 247–253
  models of, 272–275
Neuropsychology
  models in, 2–3
  cognitive, 72–76
Neurotransmitters, 21–22
Normalization, 10

Outcome
  psychosocial, 8

Personality
  and coping after brain injury, 217
  changes after brain injury, 232–236
  pre-injury characteristics, 218–221
Plateau of function
  and cerebral hemisphere, 28–30
physical deficits
  and functional outcomes, 237
  long term sequelae of head injury,
    255–256
Psycholinguistics
  and agraphia, 72–77
  and alexia, 49–53
Psychosocial
  adjustment and vocational rehabilitation,
    259–260
  consequences of brain injury, 217
  deficits and long term sequelae of head
    injury, 298–300
  factors in epilepsy, 125–127
  factors in neuropsychological
    rehabilitation, 275–277
Practical intelligence, 184–185
  and real-world activities, 188–190
Pragmatics
  and communication changes after brain
    injury, 240
Pre-injury
  assests and liabilities, 217–224
  family characteristics, 222

Process model
  of cognitive rehabilitation, 272
Processing styles, 32–33, 37

Reading disorders, 56–61
Recovery of function
  and behavioral performance, 85–87
  six-phase model, 241–244

Scaffolding, 288
Seizure disorders
  and psychiatric disturbances, 123–125
  as long term sequelae, 296
  effects on developing nervous system,
    116–117
  neuropsychologic aspects, 114–122
Sensorimotor function
  anatomic organization, 27–28
  in childhood learning, 37
Synaptic organization
  and neural development, 19–21

Television viewing
  and brain damage, 93–94, 106
  cognitive effects, 103–105
Therapist
  activity in rehabilitation, 286–289
Therapeutic alliance, 250–251, 275–276

Vascular disorders, 228–229

Work
  capacity, 302–303
  critical behaviors necessary for, 263–265
  meaning of, 258–259
  pre-injury cognitive assets, 221–222
  reintegration after brain injury, 246–247
Writing disorders, 69–79